T0274283

KRAV MAGA

FUNDAMENTAL STRATEGIES

BECAUSE NOT ALL KRAV MAGA IS THE SAME® . . .

"IMITATION IS THE SINCEREST FORM OF FLATTERY."
—Charles Caleb Colton

KRAV MAGA

FUNDAMENTAL STRATEGIES

BY DAVID KAHN

YMAA Publication Center
Wolfeboro, New Hampshire

YMAA Publication Center, Inc.
Main Office:
PO Box 480
Wolfeboro, New Hampshire, 03894
1-800-669-8892 • info@ymaa.com • www.ymaa.com

ISBN: 9781594398131 (print) • ISBN: 9781594398148 (ebook)

Editing by Doran Hunter
Cover design by Axie Breen

20210928

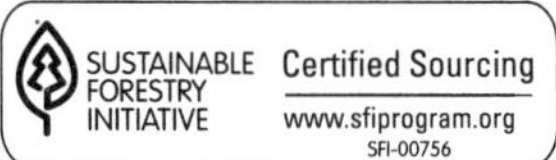

Publisher's Cataloging in Publication

Names: Kahn, David, 1972- author.

Title: Krav maga fundamental strategies / by David Kahn.

Description: First edition. | Wolfeboro, New Hampshire : YMAA Publication Center, [2021] | On cover: The contact combat system of the Israel Defense Forces. | Includes bibliography and index.

Identifiers: ISBN: 9781594398131 (print) | 9781594398148 (ebook) | LCCN: 2021937558

Subjects: LCSH: Krav maga. | Krav maga--Training. | Self-defense. | Self-defense--Training. | Hand-to- hand fighting. | Hand-to-hand fighting--Training. | Martial arts--Training. | BISAC: SPORTS & RECREATION / Martial Arts / General. | SOCIAL SCIENCE / Violence in Society.

Classification: LCC: GV1111 .K255 2021 | DDC: 796.81--dc23

The practice, treatments, and methods described in this book should not be used as an alternative to professional medical diagnosis or treatment. The author and the publisher of this book are NOT RESPONSIBLE in any manner whatsoever for any injury or negative effects that may occur through following the instructions and advice contained herein.
It is recommended that, before beginning any treatment or exercise program, you consult your medical professional to determine whether you should undertake this course of practice.

Warning: While self-defense is legal, fighting is illegal. If you don't know the difference, you'll go to jail, because you aren't defending yourself. You are fighting—or worse. Readers are encouraged to be aware of all appropriate local and national laws relating to self-defense, reasonable force, and the use of weaponry, and to act in accordance with all applicable laws at all times. Understand that while legal definitions and interpretations are generally uniform, there are small—but very important—differences from state to state and even city to city. To stay out of jail, you need to know these differences. Neither the author nor the publisher assumes any responsibility for the use or misuse of information contained in this book. Nothing in this document constitutes a legal opinion, nor should any of its contents be treated as such. While the author believes everything herein is accurate, any questions regarding specific self-defense situations, legal liability, and/or interpretation of federal, state, or local laws should always be addressed by an attorney at law.

When it comes to martial arts, self-defense, and related topics, no text, no matter how well written, can substitute for professional hands-on instruction. These materials should be used for academic study only.

Printed in USA.

For Claire, Benjamin, and Leo
In Loving Memory of Helen Brener Smith

For my fellow instructor, photographer, editor, confidant, and overall great friend
Paul Karleen

In memoriam of krav maga pioneer Alan M. Feldman

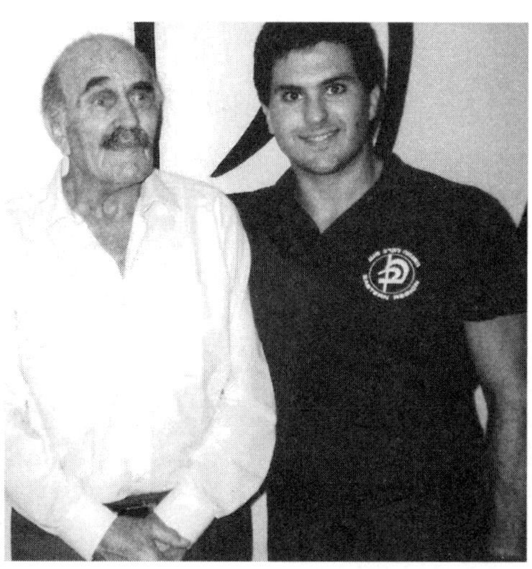

An Israeli Krav Maga blessing
The Book of Psalms, chapter 144:1

לדוד ברוך יהוה צורי המלמד ידי לקרב אצבעותי למלחמ:

"A Psalm of David. Blessed be the LORD, my rock,
Who trains my hands for war,
And my fingers for battle."

Also by David Kahn

Krav Maga: An Essential Guide to the Renowned Method—For Fitness and Self-Defense

Advanced Krav Maga: The Next Level of Fitness and Self-Defense

Krav Maga Weapon Defenses

Krav Maga Professional Tactics

Krav Maga Defense: How to Defend Yourself against the 12 Most Common Unarmed Street Attacks

Krav Maga Combatives

Contents

Foreword: Col. Corey L. Britcher

As a martial artist for over thirty years and a Law Enforcement Defensive Tactics Instructor, I am constantly looking for that program that will take my officers to the next level. When I was promoted to colonel and took the helm of the Bureau of Law Enforcement, one of my first priorities was to revamp our program. At that time, approximately 99 percent of our use-of-force incidents were hands-on with a violator, and many times the officer ended up getting injured. Upon closer examination, officers were reacting to an attack with a simple defense and then waiting for the next attack. Additionally, the tactics were difficult and, without constant practice, needed to be retaught every year. There had to be a better way.

I had always been impressed with krav maga but never had the opportunity to train in the system. Upon learning that there was a Police Krav Maga® program, I immediately set out to find out about it. Enter David Kahn. When I reached out to him, he explained the program and offered to come to Pennsylvania and run a course. That was in 2014. Now, as a Level-2 Police Krav Maga and Civilian Krav Maga instructor, I am hooked on the program. Not only are the techniques effective, efficient, and easy to retain, the kravist mind-set is also something that is missing in most law enforcement programs. The concept of (use-of-force compliant) retzev turns an officer with basic skills into a winner. This mind-set allows the defender to overwhelm the attacker and successfully take the individual into custody while limiting the risk for injury to all parties.

I cannot say enough about the level of instruction that David Kahn offers, the krav maga system, and the information within this book. *Krav Maga Fundamental Strategies* is a must-read for any dedicated kravist.

Col. Corey L. Britcher, Ret.
Director Pennsylvania Bureau of Law Enforcement
Fish & Boat Commission

Foreword: Paul Karleen

Why a book on krav maga strategies? To answer that I need to begin with a few personal reflections. For a number of reasons, nearly a decade ago I sensed the need to acquire some skills to enhance my own physical safety and that of my family. The online information I found about Israeli Krav Maga as taught in a nearby facility intrigued me. So, I signed up, not knowing the impact this would have on my life. As I got more and more into training under the superb instruction of David Kahn, I learned quickly that I would be improving my physical conditioning. And I felt a new sense of empowerment at being able to execute techniques as I practiced with my partners. But, most importantly, new ways of thinking gradually started to come in alongside increased technical proficiency: I started to acquire an ability to assess what was going on around me wherever I found myself—in a store, in a parking lot, in a crowd at a ball game, or simply walking in our neighborhood—and envisioning what I would do if danger came my way. "How would I respond if those three people suddenly jumped me?" "What would I do if that guy over there was armed and hostile?" "Would a kick be the best tool?" "How many punches could I land?" "What if he's had some self-defense training?" "Maybe I should just retreat." I was connecting my everyday situations to the techniques I was honing. I was planning.

No one reading this book should miss the fact that Israeli Krav Maga was born from real-life, deadly situations in Eastern Europe and refined in the struggles of what was at that time the young modern state of Israel. As someone who has recently been in that country, I can attest to the presence of a constant condition of alertness that is still there. The nation has both the tools to defend itself and plans that will enable it to survive. Grandmaster Haim Gidon's krav maga carries in its history and philosophy the key components of 1) physical techniques and 2) the ability to apply these techniques successfully to situations. In a real sense, Israeli Krav Maga provides a metaphor for survival in life: be prepared the best you can for what can happen and be equipped to face those challenges.

David Kahn, as a lifelong student of Grandmaster Gidon, long ago established himself through teaching and writing as a highly effective teacher of techniques and one of the world's premier exponents of krav maga. In recent years, David has turned his attention to identifying the features of street violence situations and how Israeli Krav Maga can best be used to meet threats and attacks effectively. In this book, we have the results of his thinking—a viable set of strategies for krav maga (and, indeed, for any systematic approaches to unarmed self-defense) that will enable you to assess, plan, and envision your responses to situations. They constitute David's latest and best insights into the problem of "What would I do if … ?" These strategies match techniques to real-life situations and are the icing on the krav maga cake.

This is a book about *thinking* as embedded in the IKMA curriculum, and particularly *thinking the right way,* so that you are kept from harm. As Shakespeare put it, "All things are ready, if our mind be so."[1] Successful self-defense comes from both physical training (techniques) and mental training (strategic thinking). These chapters are designed to sharpen your mental approach to self-defense. Learning effective techniques is important; being able to use them effectively *at the right time* is just as important. Techniques alone won't carry the day—you have to train for the situations where they are needed.

The preceding book in this series was *Krav Maga Combatives: Maximum Effect.* That volume stressed that successful unarmed defense is centered on choosing the best technique and then executing it properly—in such a way that the attacker is repelled, and you are kept safe as you carry out the technique. This book on strategy now takes us a step further: we have to be able to use the most effective technique *for a particular situation.* To do this well means that we have thought *ahead of time* about what we would do in a situation and have *built that into our physical training.* This means that I have to train in such a way that I mentally anticipate being ambushed when I am walking through a crowded parking lot, or expect that a single attacker may very well be accompanied by one or more friends, or that, if someone tries to stab me, he is likely to come at me over and over.

Look up "strategy" in a dictionary and you'll find that one of its synonyms is "preparation." Wise Benjamin Franklin once said, "By failing to prepare, you are preparing to fail." I definitely do not want to fail when confronted with a situation where I can be injured or even killed. But preparation in this volume is primarily in our heads as we ask ourselves, "What will it take for me to be ready for an ambush, for multiple attackers, for a sucker punch, for someone who tries to take me to the ground . . . ?" and on and on. There is not much detail in this book about the features of the techniques themselves. Instead, we assume that you already know techniques or are in the process of learning them. Here we want you to learn to apply them in particular situations. In krav maga training, we prepare initially through practicing techniques. But we don't start thinking about how and where we will use them until after we have acquired a certain degree of physical proficiency. This book will help to get you to that level—*the how and where.*

Thinking strategically means that I calculate the likelihood that something bad can happen to me. This is not pessimism, but realism, especially in the day in which we live. Thinking strategically is the opposite of having my head buried in the sand. As corrections officer and martial artist Rory Miller has said about strategy, "Here's a rule of life: You don't get to pick what bad things happen to you."[2] If I anticipate the worst and prepare for it, I will have no difficulty in coming out on top in a situation of lesser gravity.

Effective strategic krav maga thinking comes from two acquired skills:

---

1. William Shakespeare, *Henry V,* Act IV, Scene 3.
2. Rory Miller, *Meditations on Violence: A Comparison of Martial Arts Training & Real World Violence* (Wolfeboro, NH: YMAA Publication Center, 2008), 4.

1. Anticipation during physical workouts of what I as a defender will do—*I build my strategy into my training*. In other words, part of my strategy is ingrained in my mind and is expressed through my practiced physical response. I learn to move and act defensively in ways that correspond to what is presented to me, and I can do it *without thinking*. So, for example, I learn in defending against a knife thrust how to move my hands and feet and how to take away the knife, but I also learn that my attacker is not likely to stop with one jab—he is likely to stab over and over until I am out of commission. I therefore build such thinking into my execution of the technique itself, practicing it with my training partner until it is second nature.
2. Development of the ability to *rapidly assess situations as they present themselves*. I will have acquired the skill of evaluating an attack against me—on the spot—and comparing it to situations that I have already previewed in my mind. I am thus able to compare in real time this new state of affairs to situations I have previewed, and my subsequent physical actions come as a result of my assessment of what I am facing.

In either case—whether through training that facilitates instinctive responses or through development of rapid evaluation skills—I am relying on strategic approaches.

So read, enjoy, and put some icing on your own self-defense cake!

—Paul Karleen, Ph.D.
Senior Instructor IKMA (Gidon System)

Acknowledgements

I cannot say or write enough about my gratitude for Grandmaster Haim Gidon's investing his krav maga knowledge in me. The krav maga as taught by the Israeli Krav Maga Association (Gidon System), henceforth referred to as IKMA, is simply the best krav maga in the world. I, and a growing legion of others, understand why krav maga founder Imi Lichtenfeld vested his faith in Haim to advance and improve krav maga as head of the IKMA system. Once again, many of the tactics you will see in this book are courtesy of Haim's unique understanding of Imi's thinking and what krav maga must be.

Supporting Grandmaster Gidon are the highest-ranking sixth dan and fifth dan Israeli Krav Maga instructors: respectively, Ohad Gidon, sixth dan; and Noam Gidon, Yigal Arbiv, Steve Moishe, and Aldema Zirinksi, all fifth dan. These men represent the best of krav maga professional instruction. One will not find finer krav maga fighters and instructors in the world.

My great friend Paul Karleen, a fellow instructor and mentor who has selflessly taken thousands of krav maga photos—some of the best I've ever seen—helped me edit this book (Paul also helped me edit my previous book *Krav Maga Combatives*). Many of his photos appear in this work. Along with his self-defense capabilities, I find Paul's insights, as a septuagenarian, to be just remarkable. So as we finished the book, I thought, who better than Paul to write a foreword? I didn't expect such compliments and am both humbled and honored by Paul's kind but candid words. He warrants a special thanks for his amazing instructional abilities, patience, and outstanding support.

Black-belt Instructor Rinaldo Rossi, along with instructors Mike Delahanty, Don Melnick, Jeff Gorman, Frank Collucci, Paul Karleen, John Papp, Bill Dwyer, Sean Hoggs, Yu Oen, Clay Hamil, Het Hetman, Anne Mennen, Mike Hosgood, Brandon Druker, Dion Privett, Christian Stanley, Rich Kahl, Kevin Scozorro, Jonathan Sabin, Andre Kwon, Darius Davis, Marc Shneiderman, Suzanne Dougherty, Corey Jones, Adam Peterson, Devora Lapidot, and Kathyrn Badger were each pivotal in the development of our instructional materials. You all came to the rescue and I am eternally grateful time and again. A big thanks to prolific author Chris McNab along with law enforcement subject matter experts Bill Lewinski and Von Kliem of the Force Science Institute for their support. Paul Gilbert, Areyah Joseph, and Lance Hyatt are also three great supporters whom I thank. Paul Szyarto, one tough dude, deserves a superlative thanks for his support and interest in learning what actually works.

My attorney, David Schroth, is both my legal shield and sword when necessary. He can also use his personal weapons to great effect should the need arise. I deeply appreciate his legal acumen, generosity, and contributions to what we do. If you need a krav maga attorney (or a great attorney at anything else for that matter) in New Jersey, he's the guy (www.davidpshroth.com). Jon Soderberg, an older brother figure to me, and his family are dear to my heart. I thank the Soderbergs for their interest and support since my high school days. I am thankful to have Chris Cornish as a close supporter, visionary of change, and kravist in my corner.

I am grateful to my great friend MSgt. Ronald E. Jacobs, Ret., former chief instructor for the United States Marine Corps Martial Arts Program and former lead Naval Special Warfare Combatives Instructor at TRADET 2, who now holds a very special hand-to-hand combat instructional position in the government community. I am also deeply grateful to Major H. C. "Sparky" Bollinger, who is one of our top instructors and who has helped us improve the krav maga system. I am privileged to have the support of MSgt. Ronnie Groves, Ret. along with that of Army Special Forces MSgts. Dan and Josh. We are honored our krav maga is helping our military personnel enhance their hand-to-hand combat skill sets. Army CW4, Ret., Mike Reidel is another elite supporter to whom I am grateful and honored to help. I am also grateful to retired Navy instructors R., J., N., J., and S., and USAF SERE instructors TSgts. Mike and Ben.

I thank the following additional United States Marine Corps personnel: Lt. Col. Joseph Shusko, Ret.; GySgt. Gokey, Ret.; MGySgt. Urso, Ret.; and Lt. Col. "Tonto" Ardese, Ret. Thanks also to Sgt. Ben Perkins of the Royal Marines, along with 1st Sgt. Johnson and Maj. Lanzolloti of the United States Air Force for their support. Once again, Maj. Sean Hoggs, Ret., is an amazing supporter of our system and provides invaluable insights on training and life. I thank all of the fighting men and women of the United States military and Israel Defense Force for protecting our freedom. They collectively merit a profound thank you for their service.

Sgt. Maj. Nir Maman, Ret., former LOTAR lead counterterror instructor, krav maga instructor, and IDF Infantry and Paratroopers Ground Forces Command Soldier of the Year, 2009, possesses many unequalled professional insights and offers specialized training expertise as only he can provide. Nir has improved the IKMA system immeasurably. I also have the benefit that Nir is one of my greatest friends. Eyal E. and Dima G. are also great friends. They add to our understanding of the Israeli method of defensive measures and close protection. Anthony Caudle is also a great supporter and I thank him for his continued interest.

I am indebted to the Hauerstocks for their *sabra* hospitality in my many visits to Israel and to my good friend Shira Orbas, along with her wonderful family. I offer special thanks to Master Kobi Lichtenstein and his organization for their hospitality. Thank you to the IKMA board of directors and all IKMA members who have welcomed and trained with me over the years. Once again, this book would not be possible without the expert training, support, and inspiration of krav maga's backbone: the IKMA (www.facebook.com/gidonsystemkravmaga/).

Two of the first American krav maga instructors, senior instructors Rick Blitstein and the late Alan Feldman, were redoubts of support and special reservoirs of krav maga knowledge. I am always grateful to Rick for sending me on the correct krav maga path.

Our good friend in Poland, Kris Sawicki, keeps the IKMA at the forefront in Europe. I am grateful to all our students at our IKMA United States Training Centers (www.davidkahnkravmaga.com and www.israelikrav.com). I am indebted to many other IKMA affiliates, friends, and supporters, along with our network of fellow in-house instructors, including Darcy Howlett, Ray Lucas, Roy Shields, Ronnie Allen, Alex O'Neil, Jeremy Shank, Charles Smith, Dustin McGee, Kim Delesoy, and Sarah Mantz. Instructor Cory Davis along with his lovely wife Sheena keep krav maga training at its best on the Alaskan Final Frontier. Chet Barnett also merits a thanks for his continued interest and support in wanting to see krav maga "done right." Thank you to Al Ackerman and Darren DeSalvo for their terrific support.

We have a wonderful supporter in ABC star reporter Rick Williams, along with all those instructors in the pipeline. Jason Weber is a great partner, superb martial artist, and instructor, and I deeply appreciate his encouragement and support. Jason is one of the few instructors to whom I'd entrust my sons. Steven Feldstein is one of my favorite training partners and people; I thank him for his generous support and interest along with the world-renowned golf instructor Joe Mayo.

Officer Al "Poodie" Carson is family to me and has helped me to change the way NFL players approach the "hands" game. Poodie is one of a kind and truly a pillar of support. Vince Pecora, may he rest in peace, merits a special thank you for his wonderful support and generosity. I am once again grateful to All-Pro NFL players Aaron Donald (2017 and 2018 Defensive Player of the Year) and Khalil Mack (2016 Defensive Player of the Year)—two of the toughest, most committed, and most athletic men one could know. NFL Guard B. J. Finney and Tackle Chris Hubbard are consummate pros and great champions of Krav Maga Football Combatives. My law school friend NFL agent David Canter and NFL agent Tyler Urban are appreciated for their support and professional insights. I would also like to thank Princeton University Football Head Coach Bob Surace (and congratulate him once again on Princeton's legendary 10–0 season, with more to come!) along with the indefatigable Coach Steve Verbit and the rest of the Princeton coaching staff for their interest in and support for our Football Combatives training. My former teammate Keith Elias and Coach Rod Marinelli are also thanked for their enthusiam and support.

Justice Mitchell, continue to do "justice" to our approach and method. Doreen and Steve Laskiewicz are amazing bastions of hands-on marketing support. They are all great friends and the best krav maga marketing minds I'll ever know. Justice and Steve are true kravists. Sorat and Alexander "Lex" Tungkasiri are family to us in no uncertain terms. My son Benjamin, along with his best pal "Lex" and my other son Leo, all budding kravists, beat me up as they should.

Instructor Enrique Prado deserves a big thanks for his support. I am also grateful to Kim and Oliver Pimley for their dedication. As ever, the Tenenbaums and Goldbergs remain pillars of my life and *mishpachat.* Photographers Paul Karleen and Brandon Jones (http://www.truestill.studio) did a superb job, and their amazing professionalism and skills helped make this book what it is. Nancy Fury is kindly thanked for her demonstrative faces and terrific support.

A special thanks on both a personal and professional level to all of our friends and supporters in the law enforcement community, including Det. Gioscio; Director Masseroni; Officer D'Antonio; Sgt. Corey Jones; Capt. Miller, Ret.; Sgt. McComb, Ret.; Sgt. Klem, Ret.; Sgt.

Oehlmann; Sgt. Rayhon; Sgt. Rich Ashkar; Lt. Critelli; Lt. Maniace; Lt. DeMaise; Lt. Wolf, Ret.; Lt. Cowan; Lt. Boland; Chief Trucillo; Capt. Capriglione; Lt. Miano; Lt. Peins; Officer Vaval; Lt. Vacirca; Officer Miller; Capt. Maimone, Ret.; Lt. Cowan; Corp. Barr; Capt. Savalli, Ret.; Deputy Chief Strother; Deputy Director Strother; AVP Ominsky; Duncan Harrison; Chief Lazzarotti, Ret.; Director Paglione, Ret.; Lt. Colon; Sgt. Hayden, Ret.; Officer Johnson; Special Agent-in-Charge Hammond; Director Murray; ATSAIC/RTC Meissner and his instructors; Special Agent Crowe; Deputy Director Newsome; Special Agents Schroeder and Belle; Special Agents Gettings, Love, Clark (Ret.), Nowazcek (Ret.), and Baucom; Special Agent Crowe; Captain Laskiewicz; Sheriff Smith; Sheriff Kemler and the entire Mercer County Sheriff's Office; Chief Werner; Lt. Medina; Officer Hobson; Sgt. Lopez; Sgt. Gill; Lt. Watson; Lt. Rabinovitz; Officer Hosgood; Lt. Finicle; Chief Sutter, Ret.; Chief Morgan; Lt. Maurer; Officer King; Officer Donnelly; and my entire hometown Princeton Police Department along with Local PBA 130, Princeton University's Public Safety Department along with the many other law enforcement professionals with whom we have the honor of working. Col. Britcher, Ret. and his agency merit a special thanks for his stellar support and sponsorship within the PA law enforcement community and for his great assistance in our instruction.

I thank security expert Steven Hartov, one of my favorite authors and good friends, for his personal and professional support. I am grateful to Drs. Steven Gecha, Jeffrey Abrams, Stephen Hunt, and Bruce Rose, as well as massage therapist Autumn Magee and Denise Valdes along with PT Jennifer Kole for continuing to hold me together. Thanks to Jerry Palmieri for his conditioning advice, along with "Doc" Mark Cheng. Former Marine Matt Brzycki made a huge impact on my later krav maga training with his recommended high intensity training program and wrestling insights during my time at Princeton University.

I am fond of stating that good tactical minds think alike. To that end, I would like to compliment and recommend some fellow YMAA authors and renowned self-defense subject matter experts. At the top of the list are Rory Miller, Loren Christensen, Lawrence Kane, Kris Wilder, and Joe Varady. These guys possess some of the keenest street insights and hard-won experience in the ugly business of self-defense. I highly recommend their works. Their practical, street-oriented approaches dovetail well with krav maga thinking. I would also like to thank the superb YMAA publishing group headed by David Ripianzi and including Tim Comrie, Doran Hunter, and Barbara Langley for their truly outstanding sponsorship and support.

My family—especially my wife Claire—patiently and lovingly endures my nonsense. When hearing of another book on the docket, my father always supplies a hearty "good, good!" along with my stepfather Ed's encouragement. My uncle Harry always told me to hit him first, hit him hard, and hit him without stopping. My mother proudly adds it to the pile of my previous books on the living room table. Benjamin and Leo are the next generation of kravists. May they always stand for all that is good about krav maga and, most importantly, the good citizenship Imi's system promotes. I hope my sons pursue Grandmaster Gidon's krav maga to ensure that the next generation benefits.

Introduction

We are proud to present *Krav Maga Fundamental Strategies.* This book's goal is to dive deeper into krav maga's core self-defense strategies and fighting insights. Importantly, these practical, battle-tested stratagems are equally applicable across the spectrum of martial arts and fighting systems. We thank the many readers, kravists, and other self-defense enthusiasts who are interested in this seventh book of the line. Hopefully, it will remind all martial-arts practitioners of the epicenter of their studies: not just mastery of core basic tactics but an overall strategy to escape a violent encounter unharmed. Perhaps this book will also help rekindle the fire of advanced martial artists and masters to rethink and once again inculcate the tactics and principles that are most likely to work when (self) de-escalation, avoidance, escape, and—if necessary—counter-violence is required.

Israeli Krav Maga self-defense can be summarized as the fierce, optimum orchestration of counterviolence designed to prevail against any aggressor. General principles are applied and customized to meet the needs of a particular situation. A few mastered "families" of krav maga tactics are highly effective against the overwhelming majority of threats and attacks. By design, krav maga defenses largely harness instinctive adaptable gross motor movements to contend with the unpredictability of an attack. Each defense combines deflections and redirections, evasive body defenses, and simultaneous or near-simultaneous counterattacks against vulnerable anatomy with extreme prejudice delivered to overwhelm an attacker. Most importantly, krav maga self-defense is devoid of any rules. The system conforms to your strengths; you need not conform to the system. This is, in part, the genius of how founder Imi Lichtenfeld built krav maga. Grandmaster Gidon continues to improve the foundations of krav maga and evolve the self-defense and fighting system.

Good tactical minds think alike. Whatever your martial-arts or defensive-tactics background, hopefully, the following material can add some additional defensive solutions to your repertoire. Our goal is to augment your capabilities—to add additional arrows to your proverbial quiver. In the interest of providing a concise approach, I have tried to summarize here many essential topics from my previous six books: *Krav Maga* (2004), *Advanced Krav Maga* (2008), *Krav Maga Weapon Defenses* (2012), *Krav Maga Professional Tactics* (2016), *Krav Maga Defense* (2016), and *Krav Maga Combatives* (2019).

This book draws on materials from nearly every level of the curriculum. All the tactics you will read and evaluate are linked to our previous books and video materials. Notably, several weapon defense series photos provide a preview of the forthcoming book *Krav Maga Weapon Defenses II.*

While my objective is focused heavily on presenting krav maga's fighting insights, I believe providing access to short overviews of krav maga's emphasis on avoiding and preventing violence is paramount. Furthermore, I believe it would be both unprofessional and irresponsible as well as fail to do the IKMA curriculum justice were I not to include a summary of Israeli Krav Maga's approach to conflict avoidance, De-escalation Education™, and de-confliction, and escape. Violence avoidance and prevention are, without question, the best collective pre-conflict and post-conflict survival practices. Remember, the only violent battle you are sure to win is the one you avoid.

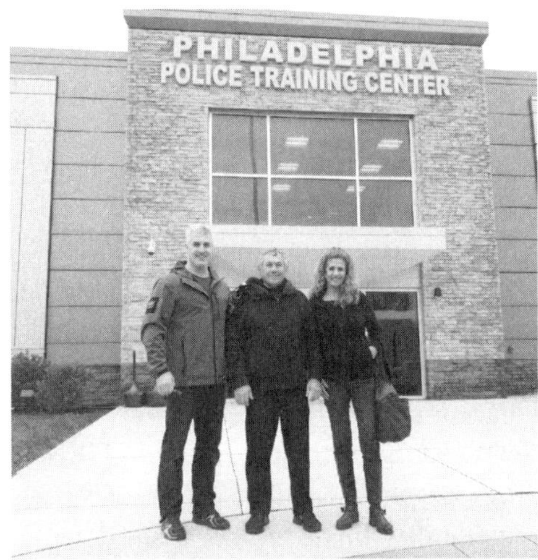

David Kahn, Grandmaster Haim Gidon, and Michal Gidon.

As the highest-ranking krav maga instructor in the world, Grandmaster Haim Gidon continues to evolve and improve the defensive system. Krav maga founder Imi Lichtenfeld appointed Haim as his successor and in June of 1996 awarded him his eighth dan (black belt). As he honored Haim, Imi simultaneously declared that ninth dan and tenth dan (red belt) were to come. Imi knew Haim would improve the krav maga system and, to be sure, Haim has. The Israeli Krav Maga Association (IKMA), headed by Grandmaster Haim Gidon, is krav maga's original governing body and is recognized by the Israeli government.

After Imi's passing in 1998, Haim followed in Imi's legendary footsteps and became the highest-ranking krav maga instructor in the world. He is the only current krav maga instructor to receive an eighth dan awarded directly by Imi. As Haim improves the system weekly in his gym in Netanya, Israel, he follows Imi's fundamental tenet that krav maga must work for all types of defenders. Constant improvement, evolution, and tactical flexibility make Israeli Krav Maga a phenomenal fighting and self-defense method. Israeli Krav Maga's pledge (and this is one of the keys to its brilliance) is that it can teach nearly anyone to successfully defend against proximate violence.

The study of real-life encounters sometimes necessitates modification or revision of tactics and the addition of new ones. Importantly, while certain krav maga defenses are specific, especially those against weapons, the application of these defenses must be adaptable to accommodate a violent situation's volatility. In short, we apply general principles and then customize them to meet whatever threat your opponent presents. Once again and most emphatically, krav maga emphasizes that there are no rules in a potentially deadly encounter so that you can make the best use of your capabilities to survive and escape unharmed.

Regarding the future of krav maga, dubious claims seem to constantly surface about krav maga's origins and evolution. Doesn't it make sense that the original governing body of krav maga, the IKMA, through its professional committee of the highest-ranked Israeli instructors, would be best able to develop the system to meet today's most modern threats? Moreover, we do not approach our specific krav maga training as an exercise program or fad. We do not just make up tactics for the sake of being different or putting a personal spin on the system to sell it to the public. The tactics and strategies we teach are designed by no-nonsense, tactically minded people, who are (forgive the pun) deadly serious about safety training. For those who convert these tactics and strategies for your own use without attribution, you know who you are. We know who you are as well.

Civilian Krav Maga Tactics

Security-minded civilians master krav maga to construct a defensive shield against violence, *not to develop an offensive capability to perpetrate violence.* Krav maga training's goal for civilians is simple: to deliver you from harm's way using autonomic responses that both harness and hone krav maga's instinctive tactics. The tactics become not second nature but first nature.

The ultimate goal is that you never hesitate about resorting to overwhelming, optimized counterviolence in the face of an unavoidable threat or attack. When there is no other choice but to defend yourself, you may be compelled to maim, cripple, and even use lethal force against an attacker, but only if under the totality of the circumstances such defense measures are legally justifiable. In actual fights, the combatants, even if they have formal training, often dispense with any complex learned training and resort to primitive combative tactics fueled by anger and bloodlust. The depth of violence will largely depend on the participants involved and how quickly animal instincts hijack the situation. In krav maga, breaking bones, injuring ligaments, and destroying an eyeball are optimized and emphasized both tactically and strategically to end the attack—provided these debilitating tactics represent proportional force. Women are often victims of violence and crime because the assailant thinks he can get away with it without injury to himself. Krav maga is designed to exact a steep physical toll on anyone who will not listen to reason and is intent on harming you.

In the basest, most primal sense, when faced with a life-threatening situation, the kravist understands how to inflict terrible, debilitating wounds on an adversary. There is no pity or compassion in a self-defense situation, but only if, once again, the counterforce is legally justifiable. In general terms, the party who significantly damages the other party first usually prevails, provided he presses the counterattack home to neutralize the threat.

The Language of Krav Maga

Throughout *Krav Maga Fundamental Strategies* the following terms will appear. Once you understand the language of krav maga, you can better understand the method.

Combative: Any manner of strike, takedown, throw, joint lock, choke, or other offensive fighting movement.

Deadside: Your adversary's deadside, in contrast to his liveside, places you behind his near shoulder or facing his back. You are in an advantageous position to counterattack and control him because it is difficult for him to use his arm and leg furthest away from you to attack you. You should always move to the deadside when possible. When executed properly, this will also place the adversary between you and any third-party threat.

Kravist: A term I coined to describe a smart and prepared krav maga fighter.

Liveside: When you are in front of your adversary and your adversary can both see you and use all his arms and legs against you, you are facing his or her liveside.

L-parry: A defensive arm movement that leads a defense by delivering a mini-forearm chop to an incoming attacker's arm. The defensive rotational arm movement is best delivered when the deflecting arm is bent 70 or so degrees to optimally extend the arm.

Nearside: Your adversary's limb closest to your torso.

Off-angle: An attack angle that is not face-to-face.

Parry: A redirection of an incoming strike.

Retzev: A Hebrew word that means "continuous motion" in combat. The backbone of modern Israeli Krav Maga, retzev enables you to move your body instinctively in combat motion without thinking about your next move. When in a dangerous situation, you'll automatically call upon your physical and mental training to a launch seamless, overwhelming counterattack using strikes, takedowns, throws, joint locks, chokes, or other offensive actions combined with evasive action. Retzev is quick and decisive movement merging all aspects of your krav maga training. Defensive movements transition automatically into offensive movements to neutralize the attack, affording your adversary little time to react.

Same side: An arm or leg directly opposite that of an opponent when you are facing each other. For example, in this situation your right arm is "same side" to his left arm.

Stepping off the line: Using footwork and body movement to take evasive action against a linear attack such as a straight punch or kick. Such movement is also referred to as breaking the angle of attack.

Tai sabaki: A 180-degree or semicircle step executed by swinging one leg around behind yourself. Often used to create torque on a joint to complete a takedown or control hold.

Trapping: Occurs when you pin or grab the adversary's arms with one arm, leaving you free to continue combatives with your other arm.

The Optimum Use of This Book

In this seventh book we continue to expand the reader's understanding of self-defense and fighting at the beginner, advanced, and expert level of Israeli Krav Maga tactics. This book is designed for the responsible, security-conscious civilian to enhance his or her chances of surviving an unavoidable violent encounter without sustaining serious injury. These techniques derive from my translation of the IKMA guidelines. Some of the photos included to help illustrate and undergird the principles portray partial technique execution. A significant number of the full techniques, along with step-by-step descriptions, have been included in previous books and will be included in forthcoming ones.

Developing a personal defense strategy solely grounded in proven tactics is essential. While targeting your adversary's vulnerable anatomy is always a key to winning a violent encounter, many situations require some specific defensive-priority and reaction stratagems. One indisputable self-defense tenet is to get off the line of an attack. Another crucial strategy is to optimally deflect or redirect a weapon for maximum control and subsequent confiscation. If you are faced with multiple (un)armed adversaries any coherent strategy can be rapidly taxed to its limit. In other words, any built-in margin for error is drastically reduced. Therefore, you cannot simply rely on what your untrained instinct tells you to do. Instead, krav maga dictates that you harness your natural instincts and training, and optimize your inbred survival mechanisms. To survive an unavoidable violent onslaught uninjured, you must internalize a few core interrelated and interdependent fight strategies. Your self-defense path must become first nature through correct mental and physical training. Hopefully, this book will combine with any previous professional self-defense knowledge to enhance your personal survival blueprint.

The most advantageous use of this book is to practice each principle as presented under safety-observant training conditions. It cannot be overemphasized that Israeli Krav Maga relies on a few core self-defense strategies and tactics adaptable to thwart most violent encounters. Obviously, no book is a substitute for hands-on learning with a qualified Israeli Krav Maga expert instructor. Be sure to thoroughly vet any instructor with whom you decide to train. I will hazard a guess that instructors who complete three-day civilian "krav maga" certification courses without serious, legitimate prior krav maga experience are suspect, as is someone who purchases a purported krav maga black belt every year. The same goes for an organization that sells a black belt to such an individual. **BECAUSE NOT ALL KRAV MAGA IS THE SAME. . .®**

Best Use of Training Partners

The importance of a determined training partner who is prepared to challenge and attack you cannot be overstated. The reality is that committed attackers are not going to stop the attack until you stop them. Obviously, in training, one must not injure one's training partner, so strict control of combatives and range must be honored. At the same time, the attacker does not give up until the defender correctly attacks using anatomical targeting that would debilitate the attacker.

In large part, the difference between professional training and amateur training is the intensity and commitment of a realistic simulated attack. Note that when participating in a higher level of training, real attacks can be orchestrated; *however using real knives and live firearms is neither recommended nor wise*. The internet is replete with true-life videos of the most common attacks, from the push to heinous killings. Realistic training examples include retracting the arm used in a punch or knife attack to immediately attack again, choking at 100 percent, swinging 100 percent at the attacker's head with a padded glove or with a foam baton, and yanking back one's replica gun-wielding hand as a gunman would, should someone try to disarm him (such as when a defense is initiated).

Foremost, in learning krav maga, as skill levels permit, a partner must simulate the intensity and barbarity of a concerted attack. This is one of the first and most important lessons Grandmaster Haim Gidon taught me. This distinguishes the Israeli Krav Maga taught by Haim, his top instructors, and his students. In my opinion, the level of training in Haim's gym is unsurpassed in the krav maga world. For sample videos check out Grandmaster Gidon's Facebook page (https://www.facebook.com/gidonsystemkravmaga/). There are myriad videos in the marketplace of people grunting and showing aggression, but the attack is often timid, uncommitted, and unrealistic. One cannot improve without realistic training and tactics that represent the realities of a determined attack. It is that simple.

Israeli Krav Maga Self-Defense Strategy Insights

This book provides select fighting-concept summaries from my translation of the IKMA curriculum. Many of these updated insights have never before been published. While I explain these as krav maga doctrines and principles, *any* tried and proven self-defense framework is likely to incorporate them. In other words, in this book, wherever I have used "krav maga," one might easily and accurately substitute the words "practical self-defense."

Real violence is horrific, shocking, ghastly, gruesome, and sickening to assign just a few adjectives. Those who have experienced concerted, injurious violence understand this observation well. If you are fortunate never to have experienced serious violence, the importance of viewing and digesting videos of real armed and unarmed attacks cannot be impressed on you enough. Videos of prison violence depicting nearly every conceivable type of unarmed and edged-weapon assaults along with group attacks are especially informative and sobering to watch.

Your mind-set must be to survive and escape unscathed—this is what it means to "win" in krav maga. Remember, while it is true that in a significant number of violent altercations combatants often know one another, in a street confrontation you'll likely not know anything about a looming adversary. Even if he lacks bad-ass tattoos, is diminutive, looks like a bookworm, or is otherwise unimposing, he should not be taken lightly—what you don't know about someone's intent and capabilities can get you seriously injured or killed. My personal approach is to consider that any person who challenges or confronts me could be trained and dangerous. This thinking reinforces my resolution to avoid physical confrontation even at the expense of my ego or the social indignity I might experience.

Assuming there is someone out there better trained, stronger, faster, and more physically capable also dovetails with my strategy of expecting the unexpected. Keep in mind further that if you have no avenue of escape, you must up the ante by, for example, jamming a finger underneath an attacker's closed upper eyelid and then screwing your finger deep into an attacker's eye socket to exert maximum damage; arguably this could change the level of return violence he might try to visit on you. Despite your defensive capabilities, though, remember that anyone who will not work with you to de-escalate, de-conflict, or let you escape could cause you serious injury or death. That is why krav maga is designed to be so brutally efficient when necessary.

Throughout the book for brevity and ease of reading, I have listed some of the topical and sub-topical IKMA wisdom in bullet-point format.

The Strategy of Training to the Proven Threat Categories: Incorporating Select Statistical Observations

The following summary statistics are helpful in understanding violent trends and, hence, to train to the threat. In other words, when training time is limited (as it is for most people), it is logical to determine what the most common attacks are and plan your training accordingly. Keep in mind that studies indicate that 85 percent or more of the world's population is right-handed. Therefore, you are more likely to face a right-handed threat or attack.

In 2018, FBI statistics reported that the following types of weapons were used in U.S.-based aggravated assaults. These statistics are relatively consistent over the last decade:

- Personal weapons:[3] 25.2 percent
- Firearms: 26.1 percent
- Edged weapons: 17.3 percent
- Other weapons: 31.5 percent

The 2018 FBI statistics report that the following types of weapons were used in U.S.-based robberies. These statistics are relatively consistent over the last decade:

- Personal weapons ("strong arm"): 42.8 percent
- Firearms: 38.5 percent
- Edged weapons: 8.3 percent
- Other weapons: 10.4 percent

With these attack and robbery threat statistics in mind, might it not make sense to allocate your training time accordingly? Obviously, weapons threats require serious training time and should not be neglected. In other words, wouldn't it be wise to focus on training scenarios that mimic, for example, facing a strong-arm robbery threat from personal weapons roughly five times more than the threat of an edged-weapon robbery? And for aggravated assaults, isn't it logical to focus one quarter of your training time on defending against personal weapons and a little less than one fifth of your training time on edged-weapon attacks?

3. Personal weapons are any parts of the human body, such as hands, feet, elbows, knees, teeth, and the crown of the forehead.

Chapter 1

Disengagement Strategies

The most important virtue krav maga can teach you is not to use krav maga—unless you truly have no choice. Many fights begin with social violence or a situation from which you could simply walk away. A moment of socially stoked anger can literally cost you everything. Conversely, not acting can also cost you dearly—including your life. When facing the specter of social violence, how do you best avoid it? How do you walk away without feeling emasculated, de-fanged, or that you backed down? Ultimately, how do you disengage while maintaining your pride and dignity?

Emotional control is krav maga's staunchest pillar. While such restraint is perhaps the most difficult tactic to learn and employ, it may be the most important. Despite any indignation or effrontery you may experience, you need to prioritize de-escalation, de-confliction, and disengagement. Of course, this is more easily said than done. Humans have subconscious ideas governing social violence that revolve around a vestige of rules where physical mayhem or death *is not* the preferred outcome. Alternatively stated, the typical contest where someone gets taught a lesson by asserting social dominance through either intimidation or physical force usually does not involve grave injuries or murderous intent. In stark contrast, raw violence is the use of physical force without constraint and where mayhem or death *is* the preferred outcome. In every book we produce, along with every class we teach, we try to emphasize krav maga founder Imi Lichtenfeld's wisdom in his own words. Imi stressed that the "most necessary thing is to educate you—and that is the hardest thing—to be humble. You must be so humble that you don't want to show him that you're better than him. That is one of the most necessary things for pupils. If a pupil tells me, 'I fought him and beat him,' it's no good."[4]

The bottom line is that some people will tolerate impudence and abuse while others will not. Ultimately, those who will brook no challenges may have a shorter or longer fuse, but, with enough provocation or an actual threat, it will ignite. A large part of your "awareness" is understanding your personal capacity and limits. Obviously, the amount of verbal or

4. Julia M. Klein, "Don't Get Hurt," *Philadelphia Inquirer*, April 9, 1984.

physical abuse you will accept or what actions cross your proverbial line on the concrete, carpet, mat, grass, gravel, or snow is your decision. Paramount is knowing where the line is for you. You can push the line back (assuming a verbal or gestural provocation—not a physical assault) by using a self-recognition or self-evaluation tactic. This means that you recognize your vulnerabilities, accept them, and create effective coping or deflecting mechanisms. You can then prevent a hostile person from baiting you into reacting as an excuse to commit violence against you.

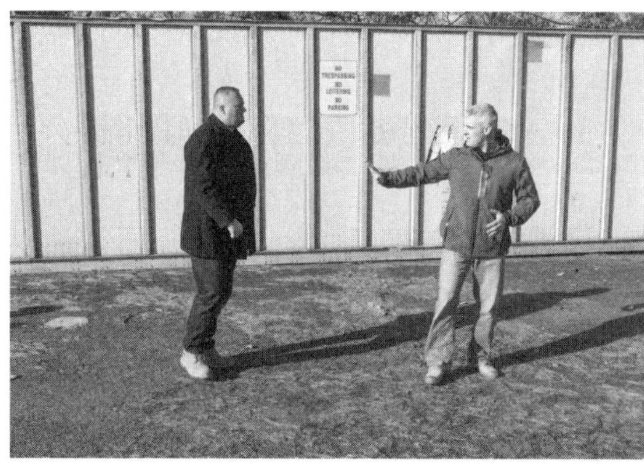

An attempt to de-escalate a situation and walk away.

Both Imi and Grandmaster Gidon underscore that "the hardest thing is to be humble." Emotions must be contained, moderated, and controlled. Most importantly, you must recognize impending social violence to prevent it from controlling your immediate future. Imi understood that true power rests in self-control. If you can swap angry emotions with alternative calm emotions, your anger will release or dissipate, preventing aggression and violence. This cognitive restructuring is the key to any anger management strategy. To be sure, learning emotional competency is a process that requires effort and practice. Without question the ability to ignore hostile language and words is not easy. When you can control yourself, you are best prepared to try to control the vortex of chaos surrounding you in a conflict. If you want to avoid conflict, you must master yourself.

Simple logic dictates that if a verbal attack is unfounded or doesn't have truth behind it, you have no reason to become upset about it. Of course, once again, this is easier said than done. When an aggressor attempts to slam one of your "go" buttons or yank one of your triggers, you should be mentally prepared for it because you have practiced an appropriate non-hostile response. Methodically harnessing and controlling your breathing is universally known to be instrumental in developing this invaluable capability. Usually the process of a deep inhale with a four-second hold, followed by a two-second pause, followed by a four-second exhale, works well. If you are confident that you can physically subjugate another another person, you have the ultimate supremacy. The key is not to feel compelled to exercise power. This avoids legal entanglements that could cost you a small fortune, not to mention your liberty and the stigma of being a convicted felon.

Understanding the Difference Between Anger and Rage

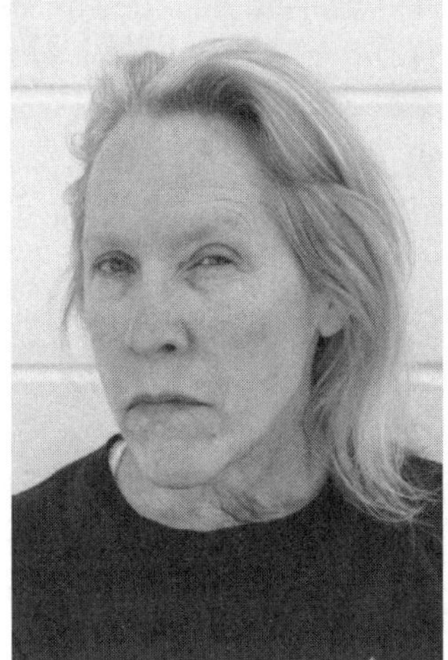

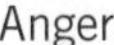

Anger.

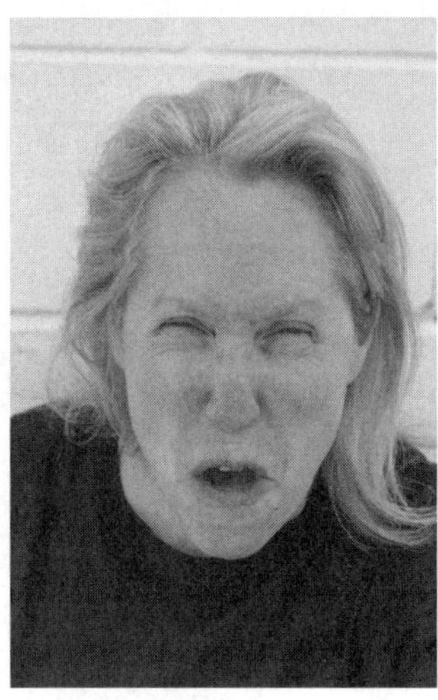

Rage.

Anger is a state of incremental arousal. Emotions govern everything when a hostile person attempts to dominate you. They immediately hijack reason. When your heart rate rises just ten percent, any disputed truth becomes less and less relevant. The altercation devolves solely into a matter of winning or losing. People often ramp up their anger threshold to anger's pinnacle—rage. The difference between anger and rage is that the latter is the supreme form of anger, where someone has discarded any social or legal inhibitors about using violence. Someone who is enraged is no longer attempting to peacefully negotiate. Physical violence is highly likely. Hot rage is a term applied to someone on the precipice of violence. This point of no return can be egged on by onlookers or a need to look tough and not back down in front of observers.

In my research on anger, I read an informative article entitled, "Anger Is Temporary Madness: The Stoics Knew How to Curb It" by philosophy professor Massimo Pigliucci.[5] Among Pigliucci's insights, which draw from the Stoic philosopher Lucius Annaeus Seneca, is that mankind has long understood the vicissitudes of anger and its consequences. Seneca's *On Anger*, written in the first century CE, posits that anger is a temporary madness. Even when anger might be justified, Seneca emphasized that one should never act on the basis of emotion because, though "other vices affect our judgment, anger affects our sanity: others come in mild attacks and grow unnoticed, but men's minds plunge abruptly into anger." Seneca concluded that anger's "intensity" was in "no way regulated by its origin: for it rises to the greatest heights from the most trivial beginnings." Another Stoic philosopher, Epictetus, admonished: "Remember that it is we who torment, we who make difficulties for

5. Massimo Pigliucci, "Anger Is Temporary Madness: The Stoics Knew How to Curb It," getpocket.com, n.d., https://getpocket.com/explore/item/anger-is-temporary-madness-the-stoics-knew-how-to-curb-it?utm_source=pocket-newtab.

ourselves—that is, our opinions do. What, for instance, does it mean to be insulted? Stand by a rock and insult it, and what have you accomplished? If someone responds to insult like a rock, what has the abuser gained with his invective?" (Though some people do talk to plants.)

Recognizing Your Own Triggers

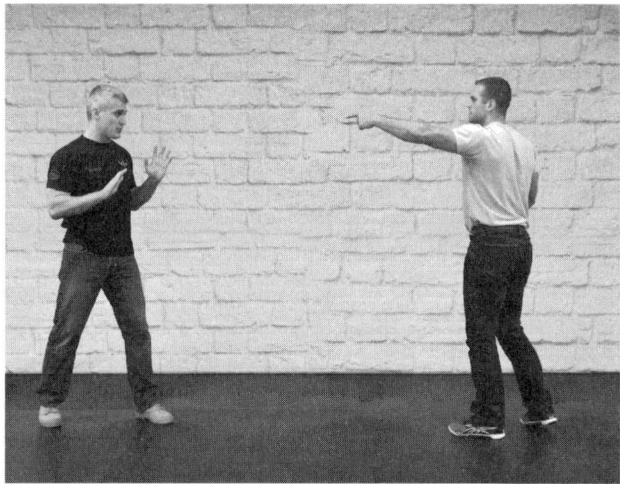

A finger-pointing trigger.

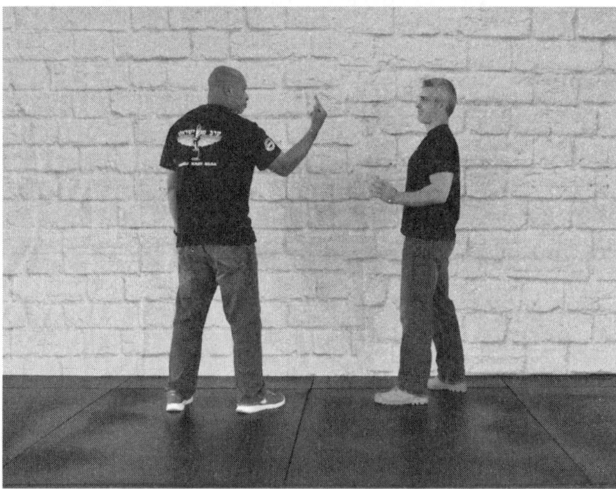

A rude-gesture trigger.

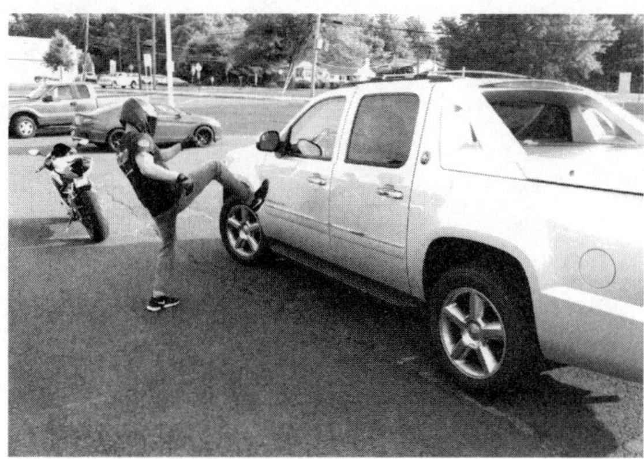

A trigger of someone kicking your vehicle door in a road-rage incident.

Aggressive people have triggers that strongly pull them toward violence. Triggers, either verbal or visual, are environmental cues that draw on past mental programming to automatically and unconsciously activate a hostile response. When a trigger is activated, you may react as though your survival is at stake when it is actually not. A triggering event enables an individual to dispense with social mores and rules: he is free to act on his impulses or desires. A triggering event might involve (1) fear for one's safety, (2) frustration, or (3) not getting one's way. It might also be a prompt to use bullying or intimidation skills such as racial or cultural slurs. Try to provide a potential attacker a way out that does not humiliate him. This balancing act requires you to show no fear but offer mutual common sense that a fight is not what you want. However, be prepared that a peaceful outcome will not necessarily be what the attacker wants.

Handling Aggressive People Through De-escalation Communication™

Krav maga advocates, when possible, compassionate non-violent conflict resolution. Founder Imi Lichtenfeld emphasized handling a threat with graceful non-violent tact whenever feasible. Imi stressed the need good for citizenship above all else—obey the law and adhere to the overall social norm of considerate behavior. This obeisance, the foundation of civilized behavior, unfortunately breaks down all too often. Most violence is of a social nature—the kind that you can avoid. Moreover, the ugly fact is that 62 percent of all violence is committed between two people who know one another.[6]

Obviously, you cannot simply wish away a possible violent episode to avoid it. This form of denial lands people in deep trouble when they are attacked and freeze, thereby having to absorb the assault. Recognize there are violent people who will attempt to harm you. Sometimes, fortunately, you can change this dynamic by providing a non-violent solution.

6. https://www.bjs.gov/content/pub/pdf/vvcs9310.pdf.

A kravist recognizes how to influence or dictate an encounter to prevent violence. Taking control of an interaction means immediately hijacking the aggressor's script, stopping his machinations at their inception.

To prevail in a potentially violent situation, your savvy in managing and manipulating human behavior is more important than your combative capabilities. The only fight you are sure to win is the one you avoid. Whenever you interact with somebody, on some level you benignly manipulate their behavior and are benignly manipulated in return. About 70 to 90 percent of communication is non-verbal and interpreted through body language.[7] Only the last 10 percent of communication is based on the actual words you use to convey your thoughts. In short, your ability to avoid fights is largely dictated by your capability to psychologically manipulate an adversary's behavior through your body language and tone of voice, as well as your ability to select words to your advantage.

Achieve this good outcome by presenting a composed, controlled, and engaged deportment that allows *you* to own the situation. Exhibiting poised conduct throws off an aggressor's targeting radar. If you are contending with a highly agitated individual, a calm demeanor can nudge an aggressor toward a calm emotional equilibrium more quickly. Of course, when you cannot walk away or escape, as a last resort you must be prepared to inflict severe physical damage.

There are two types of aggressors: reckless aggressors or hotheads and professional aggressors who are either bullies or predators, or both. Thwarting a professional aggressor requires establishing a different set of rules than the ones he seeks to impose. To be sure, aggressors and predators recognize that any failure to defend smaller boundaries presents an opportunity to encroach on larger ones. For example, a sexual offender will often touch a potential victim's arm to see how the victim will react: meekly or assertively. A meek response encourages him to pursue his goal; an assertive response can repel his advances.

Kravists don't shrink from defending their morally grounded positions. We strive to do it with confidence, dignity, and civility. Equally important, a kravist should make the choice to walk in the path of peace even when preemptive counter-violence might be legally justified. In short, if you ransom your social or safety boundaries, self-deprecate, and assume a submissive posture, someone bent on testing your mettle will be all the more encouraged.

Danger recognition often presents subconsciously. When you sense and feel danger signals, that is your intuition at work; it is part of your naturally embedded learning/logic system. Listen to this innate warning mechanism. Research suggests that when information remains at a subconscious level it is analyzed at a faster and more thorough pace than your consciousness can dissect and process. In sum, your intuition is your biological subconsciousness that collectively harnesses all of your senses, including sight, sound, touch, taste, and smell. Therefore, mind it (forgive the pun) and certainly do not ignore it.

Keep in mind that awareness is not simply physically scanning for indicators of a potential problem; it is an appraisal by all of your senses including that sixth sense in your gut.

7. https://ubiquity.acm.org/article.cfm?id=2043156.

That gut feeling should automatically make you pause and analyze why you feel endangered. Awareness of your surroundings, of others, and of yourself must all work in concert to hone your defensive plan.

One of the best ways to diffuse a potentially violent situation is to find or establish common ground with an aggressor. Accordingly, while creating physical distance is always best to thwart violence, narrowing psychological distance can also help.

Remember, though, that what you *say* and what a person may decide to *hear* can be very different. Moreover, using a condescending tone with a potential aggressor is a sure-fire way to further draw his ire. You must earnestly demonstrate that you value a peaceful solution. Neutral eye contact underscores that you are listening and sincerely communicating with him. There is a vital distinction between assertive versus aggressive eye contact. Assertive eye contact maintains your boundaries while aggressive eye contact issues a challenge. When signaling your ability to stand up to an aggressor, adopt a neutral but confident facial expression and punctuate your message with a De-escalation Communication stance while speaking clearly and forcefully. Shawn T. Smith provides a nice summary of the importance of how you project your solution in his excellent book *Surviving Aggressive People*: "People act on what they perceive. If there is no other option apparent to them than perceived hostility, they will proceed in kind with hostility. Even a threat of severe counter-violence does not always dissuade an aggressor from pursuing violence if that's the only option he sees."[8] So, you must project non-threatening control in a best De-escalation Communication attempt.

Be mindful that a reckless aggressor may be hypersensitive, hypervigilant, or both. These states of mind might exacerbate his angst regarding anything you suggest. Therefore, roll with, and, if necessary, absorb any further emotional strikes he might launch at you. Your goal is to parry verbal abuse and get off the proverbial X to achieve a peaceable endgame. Be lithe and adaptable in any verbal exchange, similar to how you might need to physically deflect an attack. When attempting De-escalation Communication, you might consider using the word sir or ma'am using an even tone to bestow respect or sincerity in your earnest attempt to de-conflict. In addition, you might nod your head up and down to indicate that you are hearing the aggressor's message. At the beginning of a verbal onslaught directed at you, interject a phrase such as "Hey, please listen" or something to that effect to break the verbal aggressor's thought pattern. The more quickly you can apologize, explain, and de-conflict the more sincere it will appear.

If the trigger event was accidental, by validating a potential aggressor's feelings you stand a much better chance of talking your way out of violence. If you think an apology might end the situation peacefully, do it wisely without indicating subservience. A few initial De-escalation Communication responses Smith recommends:

---

8. Shawn T. Smith, *Surviving Aggressive People* (Denver: Mesa Press, 2014), 82. This informative book is a great guide for handling hostile and predatory people and goes hand in hand with the IKMA curriculum's notes on conflict preemption and de-escalation. When reasoning fails, Smith recommends krav maga as a great personal defense system.

- "Please tell me if I understand. You're upset that . . ."
- "I would be angry as well if . . ."
- "I understand why you'd be angry . . ."

Putting yourself in the other person's proverbial shoes can often go a long way toward finding mutual ground to resolve a fractious situation. Remember the shibboleth of do unto others as you would have others do unto you. Note that if you are dumbfounded about what to say or how to respond, simply keep listening instead.

Open-ended questions keep the aggressor talking. Remember, the mind has difficulty performing two tasks at once. His verbal engagement with you hampers his ability to physically attack you. Moreover, if you are successfully de-escalating the situation by genuinely addressing his issue, he will be less likely to attack. If an aggressor won't allow you to interject or make suggestions, here are a few strategic phrases presented by Smith that might capture his attention or break his rant:

- "Tell me if I have this correct . . ."
- "It seems that you feel ________ because ________ ."
- "Are you saying that you think ________ because ________ ?"

The key to empathy in a volatile situation is attempting to understand the problem from the aggressor's point of view. Therefore, empathy is a bedrock principle in:

- convincing an aggressor that you're attempting to act in his best interest and not as an adversary.
- ensuring that you focus on the true problem from his point of view. Present yourself as a problem solver rather than an aggressor. Lay the groundwork for a peaceful resolution by offering options.
- establishing common ground to develop a solution. Listening, empathizing, and De-escalation Communication responses are all dictated by the aggressor's current state of mind. As in a fight, timing is crucial.

Smith makes some additional great points:

- Verbal confrontations also involve something like fight timing: speaking earlier than opportune runs the risk of antagonizing the aggressor, while not responding quickly enough might suggest to him that you're not interested.
- Requesting information makes it possible to truly recognize a problem and helps to avoid making assumptions about how somebody feels or should feel.
- When asking a hostile individual to confirm your perceptions of what he is saying, you'll allow him the opportunity to correct or modify your paraphrase or reiteration of his problem without arguing about it. In doing so, you demonstrate a genuine commitment to understand.

- If the aggressor agrees with your statement summarizing the situation or corrects it, either way you have laid the groundwork for trust.

Criminals may test you by using incremental transgressions. These might include asking for snippets of personal information, patting you on the shoulder, or grabbing your arm to gauge your initial reaction. Smith categorizes seven testing rituals:

- overaccommodation with an offer to help or engage
- getting a foot in the door
- violating personal space and social conventions
- exploiting sympathy and guilt
- exploring insecurity by dispensing insults
- intimidation and exploiting fear
- distraction by information overload

Another of Smith's important observations is that successful predators become immune to a victim's protests.

It is vital that you distinguish between spiteful or unkind language versus threatening language. Smith points out that insults are a bid to change the balance of power. Threats should be taken seriously because they are a window into the aggressor's intentions. That can also provide a tactical advantage. If an aggressor is still spouting and thinking about causing harm, he is still in the planning stage for you to interrupt/disrupt such a plan. Importantly, a legitimate threat is a statement of intent with no provisions or conditions attached to it. According to some FBI guidelines, a threat should be classified as real when it is detailed, specific, contains a high emotional content, and the person issuing the threat is facing a number of stressors.

Finally, Smith concludes with a nice paraphrase of krav maga founder Imi's philosophy toward developing and maintaining a position of strength. "One of the great paradoxes is that peace comes through strength. Not the brute physical strength to club a malefactor into submission, but the mental strength to recognize and respond to an attack when the stakes are still low, and the strength and ability to respond peacefully even when the stakes are high. . . The person who makes reasonable preparations against the threat is likely to avoid conflict altogether."[9]

Contending with Road Rage

Road rage: we've all witnessed it, if not experienced it. The first use of the term "road rage" is attributed to Los Angeles news station KTLA after reporting a series of freeway shootings in 1987.[10] Road rage is defined by the National Highway Traffic Safety Administration (NHTSA)

9. Smith, *Surviving Aggressive People.* 208.
10. Stephanie Buck, "Road Rage Was Invented 30 Years Ago This Summer in LA, When Gunplay Came to the Freeways," timeline.com, July 6th, 2017, https://timeline.com/road-rage-history-los-angeles-563259c3ba78.

as occurring when "a driver commits moving traffic offenses so as to endanger other persons or property; an assault with a motor vehicle or other dangerous weapon by the operator or passenger of one motor vehicle on the operator or passengers of another motor vehicle."[11] Basically, any sort of violent or aggressive behavior that occurs on a road, or involves a car, could be considered an act of road rage. So, if someone is guilty of breaking the rules of the road and upsets you, you must be capable of de-escalating yourself (of course, a generally useful tool).

Road Rage: Pounding on Your Window Example

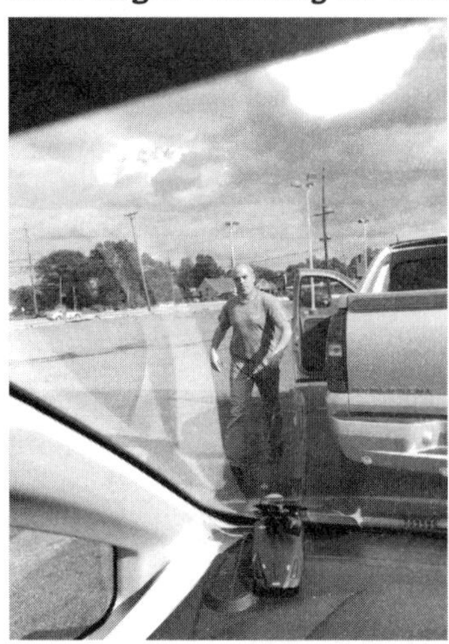

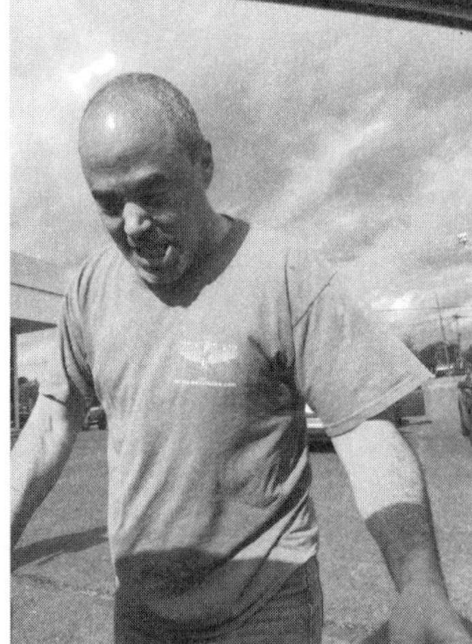

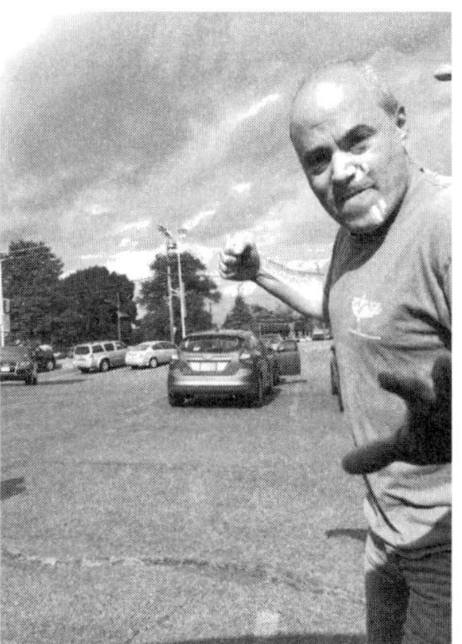

In a road-rage incident, as depicted in the photo series, an aggressor exits his vehicle and approaches your vehicle. The best course of action is to stay put and call the police. Use your phone to capture the license plate of the aggressor's vehicle along with a photo of the perpetrator. This course of action must be thought through ahead of time. Accordingly, you should practice working your mobile device's camera under simulated time pressure and stress. One way of practicing under time constraints is to have a friend walk at you from a measured distance and see if you can work your camera before the friend can reach or touch you. Another factor to consider is locating your phone under stressful conditions. Keeping it accessible and in the same place is always a good precautionary measure in case of an emergency. If possible, drive away immediately, but be prepared for the offender to follow you; hence the redoubled importance of contacting the police as soon as possible.

While aggressive driving is understood as reckless, willful, and wanton disregard of other motorists while operating a motor vehicle, the NHTSA distinguishes between aggressive driving (a misdemeanor) and road rage (a felony). Road rage becomes a felony when it involves both a *mens rea* (guilty mind) and *actus reus* (volitional [violent] act) toward another driver. Possible examples of each offense include:

---

11. Safemotorist.com, "Aggressive Driving and Road Rage," n.d., https://www.safemotorist.com/Articles/road_rage.aspx.

Non-felony
- Honking a vehicle's horn
- Shouting, screaming, and cursing
- Making rude hand gestures
- Flashing headlights or improperly turning on high beams
- Tailgating
- Cutting off another vehicle
- Deliberately driving well below the speed limit to impede another's progress
- Brake-checking (stopping short in front of another vehicle)
- Antagonistic use of horns, overuse or flashing of lights

Felony
- Forcing another driver off the road
- Intentionally ramming or colliding with another vehicle
- Exiting your vehicle to assault another driver, cyclist, or pedestrian
- Brandishing or using weapons against other drivers or pedestrians
- Shooting a gun toward another vehicle. Antagonistic use of horns, overuse or flashing of lights
- Using a vehicle as a tool to exhibit rage such as following other vehicles extremely closely, abruptly braking, or accelerating
- Singling out and aggressively pursuing another vehicle in a stalking manner
- Purposefully damaging another vehicle in any way, including striking a vehicle with a blunt weapon

According to the Insurance Information Institute, the following are the top twelve inattentive and careless actions that often contribute to road-rage incidents:[12]

1) Cutting off another vehicle
2) Tailgating
3) Failure to signal
4) Failure to yield a right of way
5) Improper and erratic turns or lane changes
6) Passing where prohibited
7) Driving in an erratic, reckless, careless, or negligent manner
8) Illegal driving on the road shoulder, in the ditch, sidewalk, or median
9) Failure to obey traffic signs, control devices, traffic zone laws, or officers
10) Suddenly changing speeds
11) Driving too fast for conditions or in excess of the posted speed limit
12) Racing

12. https://www.iii.org/fact-statistic/facts-statistics-aggressive-driving.

The following statistics,[13] compiled from the NHTSA and the Auto Vantage Auto Club, show the serious problems in America that aggressive driving and road rage precipitate:

- 66 percent of traffic fatalities are caused by aggressive driving
- 37 percent of road-rage driving incidents involve a firearm
- 50 percent or more of drivers who are on the receiving end of an aggressive behavior respond with aggressive behavior themselves

Over a seven-year period (2011–2018), 218 murders and 12,610 injuries were attributed to road rage.

2019 Road Rage Statistics

In October of 2019, The Zebra, an automotive insurance provider, conducted a national road-rage survey of American drivers while also incorporating additional previous data.[14] Some of the findings include:

- 82 percent of drivers in the U.S. admit to having road rage or driving aggressively at least once in the past year.
- 59 percent of drivers reported showing anger by honking.
- 42 percent of drivers claimed they have yelled or cursed loudly at another driver.
- 38 percent of drivers admitted gesturing obscenely toward other drivers.
- Males under the age of 19 are the most likely to exhibit road rage.
- Male and younger drivers ages 19–39 were significantly more likely to engage in aggressive behaviors. Male drivers were more than three times as likely as female drivers to have gotten out of a vehicle to confront another driver or rammed another vehicle on purpose. Roughly 40 percent of men have experienced road rage directed at them.
- Roughly 30 percent of women have experienced road rage directed at them.
- 31 percent of teenagers retaliate when they are on the receiving end of aggresion or road rage.

Notably, only 10 percent of the drivers actually called the police to report another driver's aggressive driving or road rage.

An April 2017 *New York Times* article reported that road-rage incidents involving someone who had brandished or fired a gun at another person had more than doubled since 2014. In 2016 alone, there were more than 620 road-rage incidents involving firearms being deployed. In a 2014 survey, the American Automobile Association (AAA)[15] presented some troubling numbers about American drivers who admitted to doing the following:

---

13. Safemotorist.com, "Aggressive Driving and Road Rage."
14. Taylor Covington, "Road Rage Statistics," thezebra.com, August 18th, 2020, https://www.thezebra.com/road-rage-statistics/.
15. AAA, "Nearly 80 Percent of Drivers Express Significant Anger, Aggression or Road Rage," AAA NewsRoom, July 14, 2016, https://newsroom.aaa.com/2016/07/nearly-80-percent-of-drivers-express-significant-anger-aggression-

- 51 percent (104 million drivers) to purposefully tailgating
- 47 percent (95 million drivers) to yelling at another driver
- 45 percent (91 million drivers) to honking to show annoyance or anger
- 33 percent (67 million drivers) to making angry and rude gestures
- 24 percent (49 million drivers) to blocking another vehicle from changing lanes
- 12 percent (24 million drivers) to cutting off another vehicle on purpose
- 4 percent (7.6 million drivers) to getting out of a vehicle to confront another driver
- 3 percent (5.7 million drivers) to bumping or ramming another vehicle on purpose

The Causes of Road Rage

The American Psychological Association (APA) published an insightful article called "The Fast and the Furious" examining what makes some people highly susceptible to road rage and how to best counsel these high-anger drivers to refrain from this behavior.[16] While road rage, according to the Diagnostic and Statistical Manual of Mental Disorders, is not an officially recognized mental disorder, a recognized "intermittent explosive disorder" is associated with road rage.

Psychologists note that a vehicle provides a motorist with power, protection, anonymity, and easy escape. In contrast, without a physical barrier such as when standing in a line, most people would not make offensive gestures or scream and shout. When in the safe confines of a vehicle, people let it fly and indulge themselves in the most uncivil behaviors. Environmental factors such as crowded roads and inattentive driving coupled with displaced anger and high life stress collectively exacerbate the problem.

Behavioral Therapy to Reduce Road Rage

The APA article cited a successful road-rage treatment program that was rolled out in New York state more than two decades ago. At the University at Albany's Center for Stress and Anxiety Disorders, twenty aggressive drivers referred by the local district attorney's office as well as ten volunteers who described themselves as aggressive drivers were counseled. Treatment sessions included "deep relaxation, stress-management coping skills, cognitive restructuring, and learning different ways to think about roadway events and stressors. These strategies have proven to help reduce anger and aggression, both behind the wheel and in general." The article reports that "the treatment group averaged a 64-percent drop in aggressive driving behaviors and showed marked reductions on measures of psychological distress, a standardized Driving Anger Scale, and a Driver Stress Profile. At a follow up three months later, the participants had maintained those improvements."

---

or-road-rage/.

16. American Psychological Association, "Fast and the Furious," February 2014, https://www.apa.org/action/resources/research-in-action/rage.

Here are a few practical suggestions that may help you avoid a road-rage incident:

- A simple apologetic wave can help defuse most confrontational matters.
- Conform to the rules of the road (as noted, many road-rage incidents turn into conflagrations because of ignored statutes and lack of simple driving etiquette).
- If tailgated, change lanes.
- Plan ahead for contingencies (such as through route planning and leaving adequate time to get to where you're going) to avoid making yourself susceptible to road rage.
- Aggressive horn usage is just that—avoid it.
- In short, operate your vehicle in a safe, civil manner; do unto others as you would have others do unto you.

More will be said on self-de-escalation and anger management strategies in the following sections.

De-escalating Yourself

Anger and anxiety place the body in a similar physiological state. Therefore, tactics to alleviate anxiety may also be used to defuse anger. Here is a well-accepted sequential method for defusing and managing anger or reactive aggression.

1. Emotion management starts with recognizing what the emotion is.
2. Try to identify your feelings or affect label yourself—articulate to yourself something to the effect that "I am angry" or "I feel disrespected" to prevent yourself from acting unconsciously. Doing this can calm you down and slow down automatic reactivity.
3. To reduce negative emotions, use diaphragmatic controlled breathing (deep inhale with a four-second hold, followed by a two-second pause, followed by a four-second exhale) and muscle relaxation and control.
4. Differentiate between *reacting* (irrational) and *responding* (rational) tactics.

You cannot afford to take the bait an aggressor offers. Provocation and enticement to respond are seeds of social violence. You don't need to risk putting yourself into a situation where you have to use your defensive-tactics skills only to be sued, criminally charged, and possibly incarcerated. Simply put, don't allow your emotions to hijack your reasoning. Recognize the emotional triggers a situation prompts and lock them down.

In the end, confidence—not overconfidence—in your ability to physically handle yourself in almost any situation should allow you to walk away. This was one of Imi's goals: "to walk in peace" or to walk away from social violence. Most importantly, adopt the mind-set that it is *the provocateur's* lucky day. Of course, if you are physically attacked, then krav maga is the answer.

Conflict Avoidance

Common sense and street smarts are your optimum shields to avoid violence. Truly understanding the nature and consequences of injurious violence should eliminate it as a dispute resolution option. Mental conditioning and rehearsal allow you to de-escalate or walk away (always the best solution if possible) from a potentially violent situation. In short, avoidance is often about keeping your cool, but so is every other aspect of self-defense, including de-escalation, escape and evasion, and, lastly, fighting for your life.

Impending Violence Usually Has Overt or Covert Signals

Many people who suddenly become embroiled in a violent encounter have no idea why it happened. Often, there is a buildup they did not recognize or were party to without their knowledge. A few commonsense suggestions:

- Be careful of other people's personal space.
- Do not return challenging stares.
- Be aware of kinesic indicators indicating an angry or hostile person.
- If in the wrong, apologize sincerely, but be subtly prepared for a potential attack.
- Leave any volatile or potentially hostile situation immediately.
- Social mores should readily be ignored (for example, leave an elevator if you feel threatened by someone; don't worry about the person's feelings).

Escape

Escape methods are a vital and major part of the krav maga curriculum. Wherever you are, you should have an escape plan for how you can best leave a bad situation. In other words, what is the most direct and expedited route to physically extricate yourself from harm's way? In an enclosed space, have you identified a primary, secondary, and perhaps tertiary exit?

Escape is your second choice when avoidance and de-escalation fail. Escape is different from avoidance as the aggressor has already begun his actions and you are actively fleeing. (To review, avoidance allows you to calmly remove yourself before a hostile situation begins.) Your goal in escaping is to evade physical contact and preserve your ability to successfully flee. Your ultimate goal is to find safety through breaking contact and losing any pursuers by creating no sight line, including quickly hiding or finding safety among other people. Physically escaping requires you to recognize egresses and to successfully negotiate terrain and obstacles. For example, in a potential road-rage incident, consider your driving escape options. (You should always leave enough room in front of your vehicle to maneuver.)

Terrain can aid or hamper you. High ground such as a stairwell gives you the advantage of gravity and using your strongest long-range weapons: kicks. Conversely, when fleeing up a stairway, ascending it will slow you down as you take the first steps and pursuers can close the distance. Your footing, and hence your traction and balance, can be affected by liquids (including blood), gravel, wet grass, mud, snow, and ice. Therefore, you must consciously and instinctively pay attention to your movements, shifting your balance onto the balls of your feet and altering your stance and pace. If you disable an attacker through counterassault, the attacker may have accomplices. The accomplices may be momentarily shocked by your counter-violent actions, providing you with a head start.

When running away, as noted, seek the safety of other people, using concealment as available. (Note that professional escape and evasion requires preplanned evacuation routes, safe houses, and dedicated support, among other things.) When running, focus on the physical route ahead of you. If you are part of a group, you must all act in concert: flee or fight together and act as a cohesive unit. If you decide to flee, you may also be able to turn around and ambush your pursuer. In a road-rage scenario, if you find yourself outside of your own vehicle (because you've made a tactical choice), you could momentarily escape an aggressor by running around the perimeter of your own car. In a run-around-a-stationary-car scenario, you can also use preemptive self-defense (a counter-ambush) against the aggressor by swiftly changing directions and catching the would-be assailant by surprise. However, if there are multiple pursuers, fighting a group is obviously not the best option.

Understanding One's Physiological Reaction to Threats and Violent Conflict

The krav maga curriculum considers the body's natural reactions when facing the specter of serious violence and when actually engaged in extreme violence. From a fighting standpoint, the following key points stand out:

1. Humans have three primary survival systems: vision, cognitive processing, and motor-skill performance. Under stress, all three capabilities degenerate.[17]
2. Fighting for your life is highly anaerobic. Your heart rate increases while breathing becomes slow and rapid. Blood is pulled away from your limbs to your vital internal organs.
3. Under extreme stress, a person's heartbeat can accelerate from about 60–70 normal beats per minute (BPM) to 200–300 BPM, a rate that can be reached in just a couple of seconds in a serious self-defense situation. Physical tasks, especially those requiring coordination (fine and complex motor skills), become difficult at 145–175 BPM.
4. Muscles begin to tighten as adrenaline pours into your system. In general, males' adrenaline dumps occur more quickly than females' but also dissipate faster.

17. High emotional arousal (precipitated by an emergency) speeds up gross motor movements but impairs fine, detailed movements as described by the Yerkes-Dodson Law.

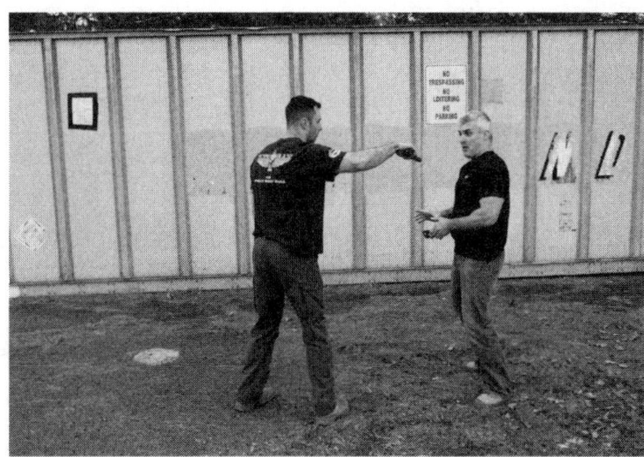

You are likely to experience physiological changes when unexpectedly held up at gunpoint.

Fear and Your Sympathetic Nervous System

Fighting in an enraged state, while boosting strength and speed, ultimately degrades a skilled fighter's capabilities. An essential difference between hard-core training and a true violent encounter is the activation of the defender's sympathetic nervous system (SNS).

Unfamiliarity with violence obviously makes facing aggression a frightening prospect. Both anxiety and subsequent fear, when triggered in a potentially violent situation, are evolutionarily designed to protect the body. Adrenalized strength coupled with a heightened internal first-aid capability are summoned. Fear triggers certain automatic human responses including physical, emotional, perceptual, and cognitive—triggering the freeze/flight/fight reaction. Fear, summoned through the SNS, creates time and distance distortions where actions may be perceived to speed up or slow down. When transformed to panic, fear can also paralyze.

The SNS forms one leg of the triad of your autonomic nervous system. The SNS mobilizes your body's nervous system fight-or-flight response. Immediate SNS activation occurs when you recognize and face imminent violence. Once activated by the perception of possible impending bodily harm, the SNS in turn activates immediate physiological changes by flooding your body with stress hormones. Your freeze, flight, or fight response hits full throttle.

The SNS is thought to counteract or hijack the parasympathetic system, which generally works to promote maintenance of the body at rest. The SNS both enables and disables. Your strength and speed increase while your analytical processing and complex motor skills decrease. Your SNS will not relinquish control until the observed threat is eliminated or you have escaped. Then the parasympathetic nervous system will reassert control.

While the SNS is not consciously controlled, it can apparently be manipulated through training and combat experience. There are four prime variables that have an immediate impact on your SNS activation level, including your:

1. perceived level of threat, ranging from risk of injury to the potential for death
2. available time to respond
3. level of confidence in your personal skills and training, especially in dealing with a specific threat
4. physical fatigue level, combined with anxiety

Once activated, the SNS causes immediate physiological changes, the most noticeable and easily monitored of which is increased heart rate inhibiting your complex motor-skill function. As combat stress increases, heart rate and respiration will increase until catastrophic physiological failure or until your parasympathetic nervous system once again assumes control.

Recall that in a crisis, your heart rate can go from a normal resting rate of about 60–70 BPM to more than 200–300 BPM in a matter of seconds. Optimal survival performance occurs when the heart rate is between 115 and 145 BPM. When your heart rate exceeds 145 BPM, your physical skills and capabilities begin to degrade. Good physical conditioning, deep-rooted confidence in personal abilities, and experience with similar situations in the past can help to keep the heart rate down, and visual- and motor-skill performance up. Stress responses include fleeing, freezing in place, posturing, or fighting—or possibly all four in some continual order resulting in counterviolence when there is no other choice. Your heart rate in response to perceived danger is crucial since once you surpass a particular rate (approximately 175 BPM), your fine and, shortly thereafter, your gross motor skills deteriorate. Once your heart rate reaches 225 BPM, you are likely to become catatonic or freeze in place, no longer capable of functioning to respond to the danger.

The following are some well-documented human responses to a violent situation:

- **Tunnel Vision**. Under extreme stress, more blood and oxygen may be delivered to your eyes, and your attention may be focused primarily on the greatest threat, resulting in a temporary loss of peripheral vision.
- **Auditory Exclusion.** As your vision takes over, your hearing will diminish.
- **Time and Space Compress** (**Tachypsychia**). Time and space will become muddled and there will be the added difficulty of judging the relationship between speed and distance. Movements may appear in slow-motion.
- **Random Distracting Thoughts.** Your brain struggles with itself to prevent conscious decision-making from interfering with the primordial flight-or-fight mechanism.
- **Behavioral Looping.** You repeat an action such as asking an assailant to stop again and again while denying that the attack is actually happening. You may delude yourself by not seeing something—however harmful—so you do not have to face it, which can get you maimed or killed.

When confronting a life-threatening situation, shock can be more problematic than fear. If you succumb to shock while under attack, you will freeze, creating possibly life-threatening vulnerabilities. Victims usually go into shock when attacked because of lack of response preparation. To avoid going into shock under stress, visualize yourself in every possible attack situation in which you may find yourself and as often as your training time allows. Optimally, you will act without thinking, using a conditioned/reflexive response. Train yourself over and over in your mind until you have effective solutions for those situations. Here are a few additional summary points:

- You must develop attack pattern recognition to close the action/reaction curve to your advantage.
- Threat recognition overcomes a startle response/processing delay and prevents your cerebral cortex (the thinking part of the brain) from hijacking the situation to instinctively, and, hence, instantaneously trigger a trained response. Confidence in one's abilities to handle a violent situation can delay the triggering of the often deleterious delayed response from SNS activation—you won't freeze in inaction.
- With threat recognition, the reaction goal is less than one-tenth of a second using honed gross motor skills (which increase following enactment by the sympathetic nervous system).
- The subconscious (instinctively trained) mind can process five hundred thousand times faster than the conscious (thinking) mind, according to Bruce K. Siddle's research.[18]

18. Bruce K. Siddle, *Sharpening the Warrior's Edge* (Belleville, IL: PPCT Research Publications, 1995).

Chapter 2

Training and Legal Strategies

Mental Training

Mental training girds you to be resolute, aggressive, and decisive. Equally important, preparing yourself ahead of time for a bad situation expedites your information assessment and processing ability. In a nutshell, mental training allows you to harness your full capabilities to achieve optimum performance. Physical and mental training are analogous to two adjoining pages of a book. While you can fold one side of the book over to only look at one page (metaphorically representing either mental or physical training), the two pages are inextricably bound together.

The importance of combined mental and physical training cannot be overemphasized. Israel is synonymous with resilience. Resilience is to never give up no matter what the odds. Krav maga is representative of Israel's defensive strategies in myriad ways. Smart tactics, precise targeting, and optimized force coupled with expert timing can defeat nearly any adversary. A smaller defender, even when outnumbered, can defeat a much larger attacker with correct strategy, application of force, daring, and fortitude.

Visualizing and practicing realistic violent situations can notch down your anxiety and stress level in a time of need. Without such preparation you are likely to experience magnified stress-induced deleterious emotions and physical effects. As noted earlier, when the body is under stress, the SNS and adrenal-cortical complexes induce physiological changes. Cortisol is a stress hormone that, when released in a significant dose, will make it difficult to remember things that are not deeply ingrained. The longer a victim remains ensconced in fear, the longer it will take for the victim to recover or react. The subconscious mind winnows the gap between reaction and action on the action/reaction power curve. Stated alternatively, the subconscious mind cannot be cognitively controlled. Hence the strategic importance of a trained instinctive/conditioned response for self-defense. Responses to violent stimuli can require from less than half a second to three times that long to register in most people. Optimally, with correct training you can respond in a quarter of a second or less—a reaction time that can be achieved by highly-trained, motivated individuals.

Mastering yourself (exerting self-control), including overcoming any and all residual doubts, is required to successfully navigate and cope with stress to create a positive outcome. Self-control or self-regulation, as we discussed, is the conscious ability to control your emotions, and hence, your behavior. Keep in mind that without training, your primitive brain hijacks your higher functions to deliver you from harm the best way it knows how. Stress seizes both your cognitive and somatic body responses.

Confidence may be thought of a mental state devoid of anxiety and doubt. A positive outcome is usually determined by how you perceive the threat, not the reality or danger of the threat in and of itself. The more you train to thwart a realistic attack, the more confidence you gain. This, in turn, reduces anxiety and fear. In training, or even in a real situation, if you do not succeed with a particular defense, be confident that you can instantly and seamlessly adapt and still defeat the threat. As they say, no plan completely survives first contact. Walk into (or walk away from) a situation with complete confidence that your skill set will deliver you from harm's way.

If you lose a physical battle, whether in practice or having survived a real situation, view it as a learning opportunity; don't castigate yourself. Grandmaster Gidon has made use of this principle to continue to improve krav maga. Since the early 1990s, Haim has had top ground fighters from all over the world visit his gym in Netanya. By having his students work against these skilled opponents, Haim has been able to develop a curriculum based on a no-rules mind-set, which has helped to make the system more complete. (Similar training on Ben Zion Street has also been conducted with blade specialists.)

Survival Stress Coping Strategies

Krav maga and similar reality-based survival systems focus on the following proven coping mechanisms:

1. *Visualize the proper response.* Visualization prepares us mentally and physically for combat. Mental rehearsal of what we may have to do if the subject makes a hostile move will decrease anxiety, allow enhanced performance, and help "tune" the nervous system for combat.
2. *Come to terms with the possibility of injury or even death.* Create a state of mind that will help to control an increasing heart rate when confronted with danger. When we encounter a life-threatening situation, we should be thinking, "This is something that I knew could happen to me. I don't like it, but I'm ready for it."
3. *Prioritize the threats.* Deal with the most immediate one first.

4. *Perform tactical breathing.* You may be aware of your dry mouth or an increased heart rate and breathing rate. If circumstances permit, try to exhale for a count of four, pause for a count of two and breathe in for a count of four. Do this several times to keep the heart rate within 115 to 145 BPM.

The human brain can be divided into two sections: the subconscious mind (limbic system) and the conscious mind (cerebral cortex system). The subconscious mind governs our primordial survival mechanisms by reacting rather than "thinking." The subconscious mind searches through past experience in a dangerous situation to identify a suitable response. While serving as the emotional center, the subconscious mind controls physical reactions (as opposed to physical actions). Subconscious reactions or "thinking without thinking" are decided within the first nanosecond of a threat. This is the foundation for krav maga's instinctive movements and tactics.

The conscious mind is our higher brain. It is chiefly responsible for higher cognition and analysis. The conscious mind engages when you have the time to assess a situation thoroughly and respond deliberately. When you are caught off guard and are overwhelmed by stress, your conscious mind shuts down. All decision-making processes transfer to your subconscious mind. As noted, your subconscious mind is basically an instinctive command response or a data bank of trained muscle memory.

Strategically, you must reduce the reaction time from recognition to reaction. *Instincts will always govern your cognitive response under stress.* Krav maga hones these instincts and recognizes that action will usually beat reaction in the action/reaction power curve. In other words, if an assailant launches at you, he has the initiative. You need to catch up. But you can and usually must "cheat" to catch up by recognizing kinesic indicators. For example, as noted previously, if you see or are confronted by someone who is clenching his hands, moving onto the balls of his feet with a forward lean, coiling a shoulder, blading the body, or stiffening the neck, these are individual or collective kinesic indicators that he may be primed to attack.

The Importance of Realistic Training

Training hardwires your brain to instinctively move your body to bypass conscious thought, thereby streamlining the self-defense process. Strategic training must attempt to simulate a real attack for you to understand the speed, ferocity, and strength a determined attacker may direct at you. Imi understood that actual violence differs greatly from choreographed training. Martial artists who have devoted many years to training have catastrophically found their skills to be inapplicable when facing a violent street-smart attacker in a volatile, violent environment.

Realistic and effective training under simulated stress allows your brain to navigate and better cope with danger. The more you engage in mental and visual training with realistic expectations and scenarios, the more attuned your brain becomes, through neuroplasticity, to performing under such conditions. Using proper visualization during training, ensure that you condition your brain to envision success while also contemplating failure and then dismissing it.

Most important, realistic training helps to alleviate fear, panic, and other sensations as you prepare your body and mind to take the proper course of action, but they must never be mistaken for a real attack. The key is to expedite or even eliminate step one, where you vizualize a proper response and step two, where you contemplate death or injury, as noted above. Additionally, people often freeze during the danger recognition and visualization response by denying they are about to be caught in a violent maelstrom. The goal of training is to streamline each of the four steps collectively, making the process first nature.

With an untrained mind and body, it's difficult to process or accept that someone else intends to do you serious bodily harm. Denial is the most common obstacle to taking appropriate action against someone about to attack you. To prevent denial, krav maga's strategy is to embed your subconscious reaction with the proverbial "(I have) been there, done that (through a training scenario)."

To avoid freezing under pressure, you must train under pressure. To begin, practice with a training partner or trusted friend. Direct your partner to simulate attack situations using extreme control to build many slow repetitions. Initially, do the mock attacks and corresponding defenses at half-speed to stay safe and avoid injury. (I recommend learning these sparring techniques under a qualified Israeli Krav Maga instructor, if possible.) Only as you develop control and a working familiarity with both the tactics and your training partner can you begin to move at full speed. Remember, the moves are designed to neutralize an attack at its inception using, when possible, preemptive strikes. If practiced without caution or incorrectly, you can easily injure your training partner.

As your training advances, your tactics must also work against determined resistance. Therefore, realism must always be injected into your krav maga training. For example, with proper safety training equipment and under a qualified krav maga instructor's supervision, punches and kicks must eventually be thrown at 100-percent speed and power in multiple salvos. The strikes must be retracted quickly and not held out, telegraphed, or overexaggerated. Similarly, chokes, grabs, and takedowns should be performed with full speed and power yet under controlled conditions.

In summary, mental and physical conditioning allows you to stave off panic and channel your adrenaline into action. To develop stress inoculation, be sure to include taxing training scenarios that are near as to real life as possible. They should create an adrenaline surge and the nervousness that are sure to come with a real conflict. These physical manifestations can quickly unnerve an inexperienced kravist, and you must develop your mental toughness accordingly.

Mental dominance over your fear and firm belief that you *will* overwhelm your attacker provide a decisive advantage in a violent encounter. Truly believe that your training will carry the day regardless of an attacker's physical size, possession of a weapon, or the fact that the attacker has accomplices. Yet confidence must not lead to overconfidence. *Do not underestimate any attacker and always expect the unexpected.* Perhaps most importantly, mental conditioning will allow you to de-escalate or walk away (always the best solution if possible) from a potentially violent situation.

As noted above, a lack of confidence can precipitate the SNS's activation. Realistic training therefore is crucial. Logically, the more you experience realistic, concerted training scenario threats, the more confident you will be in prevailing in a real unavoidable confrontation. Full-on training can also make clear that the average person's maximum 100-percent physical exertion capability is about a dozen seconds. This is particularly true when you are engaged in launching strikes in a full-on fight or grappling.

Strategically, then, you have maybe twelve seconds of maximum physical defensive effort at most before you tire and your defensive capabilities significantly erode. Krav maga recognizes the limits of human endurance with its anatomical targeting approach. Therefore, tactics must be designed to end a defensive physical altercation in just a few seconds even in a multiple attacker situation.

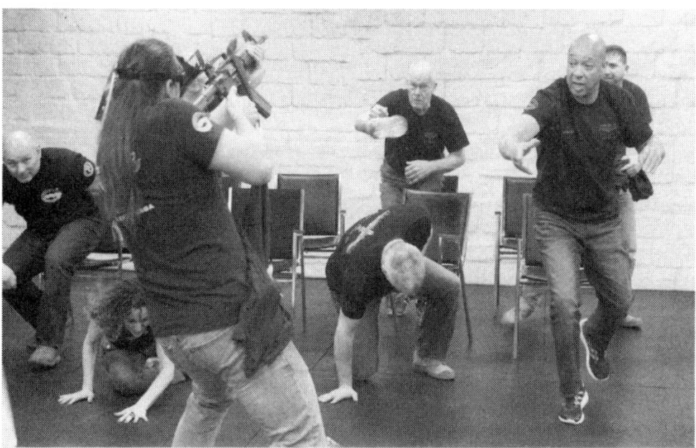

A trained active shooter group response when under stress.

Legal Use-of-Force Strategies

Almost universally, self-defense is regarded as an innate, inalienable, and individual right. Society codifies the legal right to use proportional self-defense under fairly uniform sets of circumstances. A Kentucky court's commentary in 1929 underscores this societal tenet: "The right of self-defense is not derived from any statutory enactment, but is a God-given right which man had when he was yet a savage and which he did not surrender when he came into civil society."[19] Yet, if you use counterviolence, you must believe that the stakes are real and the aggressor is playing for keeps. Equally important, you had better be able to explain what you did to an aggressor and why you did it.

19. *Morgan v. Commonwealth*, 15 S.W.2d 273, 275 (Ky. 1929).

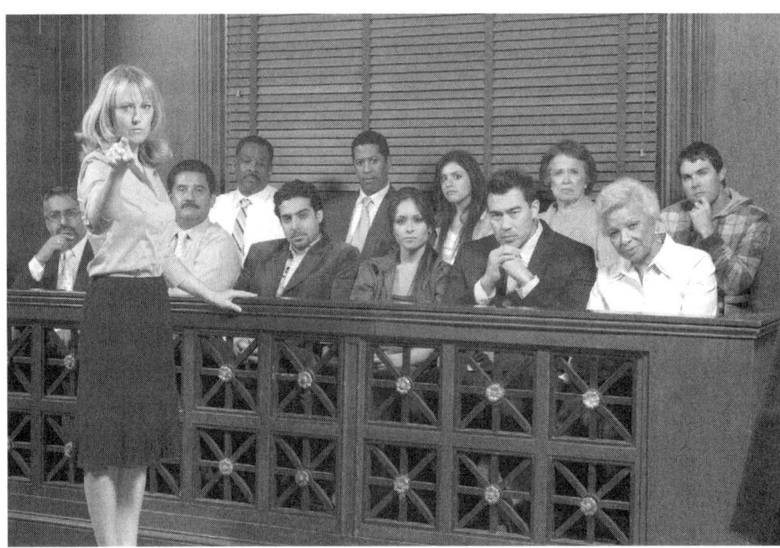

You may be put in front of a six- to twelve-person civil or criminal jury that will pass judgment on your self-defense actions. These fellow citizens may have little understanding of self-defense strategies and tactics. You will have to honestly and carefully, consistent with any prior initial statements you may have made, once again outline what you did and why you did it.

In developing a self-defense strategy to deliver you from harm's way both physically and legally, it is important to recall how and why krav maga evolved in pre-war Slovakia. Violence against Jews was visceral and deadly. Krav maga founder Imi Lichtenfeld understood that such unprovoked violence had to be met with honed, instinctive, superior counterviolence. Given the prevalent antisemitism in Bratislava, there was little or no legal recourse for those who were assaulted. Therefore, logically, any legal ramifications for using self-defense were not the highest priority; survival was. Now, thankfully, the rule of law governing violence prevails in most of the world.

While the United States Supreme Court has arguably never canonized (forgive the near pun) self-defense as an explicit constitutional right, American jurisprudence has imbued citizens with the right to self-defense based on common law. As a general rule, defendants establish a claim of self-defense when they articulate and demonstrate that (1) they were confronted by an unavoidable and unprovoked serious threat of bodily harm or death, (2) the threat was imminent, (3) the physical defensive response was reasonable or necessary and proportional, and (4) there was no legal preclusion. As applied to jury instructions, a court generally applies both a subjective and an objective analysis to what are deemed reasonable self-defense actions for a like person under like circumstances.

> **Imminent Harm**
> Imminent harm describes an articulable and demonstrable set of circumstances where you have the right to use self-defense against a physical danger presented by another. Imminent means that the time for counterforce is now; you can wait no longer. Legitimate self-defense must be neither premature (the threat must actually materialize) nor tardy (a retaliatory measure following both a completed act and disengagement by an aggressor). You must establish that you believed that objectively reasonable physical counterforce was your only option to prevent yourself from sustaining physical harm and injury. To define the matter as imminent, you must explain that a hostile party's kinesic movements reasonably indicated an attempted or incoming attack. Notably, the Model Penal Code adopted by many American jurisdictions shifts the requirement from "imminent" to "immediately necessary."[20]

Self-defense is an affirmative defense; you admit to counterattacking the aggressor or would-be aggressor. The burden of proof is on you to prove that you acted to protect yourself and *you were not the aggressor*. In other words, apparent necessity, not actual necessity will suffice. The doctrine of self-defense exonerates a person from criminal liability even though his belief in the need to use force to repel an attack is later proven mistaken.[21] To explain your actions, you need to have only a reasonable belief regarding what you believed to be the other person's actions. Understand that you may also step into the shoes of a third party to defend that party using and meeting a specific state's self-defense legal standard.

To reiterate, you need to articulate why you had no choice but to use counterviolence when faced with a threat who demonstrated all of the following:

1. **Intent** (stated or evident goal of harming you)
2. **Capability** (has the prowess or tools to harm you)
3. **Opportunity** (proximity)
4. **No preclusion** (escape was not available to you, though this requirement does not apply in American stand-your-ground jurisdictions)

---

20. MPC § 3.04 (ALI 1962).
21. *State v. Kelly*, 97 N.J. 178, 199-200, 478 A.2d 364 (1984).

What Constitutes Reasonable Counter-Force?

Once you have established a right to self-defense, your use of force will then be scrutinized. You are restricted to using only the counterforce necessary to prevent the harm. Note: There are few places in the world where disproportional counterforce will not run afoul of the law.

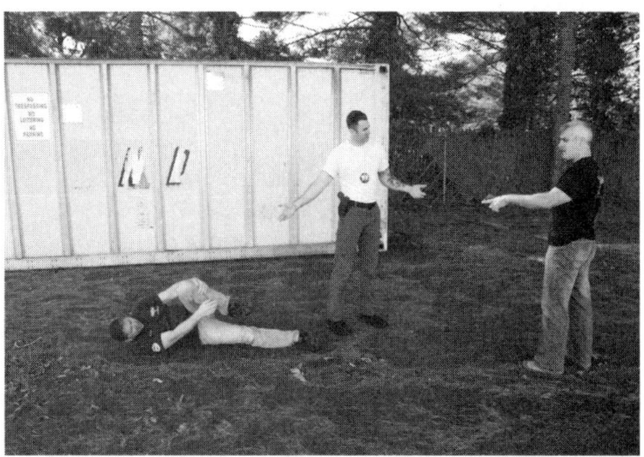

Explaining to an officer (and perhaps, later, to a jury) what you did and why you did it, in this case taking out an opponent's knee. This can be a crucial aspect in the legal process of either justifying or finding fault with your self-defense actions.

As emphasized, when civilians employ counterviolence in response to an unavoidable and imminent attack, rules govern the proportionality of "reasonable" counterforce that may be used to repel the attack. Therefore, if you use counterforce to defend against a violent threat, especially if you are a trained martial artist or fighter, you had better have a strong, and maybe even nearly a foolproof, strategy to explain and evidence your defensive actions. The type of objectively reasonable force you employed to stop the threat is paramount in assessing liability. If you batter someone, you are likely to be examined by the legal system both criminally and civilly.

You are prohibited from using counterforce that is likely to cause death or serious bodily injury if you do not believe you are in jeopardy of being maimed or killed. Should you use more force than is necessary you will lose the self-defense privilege. For nondeadly force, the law generally recognizes that a person may use such force as is reasonably necessary to thwart the imminent use of force against that person, short of deadly force.

Many factors affect what might be considered "reasonable." Your reasonable belief must approximately parallel what another reasonable person would do under the same circumstances when facing imminent danger. A few factors that determine what a person's reasonable self-defense actions were include size disparity, gender,[22] age, and terrain. In addition,

22. Women are approximately 52 percent as strong as men in their upper body and 66 percent in their lower body physically compared to men, as reported in A. E. Miller, J. D. MacDougall, M. A. Tarnopolsky, D. G. Sale, "Gender Differences in Strength and Muscle Fiber Characteristics," Eur Journal of Applied Physiology and Occupational Physiology 66(3): 1993: 254-62. https://pubmed.ncbi.nlm.nih.gov/8477683/.

whether the aggressor demonstrated fighting prowess, possessed a weapon, or had accomplices collectively weighs into any self-defense assessment. The standard of reasonable force to which you will be held will be that of a similarly situated reasonable person under similar circumstances. In other words, jurors are asked to consider a fictitious legal clone, a would-be persona in the exact same situation.

In 1846, the renowned legal scholar Francis Wharton suggested what might be considered a reasonable use of counterforce in his *A Treatise on Criminal Law of the United States.* Wharton hinted that a defender's use of proportionate counterviolence might be legally justified in incrementally exceeding the unprovoked violent action being visited on the defender. While Wharton opined that counterviolence should be "proportioned to the nature of the injury offered,"[23] when in the heat of self-defense and facing imminent harm, citizens could not be expected to exert perfect self-control. If a self-defense overreaction was not too severe and within the bounds of reason, the law would still support an action that an average juror could understand. In other words, a victim is entitled to a measured escalation of reasonable counterviolence against an aggressor. Theoretically, an assault could excuse a battery, a battery could excuse a mayhem, and a mayhem could excuse a homicide.[24]

In 1921, the U.S. Supreme Court, in *Brown v. United States*, a case involving a foreman who repeatedly shot a laborer who approached him menacingly with a knife, emphasized, "Detached reflection cannot be demanded in the presence of an uplifted knife . . ."[25]

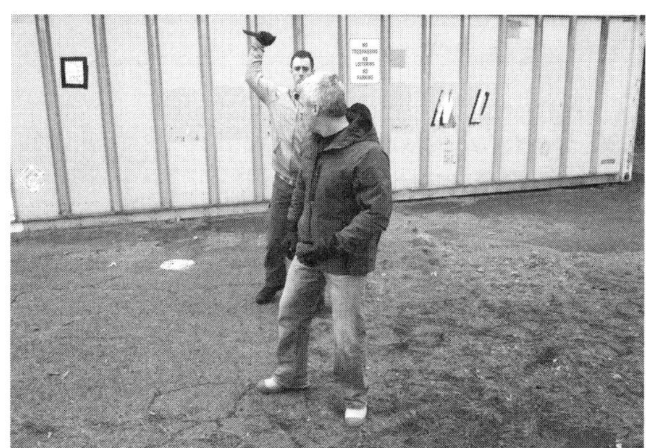

This famous *Brown* case established that any deep rational analysis of one's reactions is largely precluded in a self-defense situation. A 2007 California court case, *People v. Ross*, provides additional insight into the legal analysis of permissible reasonable counterforce:

23. Francis Wharton, *A Treatise on Criminal Law of the United States* (Philadelphia: James Kay, Jun., and Brother, 1846), 313.

24. Franklin Stockdale "Withdrawing A License to Kill: Why American Law Should Jettison 'Stand Your Ground' and Adopt the English Approach To Retreat," *Boston College International and Comparative Law Review* 39, Issue 2, Article 8, (2016).

25. *Brown v. United States*, 256 U.S. 335, 343, 41 S. Ct. 501, 502, 65 L. Ed. 961, 963 (1921).

> *The test is not whether the force used appears excessive in hindsight but whether it appeared reasonably necessary to avert threatened harm under the circumstances at the time. The law grants a reasonable margin within which one may err on the side of his own safety … since in the heat of conflict or in the face of an impending peril a person cannot be expected to measure accurately the exact amount of force necessary to repel an attack, that person will not be deemed to have exceeded his or her rights unless the force used was so excessive as to be clearly vindictive under the circumstances.*[26]

Similarly, an earlier ruling in *Hommer v. State* by an Oklahoma court took an analogous position: "It would be absurd to anticipate that a defendant could calculate a mathematically accurate quantity of force essential to do no more than repel an attack, at the moment of the attack."[27] A New Jersey court further cemented this flexible, circumstantial principle of justified force when it concluded, "Again, we do not expect people to be purely rational actors in selecting the proper amount of force to use in response to a reasonably perceived threat to their safety."[28] A 2017 D.C. case, *Parker v. State* agreed: "The law thus recognizes the frailties of human perception, requiring only a reasonable, and not necessarily correct, judgment."[29]

Therefore, the reasonableness of your actions will be determined by a jury using an objective standard of what a reasonable person would have done in your position in light of the circumstances known to you at the time you used counterforce. What this means is, what would that juror have done facing the same situation? It is from this analytical legal reasoning that liability flows. A pitfall you may face as a trained martial artist or fighter is that the jury could be influenced by opposing counsel into thinking that you must be held to a higher standard of reasonableness given your self-defense skill set. Your training will no doubt be brought to light by both the prosecution or plaintiff's attorney and similarly by your own attorney.

The public, including your average jurors, often replay action movies and police dramas in their minds to understand violence. You can only make your argument in terms of what you perceived to be a reasonably probable or actual threat. The court will make an inference about what you did from both circumstances and the evidence presented. Strategically, you must sculpt and mold this all-important inference by your explanation of your actions (assuming your actions were justified) to prevent you, the victim, from becoming the aggressor in the court's eyes. Your actions must parallel and support your statements, and your statements must do the same for your actions.

The prosecutor or plaintiff's attorney will argue that you have, by virtue of your training, a better understanding of the use of force. Strategically, it is precisely this better understanding of use of force that allows you to articulate what actions you took and why you took

---

26. *People v. Ross*, 66 Cal. Rptr. 3d 438, 445–46 (Cal. Ct. App. 2007).
27. *Hommer v. State* (Okla. Crim.App.1983) 657 P.2d 172, 174.
28. *Parker v. United States*, 155 A.3d 835, 843 n.11 (D.C. 2017).
29. *State v. Hippelwith*, 33 N.J. 300, 316-17, 164 A.2d 481 (1960) and *State v. Mount*, 73 N.J.L. 582, 585-86, 64 A. 124 (E. & A.1906).

them. Use your training and experience to your advantage as you describe what transpired to the court and justify your actions. Your instructor or martial-arts organization—with the caveats that you have used justified counterforce and your training emphasizes credible use-of-force doctrine—should be able to provide a reliable expert witness and support to buttress your actions. To counter accusations that you used unnecessary force, you might explain:

- "My reality-based training is based on ______ and used by (______[representative number of] people and ______ [representative number of] professional organizations) . . ."
- "Generally, the human body reliably moves in only certain ways, so I immediately recognized . . ."
- "Based on my training and experience, I understand the difference between normal movements and attack movements."

A Police Interview or Legal Deposition

If an interrogator describes your opponent as the "other party," in your answer you could respond for the record "the *attacker* . . . [did this] and I could not safely retreat" or "the *aggressor* would not hear reason and therefore . . ." Your word substitution shows your contemporaneous assessment of the situation when you acted and that you were not the aggressor or had not agreed to fight with someone.

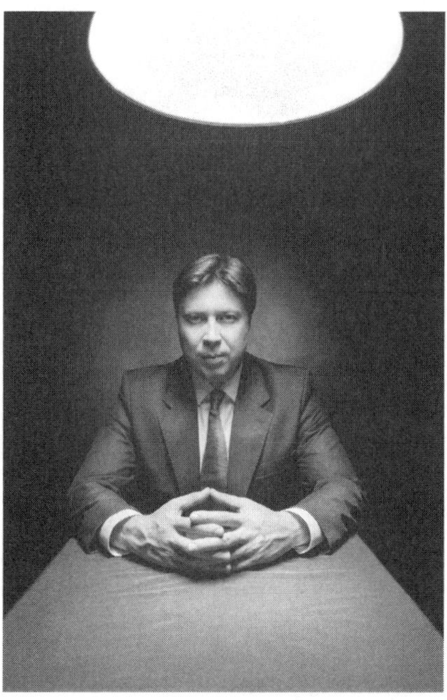

A jail-cell conference you never want to have.

You might have to answer the following questions:

- Why did you rupture the other party's testicles?
- Why did you damage the other party's cornea with a finger to his eye?
- After you kneed the other party in the groin, why did you then immediately knee him in the head?
- After gaining control of the other party's baseball bat, why did you club him with it?

The simplest and honest answer to any and all such questions is that you had to stop the threat. Your intent was only to stop the threat and not wantonly or gratuitously injure someone. Law enforcement or private security was not there to intervene and stop the attack, so you had to do it yourself and in a matter of seconds.

To recap, when defending yourself, you are only justified in using counterviolence that is proportional or commensurate with the threat. As tempting as it might be to exact retribution and physically chastise an erstwhile aggressor, you must make a deliberate conscious decision about when to cease your counterattack. In short, if you have to resort to violence to protect yourself, you must be able to explain to a jury why and how you chose your actions and that there were no reasonable alternatives. This is counterbalanced against the understanding that any given physical confrontation has the potential to kill you.

Self-Defense Does Not Require Fear on the Defender's Part

Importantly, you do not have to exhibit fear when exercising your right of self-defense. Statutes generally only require a reasonable and genuine perception of imminent harm. This is reinforced by the *Parker* court when it observed, "But if a person is confident in her ability to defend herself and does not feel afraid when she is placed in a situation where she actually and reasonably believes that she is in imminent danger of bodily harm, she would still have a right to act to prevent that harm and later claim self-defense . . . the proper inquiry is whether the defendant believed she was in imminent danger, not whether she was or was not fearful."[30]

Stand-Your-Ground Statutes

As noted, society has long allowed self-defense to justify a victim's defensive actions to avoid both criminal and civil liability. Historically, a victim had a duty to retreat, provided safe retreat was available, before using counterforce. As of January 1, 2020, stand-your-ground laws established in thirty-four U.S. states now provide that there is no duty for a law-abiding citizen to retreat from an attacker in any place where one is lawfully present. Florida set the

30. *Parker v. United States*, 155 A.3d 835, 843 n.11 (D.C. 2017).

legal bar in 2005 when it sanctioned a person to stand his or her ground in any "place where he or she has a right to be."

A stand-your-ground statute empowers a defender not to retreat when facing a reasonably articulable threat. Such a law lowers the legal threshold requirements to claim self-defense. In short, stand-your-ground laws afford the defender considerably more latitude to be proactive. Accordingly, might such statutes affect your defensive strategy in the use of krav maga? The broad answer is yes and specifically what is a permissible and reasonable measure of unarmed counterforce. These statutes largely contemplate the use of a firearm in self-defense, which is considered to be deadly force. So unarmed defensive tactics may certainly be considered reasonable when the underlying legal premises permit the use of deadly force.

Strategy: Purchase a Self-Defense Insurance Policy

The monetary cost of defending yourself for the use of legally justified self-defense will be significant. It is not uncommon for attorneys to charge tens of thousands of dollars in retainer fees for such specialized work. Therefore, you might consider purchasing a concealed carry type of self-defense insurance (CCW policy) even if you do not carry a concealed weapon. These types of specialized policies generally provide a defense fund for *any type of legally justified self-defense including the use of personal weapons.* Such a policy will provide an attorney with expertise in both criminal and civil liability matters along with additional legal costs. Equally important, a self-defense insurance policy will provide for monetary damages should a civil judgment be awarded against you. Note that some policies have set limits for certain aspects of your defense while others do not.

Mutual Combat Negates Your Right to Self-Defense

Mutual combat or combat by agreement is a term commonly used in American courts when two individuals intentionally and consensually engage in a "fair fight" while not injuring bystanders or damaging property. If mutual combat is found, no participant in it may assert a claim of self-defense. The issue then is that you could validly exert a self-defense claim only to have your vanquished opponent claim that you had agreed to fight him. If you agreed to fight him, then you cannot claim self-defense. Such a legal conundrum is presented by a Texas attorney who explained, "If you are being prosecuted for an assaultive offense, you might be able to claim that you were engaged in mutual combat. This defense could help you win your case or convince the prosecutor to drop the charges against you."[31]

Importantly, regarding such an advertisement, mutual combat is legal in only a few states, including Texas, Colorado, and Washington. Nevertheless, a clever attorney or

31. https://jerrytidwell.com/information/faq-defense-law/texas-mutual-combat-law-defense/.

prosecutor could make the case that you *willingly* participated in the violent encounter and, therefore, must be held accountable.

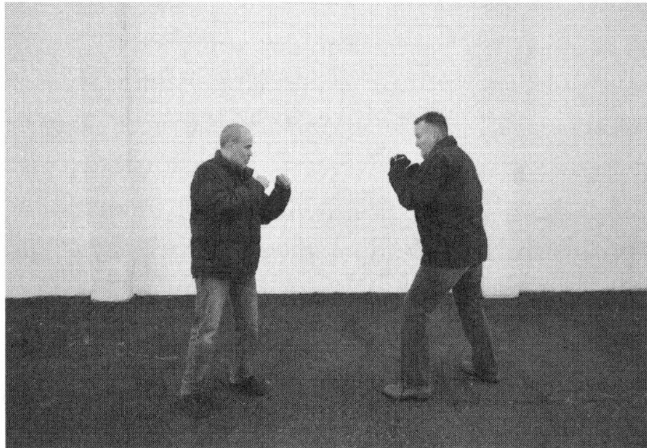

Mutual combat is illegal, prohibited conduct (except in the states of Texas, Colorado, and Washington).

Mutual combat does not have a set legal definition.[32] It can be thought of like a duel, where both participants agree in advance to fight the other.[33] According to the United States Coast Guard, mutual combat means that both participants voluntarily agreed to enter into the fight or that the participation in the fight was voluntary after the fight began.[34]

A mutual combat agreement need not be formal or express and is generally found in the combatants' behavior and actions. As one court put it, "Such an agreement may be tacit and inferred from the facts and circumstances of the case. [The] requisite agreement does not exist when one party unilaterally and dangerously escalates the previously equal terms of a fight."[35] In short, mutual combat requires a shared intent to fight, as distinguished from an encounter where one party is attacking and the other party is merely defending.[36] Legal scholar Paul Robinson summarizes: in "mutual combat both are employing *aggressive*, rather than *defensive* force, and neither actor's conduct is necessary to his defense and is, for that reason, unjustified."[37]

For a judge not to find that you participated in a mutual fight, you must prove that you did not instigate and could not avoid the violence. You exhausted all of your non-violent options to resolve the situation peacefully. In summary, regardless of whether the law requires a duty to retreat or even provides a stand-your-ground right, you were not at fault and did not agree to test your mettle against your opponent.

---

32. *People v. Ross*, 66 Cal. Rptr. 3d 438, 445–46 (Cal. Ct. App. 2007).
33. Ibid.
34. *In re Merchant Mariner's Document* No. Z-1111695, 1966 USCG LEXIS 14 at *8 (Sept. 2, 1966).
35. *State v. O'Bryan*, Supreme Court of Connecticut Sep 15, 2015 318 Conn. 621.
36. *State v. Pasterick*, 285 N.J. Super. 607, 617, 667 A.2d 1103 (App. Div. 1995).
37. P. Robinson, *Criminal Law Defenses* (1984) § 132, p. 98. (italics in text added).

Great Tactics—But Can You Legally Justify Them?

You can have many highly effective tactics, but the preeminent legal question is, do these tactics represent proportional counterforce relative to the threat? In the example below, the defender thwarts a push attempt by deflecting the attacker's arms and seizing the attacker's nearside arm for an arm-break or *ippon seo nage* type of throw variation. While this is a formidable counter against a two-handed push attempt, your defense might be viewed skeptically by a jury while deciding what money damages to award your erstwhile attacker to compensate him for his broken arm and to punish you for using such a brutal technique. The point is that you could have deflected his arms using some lesser measure of counterforce rather than breaking his arm. Of course, a legal defense can be made that you were using legitimate self-defense against a larger aggressor. Yet, why not make your legal defense easier by using a less forceful counter-tactic?

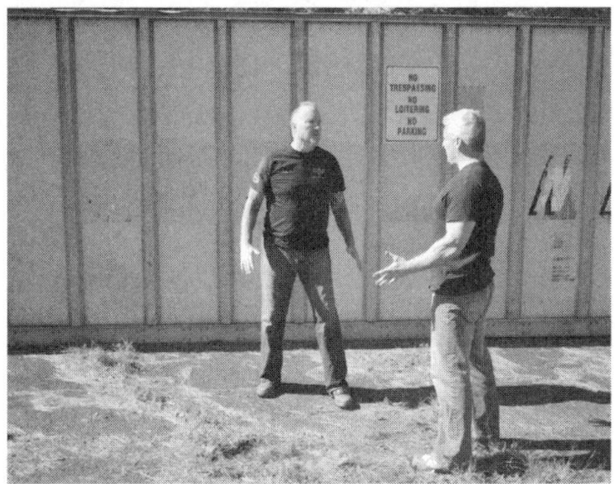

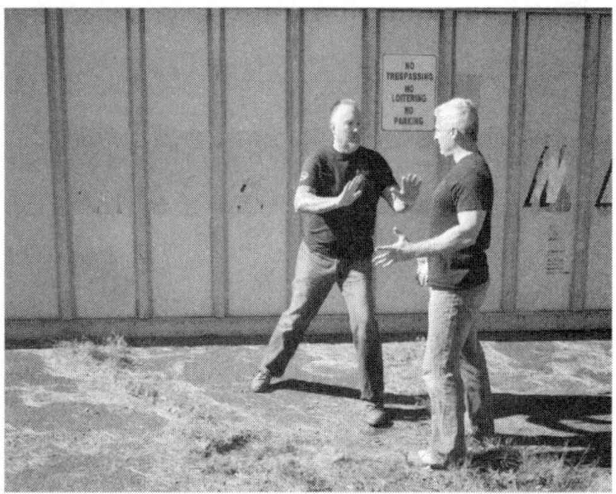

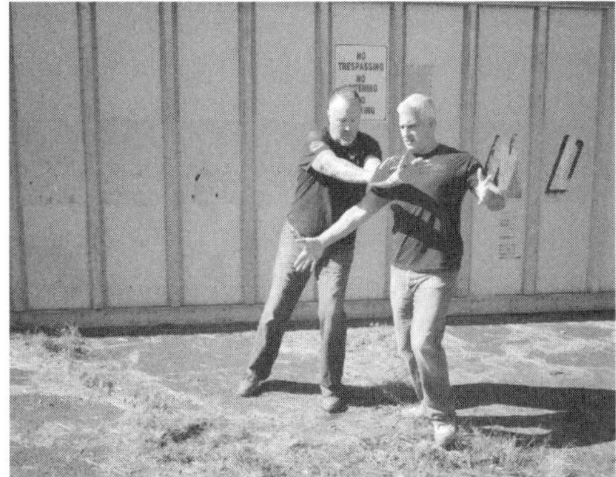

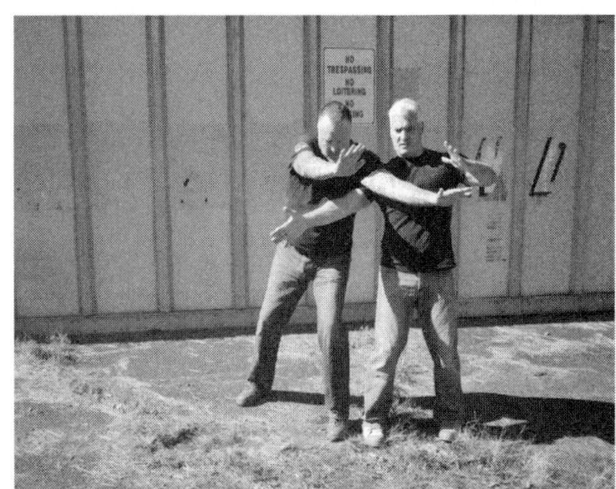

series continued on next page ...

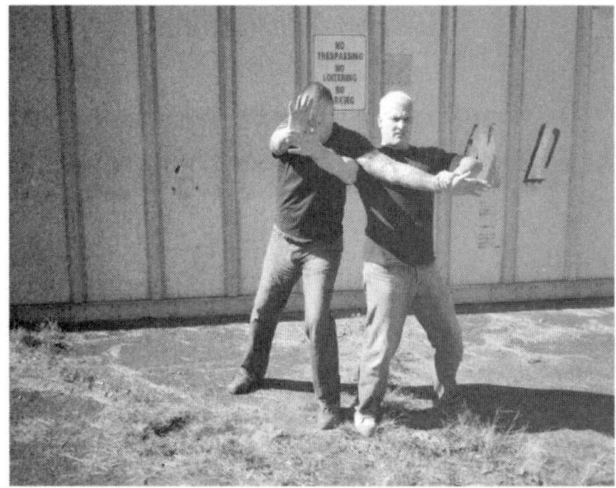

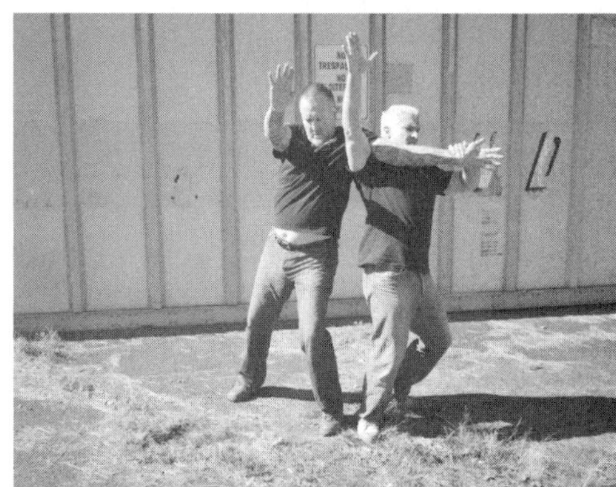

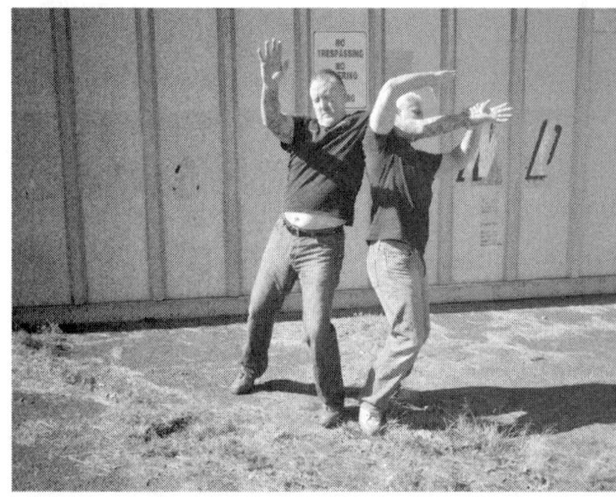

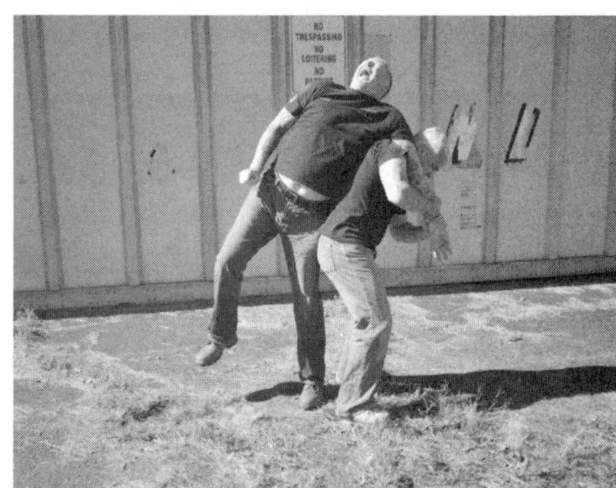

If someone were to push you, using correct timing a tai sabaki defensive step, you can sidestep the push while seizing the attacker's nearest arm to then pin it to your shoulder to execute an ippon seo nage type of throw variation.

Control-Hold Strategies

Krav maga is well-known for its brutal striking combatives and overall injurious approach to disabling an assailant. Outside of law enforcement circles, however, krav maga's highly effective control and restraint holds are not widely-known. These joint locks clamp down on an adversary to control his movement. Imi Lichtenfeld built a number of joint-lock control holds into his curriculum while being acutely aware of both moral and legal self-defense use-of-force considerations relating to tactics specifically designed to create injury. By design, these could be applied without injuring an aggressor, though, of course, they could be extended and applied more forcibly to create injury. Imi's goal was to provide a less-aggressive response if the person who grabbed your shirt was incapacitated or was someone familiar to you or simply someone you did not wish to injure. Realistically, these control tactics may not be optimal for a smaller defender against a larger, stronger attacker; however, if executed properly using correct timing, body positioning, and leverage, the tactics will work.

In the public's imagination, arm, wrist, shoulder, and leg locks have become highly popular self-defense tools. Tying an aggressor up in some form of human knot appeals to people's fantasies. Notably, a significant number of civilian- and criminal-case juries alike are disposed to think a bad actor or aggressive person can easily be subdued using a joint pressure lock or some sort of magical pressure point to (en)force good or compliant behavior. Such joint locks are, to be sure, a proven way of taking control of a violent encounter by using a form of counterviolence that is designed not to injure the opponent but rather to cause him to comply or submit. However, if the aggressor does not obey or yield to commands, the locks can also be used to injure him by hyperextending or misaligning a targeted joint.

As with all self-defense combatives, there are legal issues that arise should you apply a joint lock on someone. Not only do you risk civil and criminal charges of battery, you might also face the risk of being convicted of false imprisonment. For instance, a false imprisonment statute is readily found in New Jersey 2C:13-3 (I am using New Jersey statutes as an example, since our civilian training centers are located there). According to the NJ statute concerning false imprisonment, "A person commits a disorderly persons offense if he knowingly restrains another unlawfully so as to interfere substantially with his liberty."

In New Jersey, under this statute, if you are convicted of false imprisonment, you could face up to six months in jail and a fine of up to $1,000. Such a conviction saddles you with a criminal record. Of course, mitigating factors can lessen the charges. The length of time you detained the person, the nature and extent of the restraint you applied, along with your overall intention when you did the restraining, could possibly influence whether you face a conviction or not.

Notwithstanding these tort-liability exposures, in the event an aggressor were to grab your shirt to assert social dominance, we present in the photos below an example of a control hold that could be used. You can, of course, immediately counterattack against a shirt-grab attempt with strikes, but the curriculum provides for another option: an armlock placing the aggressor on the ground. When instructing and envisioning how such a scenario might occur, Imi suggested that this multiple-joint type of lock might be applied to a hostile drunkard, an elderly adversary, a mentally disabled person, or a family member who needs to be calmed down and controlled after grabbing your shirt, as in this photo series.

The shirt-grab defense depicted using a standing armbar shirt-grab release tactic creates tremendous pressure on the assailant's forearm, wrist, and shoulder. Breaking pressure can be applied if the defender were to step through with his front leg to sit out or to fall to the ground, landing with his weight on the aggressor's back. You'll notice that in executing the lock the defender turns his body away from the assailant to clamp down on the assailant's offending arm. This is done in such a way that should the assailant then decide to attack the defender, the defender can intercept any type of incoming strike or immediately counterattack using a straight kick as depicted in the subsequent photo series.

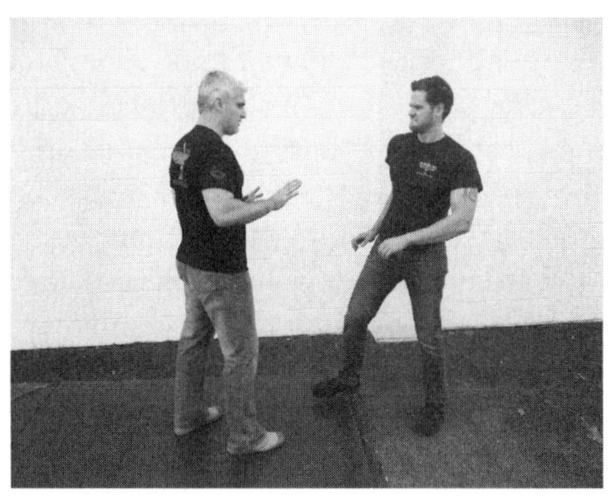

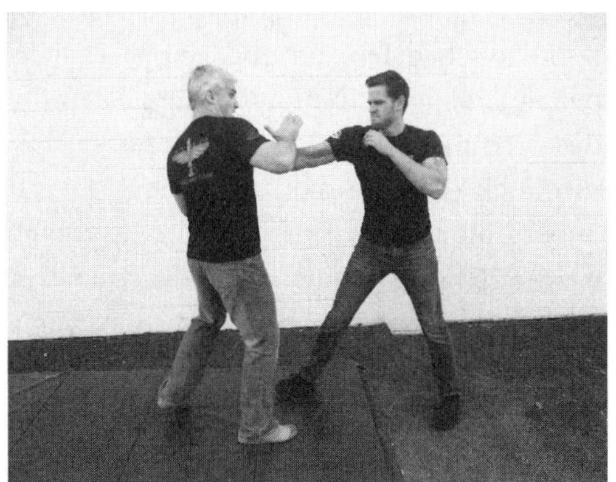

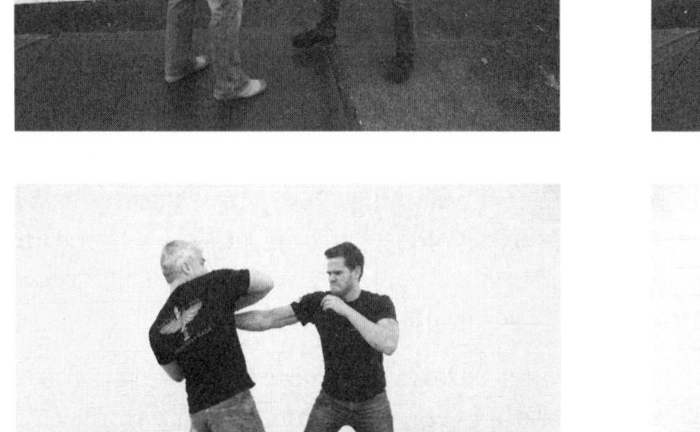

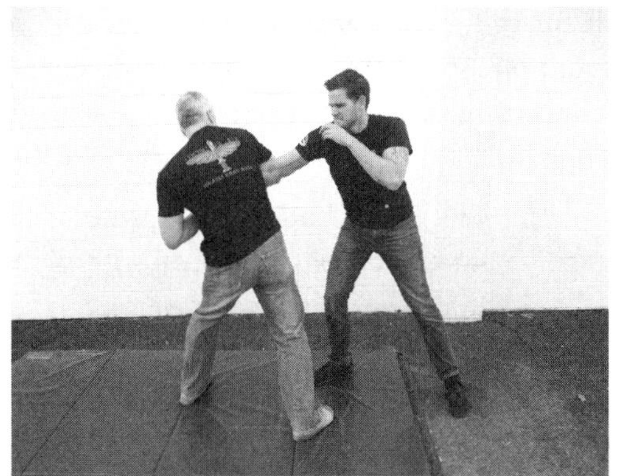

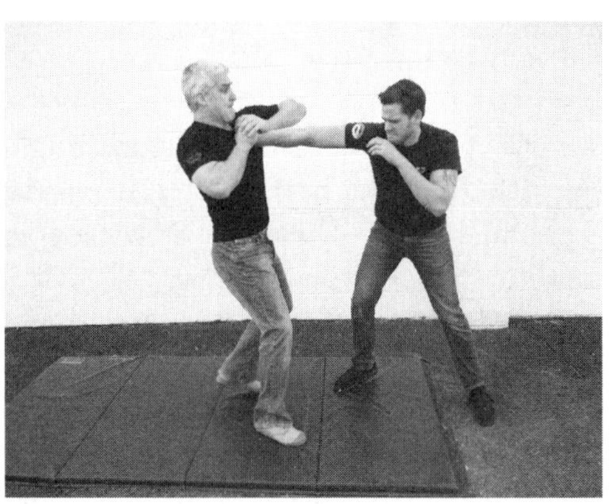

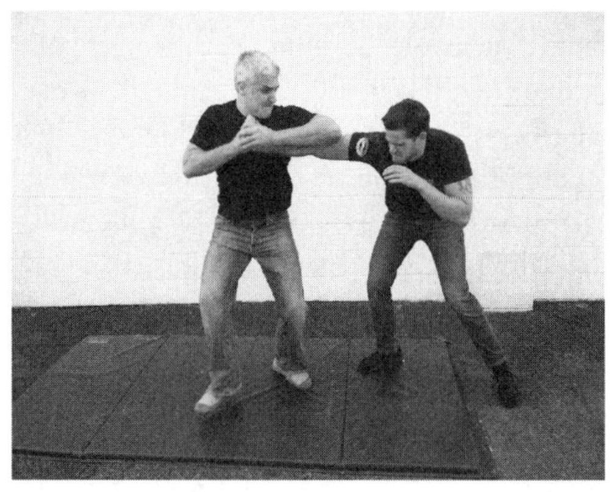

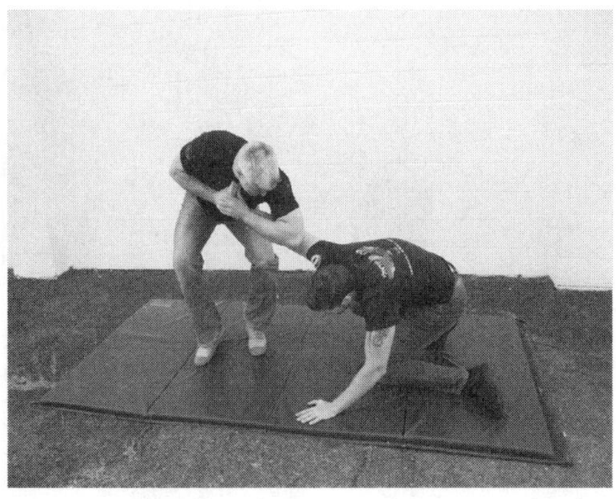

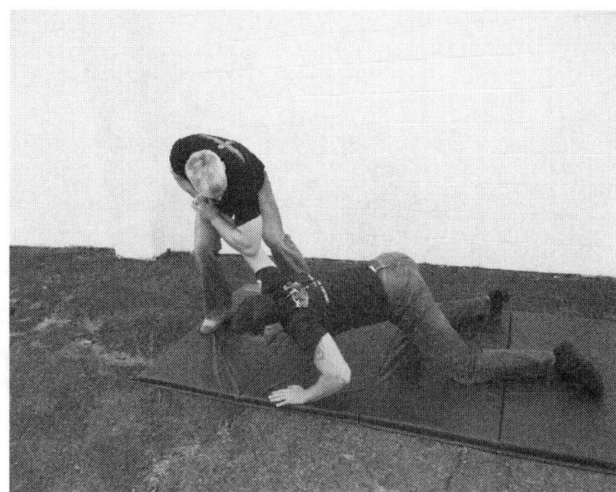

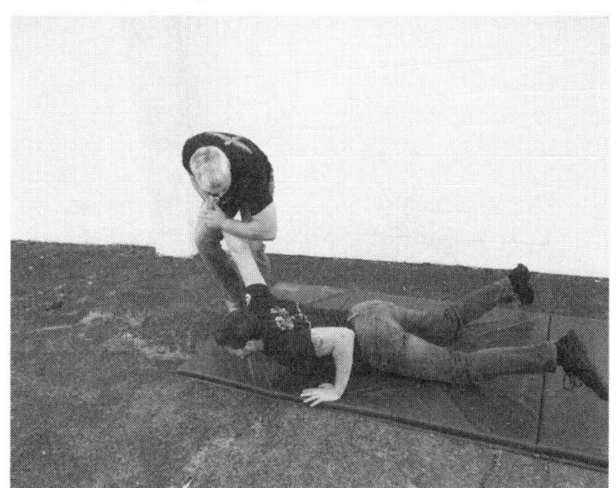

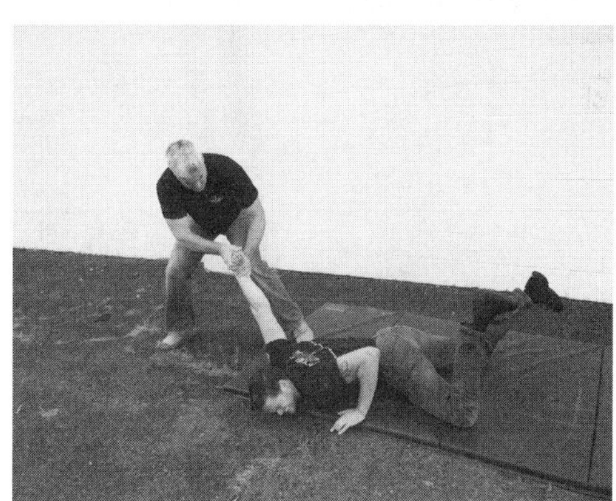

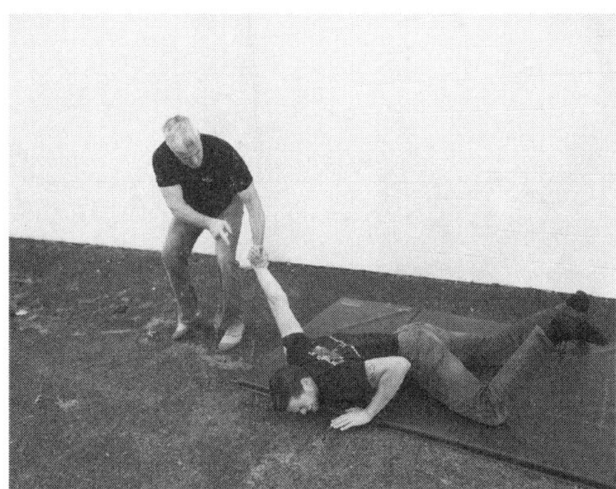

This series presents a shirt-grab control and armlock takedown variation, including a disengagement strategy telling the aggressor the incident is over. You instruct the aggressor not to get up until you have left the scene.

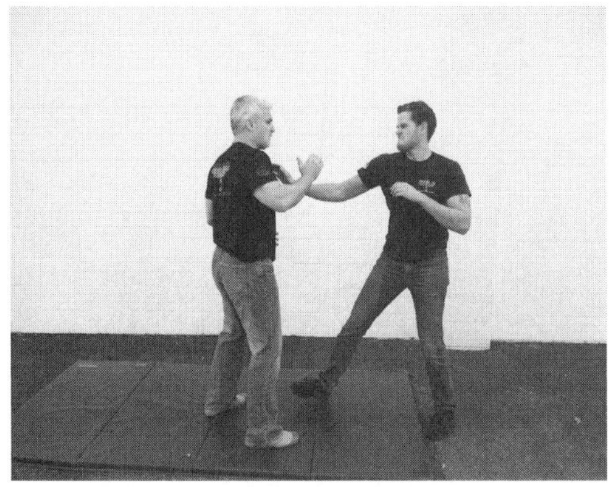

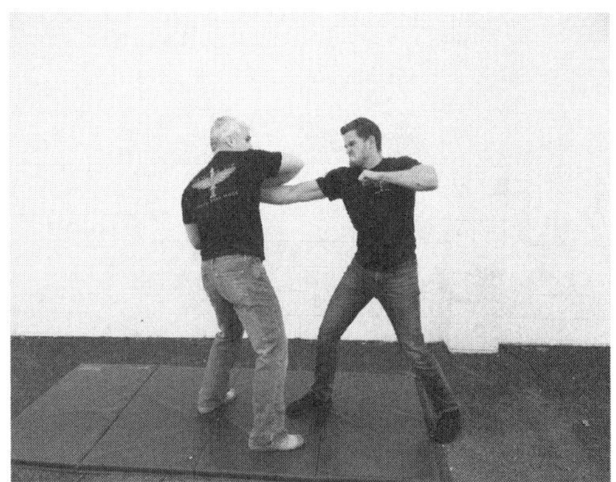

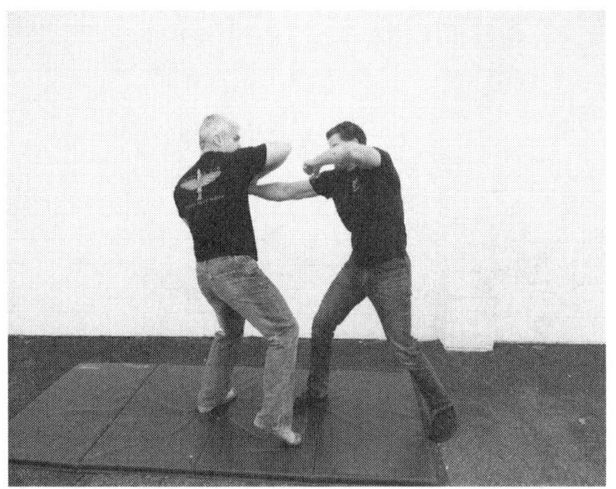

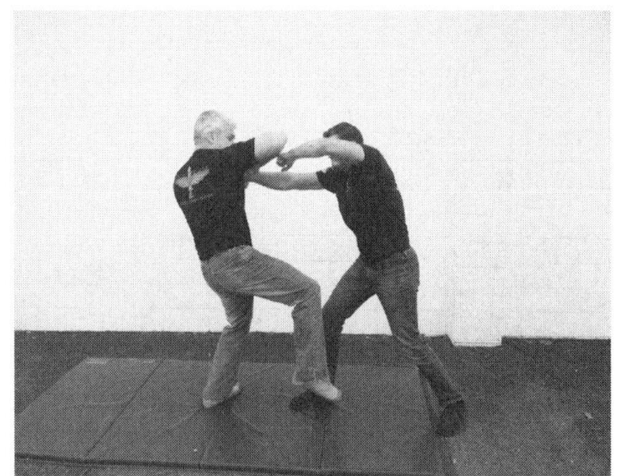

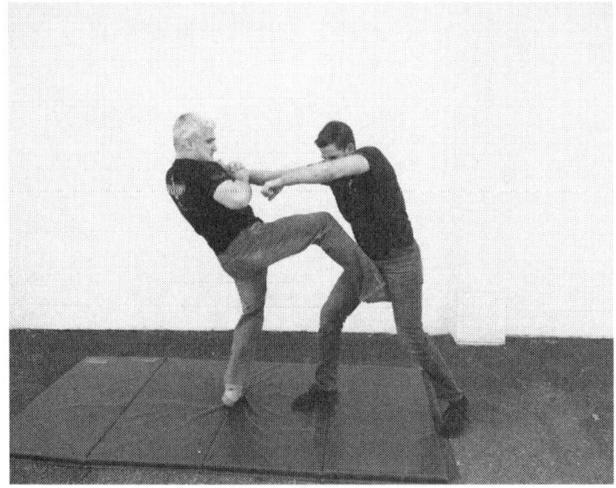

This series shows a combined shirt-grab and gunt-punch defense (similar to the previous tactic yet requires modification) while counterattacking with a near-simultaneous straight kick.

Keep in mind that you apply this lock in a standing position. Remember also that, if you feel compelled to grapple on the ground, while on the ground you are highly vulnerable to third parties attacking you, especially with stomps. As will be further examined in the "Strategies against Multiple Opponents" section, krav maga makes every effort not to go to the ground. Imi's system is rooted in this strategy because he was often outnumbered, and purposefully going to the ground, despite his champion wrestling background, could lead to serious injury at the hands (and feet) of his anti-Semitic adversaries. Nevertheless, if you feel you must drop to the ground to maximally effect the hold by using your body weight on top of your attacker, as with a standing lock, what else would you do with him?

For either a standing or ground-based lock, your attacker might realize that you are highly trained and mean business and that continued aggression would just get him injured, and so he might adopt a position of contrition and comply. Alternatively, you might have embarrassed him, and he might get up spoiling for a fight or even draw a weapon to threaten or attack you. Therefore, should you orchestrate this type of control hold, you had better have a game plan to reason any further aggression out of him.

The self-defense world teaches many formidable joint-control locks and takedowns, but often little thought is given about what you do once you have an attacker in a joint lock while standing or on the ground other than summoning law enforcement—which is nearly always the best choice. It must be underscored that anyone who has had to control or restrain a determined resisting subject ("controlee") understands the difficulty of applying minimum objectively reasonable use-of-force controls. What are you going to say to him to calm the situation down? What reasoning from a position of dominance can you offer to forestall any further violence? Perhaps you might authoritatively declare, "Hey man, I don't want to injure you. I'm going to let you go now. It's over; no more fighting." Alternatively, you can assert, "You grabbed me. If you want, we'll just wait it out until the cops show up. I have witnesses that you attacked me and I acted in self-defense. Another choice is that I can get up now and walk away. If you agree, we'll walk away and it's over." Of course, common sense dictates that you do not turn your back on this aggressor, as he may feign compliance and then attack you.

In conclusion, not only does a practical threat-analysis method enable you to avoid danger and violence, it helps you develop a legal and liability shield against arrest and prosecution should you need to use counterforce. If you have to resort to violence to protect yourself, you must be able to explain to a jury why and how you chose your actions and that there were no reasonable alternatives. This is counterbalanced against the understanding that any given physical confrontation has the potential to kill you. Even if you prevail in criminal court, you are likely to face civil proceedings. Financial penalties might include compensating the injured party for lost earnings, medical bills, pain, and suffering along with the possibility of a jury awarding punitive damages to teach you a lesson. Keep in mind that the burden of proof to establish civil liability is less restrictive than a prosecutor's burden of proof. Therefore, the plaintiff (your adversary) simply needs to prove simply that it is more likely than not that your actions caused physical injuries, mental anguish, and other losses.

Chapter 3

Defensive Engagement and Disengagement Strategies

Krav maga's overarching strategy is to adopt whatever practical measures are necessary to best deliver you from harm's way. Krav maga strives to teach you not to be susceptible to a surprise assault. The Israeli Krav Maga curriculum places a heavy emphasis on developing the ability to recognize, avoid, and preempt physical conflict. Here are six commonsense safety observations and measures:

1. The obvious and best solution is to remove yourself from the situation before an impending attack can occur. Common sense should always prevail.
2. Recognizing an attacker's (un)conscious body language, proximity, and overall behavior pattern produces decisive clues.
3. Situational awareness of whom and what to keenly observe is all-important. Recognize who or what might constitute a danger or threat.
4. Generally, human behavior is overwhelmingly predictable. Identify what are peaceful human versus threatening behavior displays.
5. Subtle cues, "tells," or "precipitators" observed in a potential assailant's behavior, especially when collectively assessed, provide an early-warning indicator.
6. Body markings, such as tattoos and clothing, can suggest someone's background, affiliation, values, attitude, and behavioral proclivities.

Being proactive overcomes victimization. If an environment projects an overall negative feeling or "vibe," heed your internal warning and take appropriate safety measures. In an unfamiliar environment, scan for threats, paying particular attention to potential assailants' proximity and hand movements. Always trust your instincts and intuition. Even a minimal amount of threatening behavioral information should be enough for you to put your defenses on high alert. Make use of your peripheral vision and constantly assess your surroundings. Note that your peripheral vision will identify movements more quickly than a narrow focus will allow. As mentioned previously, situational awareness is a compromise between being carefree and being paranoid. Most people have this innate capability. If someone acts nervously, secretively, or unnaturally and is within attack range, beware; take the appropriate defensive precautions.

Self-defense may be thought of as recovering from being caught unaware, the –5, and using superior counterviolence in the same way a criminal or sociopath intends to use violence in the attacker's assault on you. Many people are wholly unprepared to face down violence even when they see it coming. These victims of violence do not understand indicators or they do not recognize the foreshadowing "tells." An example of a "–5" situation is where you are caught at a disadvantage with your hands in your pockets as an aggressor quickly approaches you with his fists raised and clenched. Another example would be a victim engrossed in typing on her mobile device and a knife wielder attacks her.

For self-defense, the aphorism "forewarned is forearmed" is literally and figuratively on point. Keep in mind that when you are mentally focused or consumed with something such as a thought or having a conversation, you are apt to lose focus on your surroundings—a "–5" situation.

- When you are observing, remember not to use single-point focus; rather, make maximum use of your peripheral vision, combining it with a slight head swivel to see your 270- to 360-degree blind spots.
- Avoid staring at people who may concern you; be subtle with your observations.
- Fortunately, with minimum focused threat recognition training, there is a good chance you'll spot trouble and steer clear of it.

Pre-Violence Indicator Recognition

When facing street violence, you can usually identify verbal, behavioral, and physical manifestations indicating that violence is imminent. Recognize it or not—and it is decidedly important that you do—it is highly likely there will be some indicator prior to an attack. This all-important situational awareness capability allows you to avoid a "–5" situation.

- When assessing body language, evaluating a potentially hostile person is best done in combination with his physical manifestations and words.
- When nonverbal gestures do not align—someone smiling at you while coiling his shoulder and clenching his same-side fist—nonverbal gestures usually take priority in predicting behavior.
- Nonverbal gestures or "tells" should be prioritized; these are strong indicators of someone's intentions and true feelings.

Perception/Recognition

Perception enables and facilitates a defender's speed and counterviolence of action. Successfully reading hostile body language allows you to recognize an aggressor's decision to engage in violence before he physically initiates it. Recognize impending violence when it is still in the aggressor's strategy stage rather than his committed stage. By developing a honed attack-recognition capability, the kravist can suppress his stress response that might cause panic or a delayed reaction. Preventing such a vulnerable response is accomplished by overriding one's own dilatory startle response with a trained reaction. This cuts down on the action-reaction curve, which generally puts a defender at a disadvantage.

Many of the following observations and supporting photos are well-known; however, they bear emphasizing. An aggressor usually goes through two stages prior to an attack: (a) he makes the decision and (b) the decision is relayed to his limbs to initiate the attack. More will be said on this crucial self-defense aspect shortly, and accompanying photos will be offered.

Kinesic Indicators Recognition

Successfully reading hostile body language can allow you to recognize that an aggressor has decided to engage in violence before he physically initiates it. Gross motor movements often red flag someone who is adrenalized and about to explode. For example, you might need to articulate any one or a combination of the following twelve non-exclusive observations that compelled you to use a preemptive self-defense attack:

1. Fidgeting, shaking of one's limbs, muscle tremors, or clenching one's hands and teeth
2. Sweating, increased respiration or pupillary activity (dilation, constriction, and blinking excessively)
3. A forward lean
4. Moving onto the balls of the feet in preparation to attack
5. Coiling a shoulder or blading the body
6. Stiffening the neck
7. Puckering the lips or sneering
8. A change in breathing (fast-paced or measured)
9. Puffing up (as the chest expands to intake as much oxygen as possible), becoming loud to intimidate, and turning red in the face and neck (vasodilations as blood fills the capillaries)

10. Becoming pale (vasoconstriction occurs as blood rushes from the skin surface to the internal organs). This indicates an advanced stage of fear or girding oneself against an attack and is one of the surest indicators someone is preparing for violence.
11. Pupillary constriction toward something considered a threat or challenge along with momentary pupillary dilation, indicating the very moment a person is ready to act. "Looking through" a person can denote that a decision has been made to attack. Note: while pupil dilation and constriction can indicate and impending attack, an experienced fighter may turn on you without these physical phenomena precisely because he has done it before and it has become second nature.
12. Disrobing to free the arms (and legs).

An Attacker's Body Type

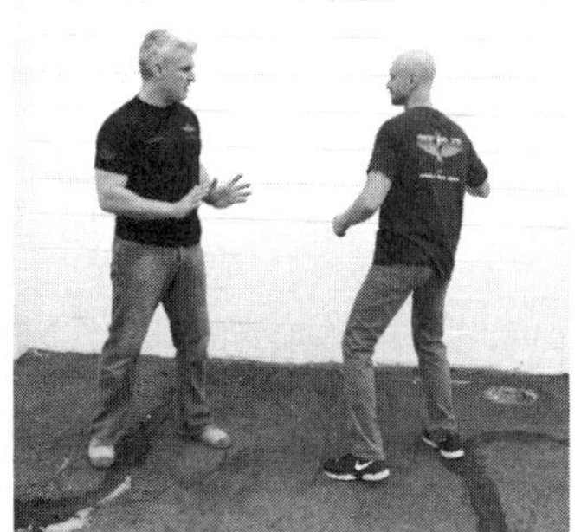

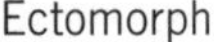

Ectomorph.

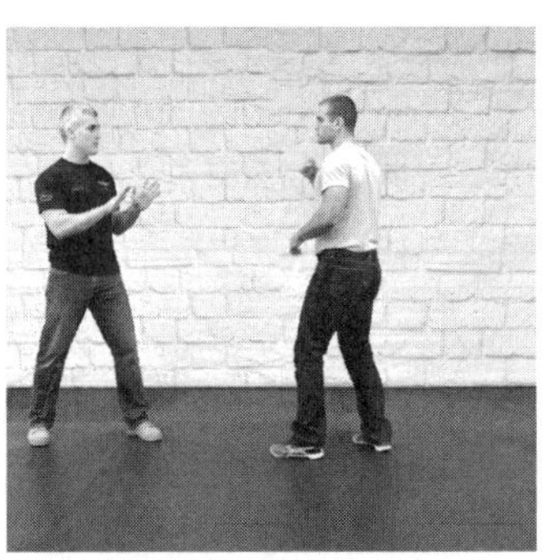

Endomorph.

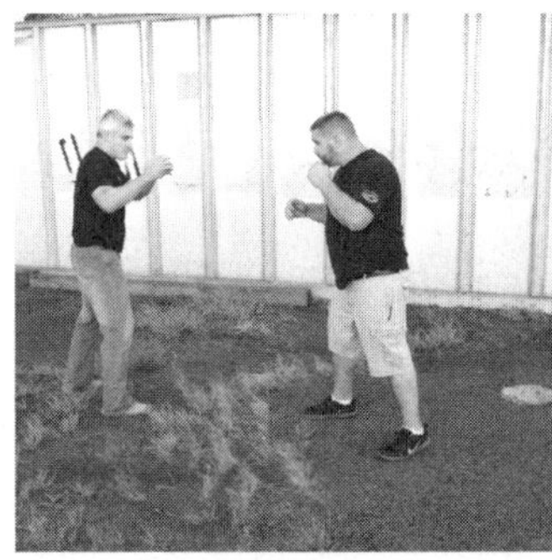

Mesomorph.

You should also observe an attacker's body type—whether the opponent is an ectomorph (skinny/lanky bone structure), endomorph (medium bone structure), or mesomorph (thick/large bone structure)—to optimize your escape/evasion plan and counterattack. A slightly built opponent is likely to move quickly and have less mass behind his strikes while, conversely, a more thickly built opponent is likely to move less quickly but with added power. A medium build opponent will be somewhere in between these respective capabilities.

Watch His Hands and Shoulders

Watching a threat's hands and shoulder movement is paramount. Neural connections are most densely concentrated between the hands and the brain. Therefore, hand gestures may most directly indicate a person's emotional state, especially aggression; clenching one's fists, for example, is an obvious sign of aggression. If you do not see someone's hands, your alert level should go to its highest. The potential aggressor could have any type of weapon, including an edged weapon, firearm, or impact weapon. You are within your rights to demand to see someone's hands. If you move in an attempt to see what the suspicious person is holding behind his back or leg, and he repositions to counter your movement to prevent you seeing from a sequestered hand, a preemptive kick may be warranted. Watching the potential aggressor's shoulders is also a reliable "tell" of his next move. Any attack will involve movement of the shoulders, including kicks and knee strikes. Nevertheless, you must train your vision to see the entire body and especially the hands to determine if they are making bellicose gestures or possibly reaching for a weapon. At the same time, you must understand the dangers of the tunnel vision you might experience.

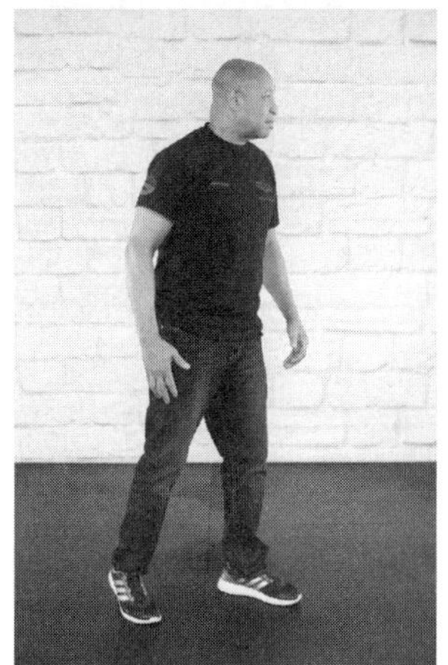

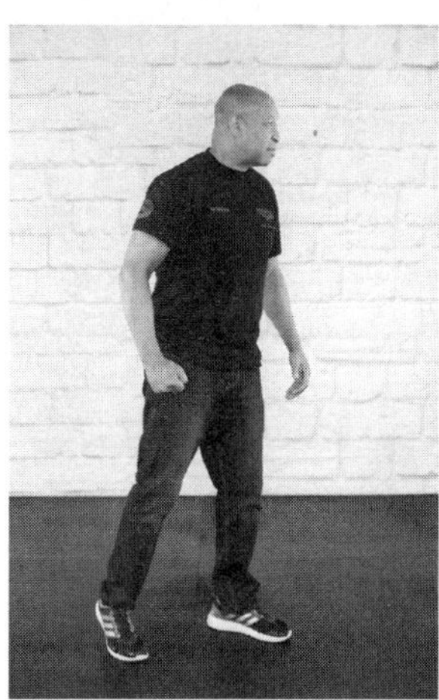

A clenched fist may indicate forthcoming aggression.

Once again, when assessing body language, evaluating a potentially hostile person is best done in combination with observing his physical manifestations and words. Awareness training would not allow anyone to come within attack range, especially if his or her hands are concealed.

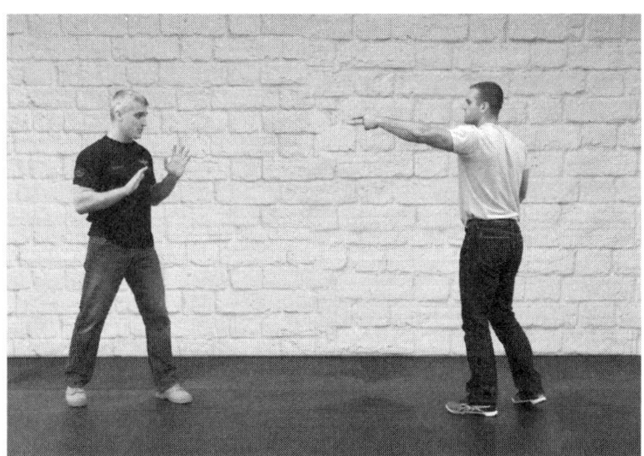

The accusatory finger, a common escalation tactic used by an adversary.

Importantly, a pointed finger can be jabbed in one's eye or poked into the body (an illegal touching and battery in most states).

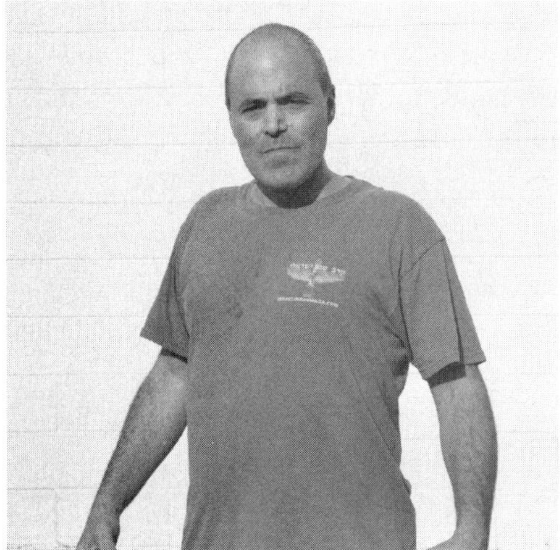

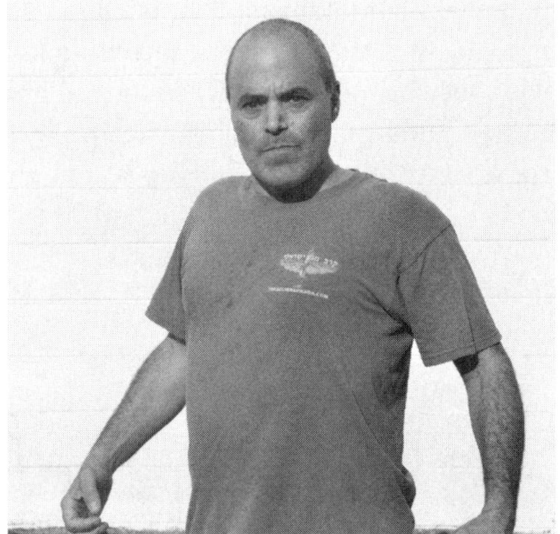

Pupillary dilation and puffing up (as animals do when displaying aggression) may indicate forthcoming aggression.

Pupillary Activity

Importantly, pupil activity functions independently of conscious control and is associated with mental activity. When someone sees something he dislikes, his pupils usually constrict. When someone reaches a conclusion, decides to act, or is surprised, the pupils dilate significantly. If an event is quickly processed as negative or hostile, the pupils change from dilated to constricted in a fraction of a second to see clearly and accurately in order to escape or defend. Recognizing pupillary oscillation can be difficult, especially with dark eyes. But it is still an indicator of possible aggression. Violence indicators also include recognizing a "giveaway" in a potential adversary's subtle physical movements or in an intuited energy shift. Physical changes result from an adrenaline dump just prior to action.

Pupillary Constriction and Dilation

Pupillary constriction naturally occurs when someone does not like something or expresses hostility. Dilation may occur in concert with other body movements, such as slightly raised shoulders and arms. Accordingly, when a potential adversary dilates his pupils, he may have made the decision to attack. Obviously, sunglasses generally thwart the ability to observe someone's eyes.

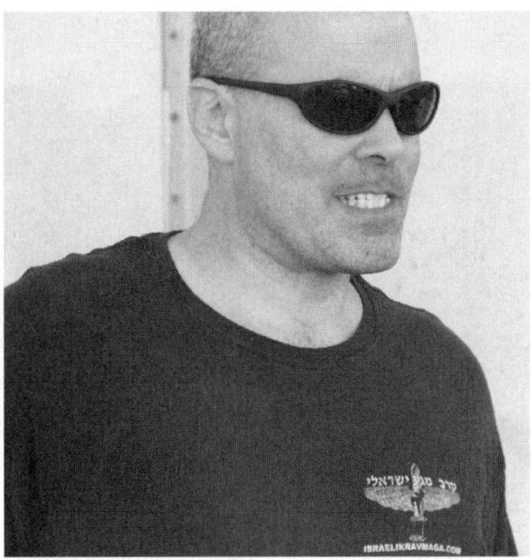

Sneering may indicate forthcoming violence.

Kinesic Indicators of Violence

A primordial sign of aggression is often present when an adversary sneers or bares his teeth. Primates expose their teeth to attack or defend. Hence, sneering is a hostile act in humans as well. Flaring one's nostrils for more air intake to oxygenate the body for flight-or-fight is also a possible sign of aggression. Also, lowering one's eyebrows can signify forthcoming aggression (a primordial signal of dominance). Gross motor movements, including clenching one's hands and teeth, often signal hostile intention. A distinct flushing or pallor of the face, a forward lean, and other indicators red-flag someone who is adrenalized and about to explode in a fit of rage.

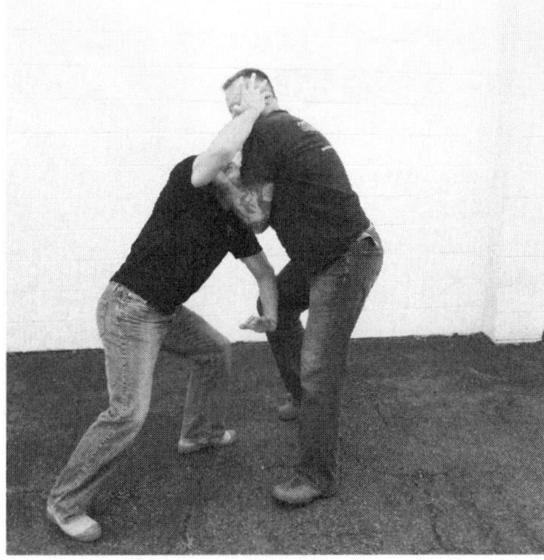

A tactile-feel example of blocking an attacker who is attempting a combined clinch and knee attack.

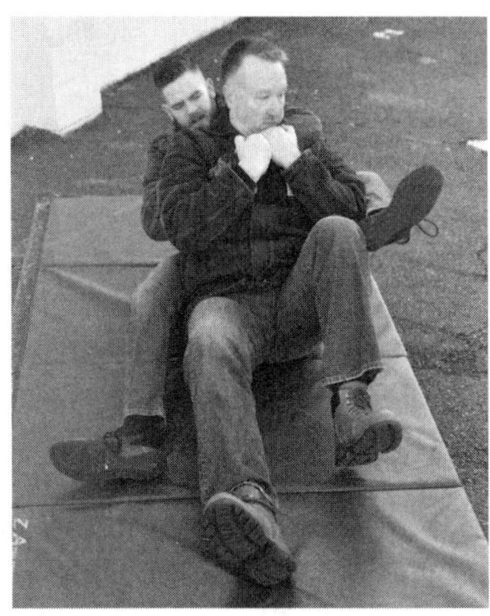

A tactile-feel example of an attacker attempting to set up a rear naked choke.

Seeing an actual strike is not the only way to recognize an incoming attack tactic. At close range and in contact with an opponent, an experienced fighter can sense the next attack by tactile feel or a shift in the opponent's body weight and positioning. In a real defensive fight, movement happens so quickly that the defender may only be able to predict the attacker's next move by feeling it. Having your hands on the attacker can help sense and, thus, indicate his next attack while also allowing the defender to counter-target vulnerable anatomy.

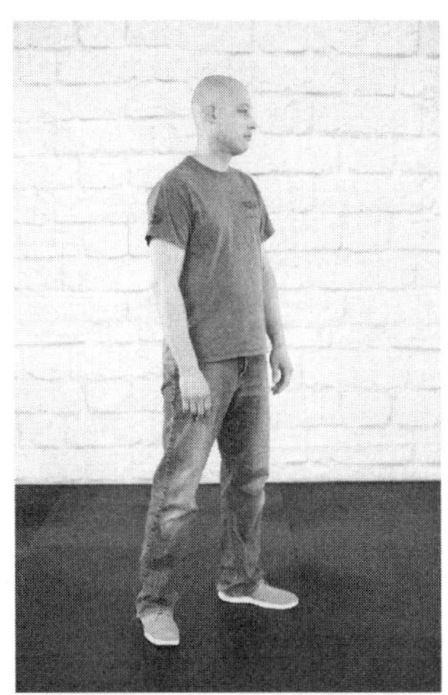

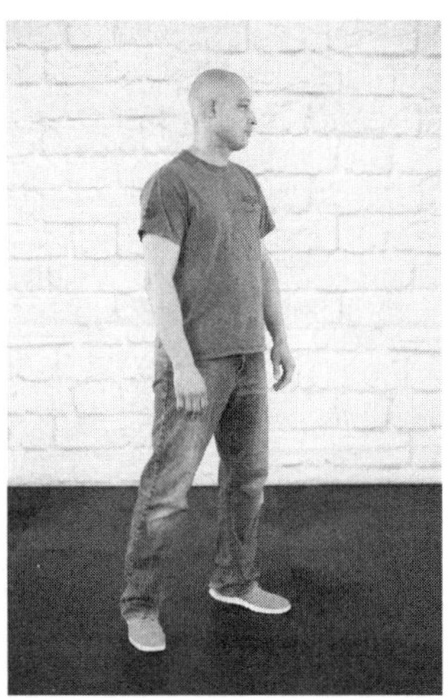

Moving onto the balls of the feet is an indicator of preparation for physical action.

If a potential adversary moves onto the balls of his feet, it is a tell-tale indicator that he is shifting his weight forward and moving into position to attack. Think about the importance of moving onto the balls of *your* feet. So be sure in any potential confrontation to subtly move onto the balls of your feet to facilitate immediate action.

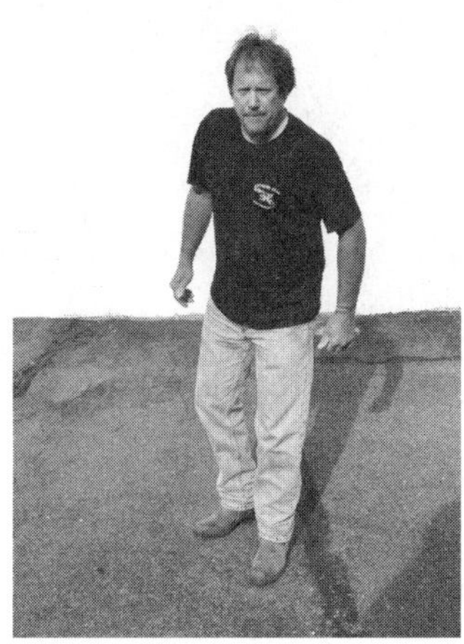

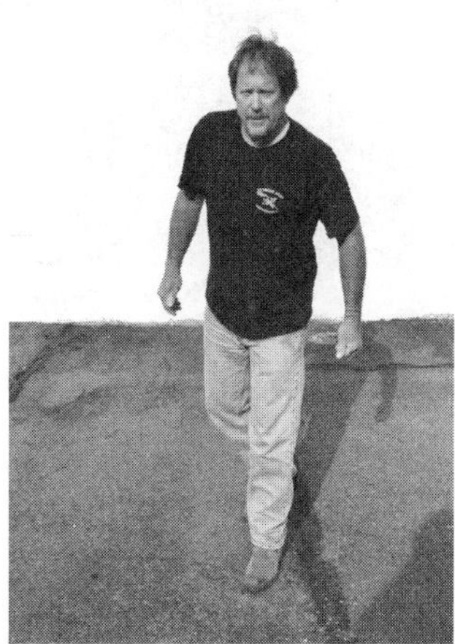

Pawing the ground (similar to many animals in a state of aggression) may indicate forthcoming aggression.

Pawing or raking the ground with one's foot, similar to what many animal species do, may be a warning sign that aggression is pending.

Target Glancing

Target glancing or focusing on a part of the body to attack may also indicate that a potential adversary is preparing to attack. These respective photo series show examples of targeting an opponent's knee and throat. Note: for law enforcement or military personnel, a potential adversary may stare at a sidearm or long-gun prior to attempting to snatch it.

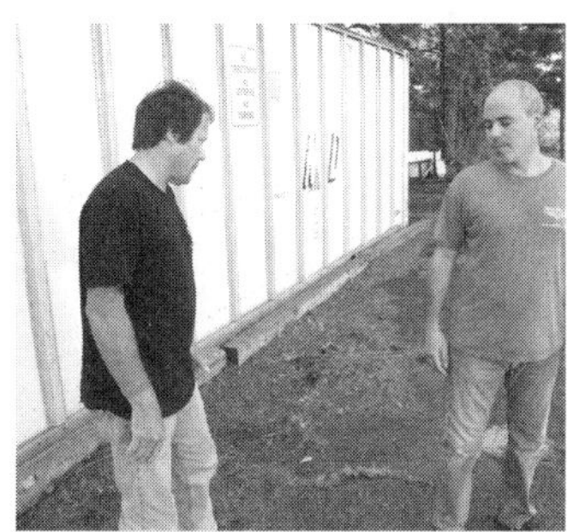

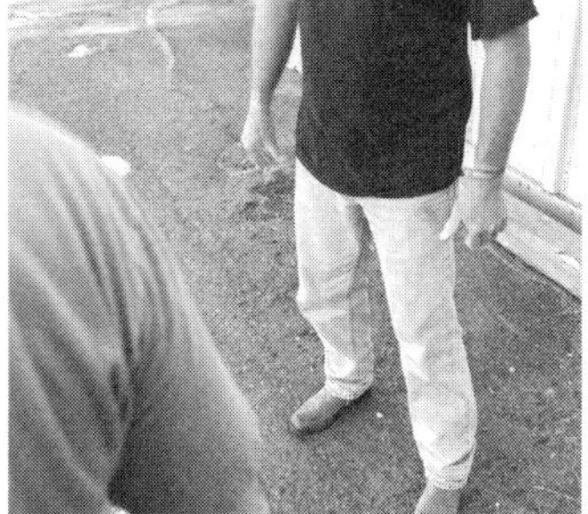

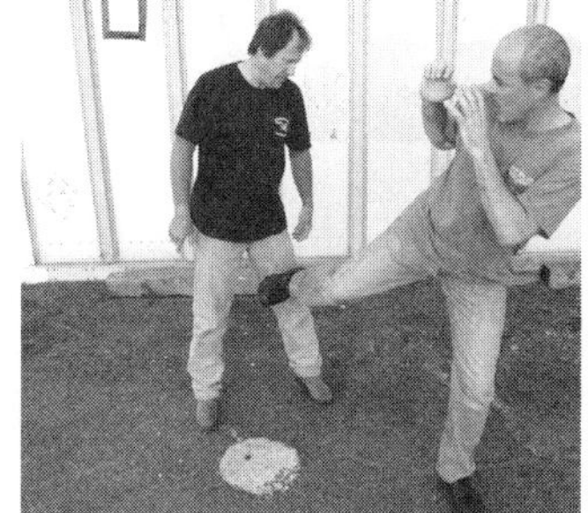

Sighting a knee for a side kick.

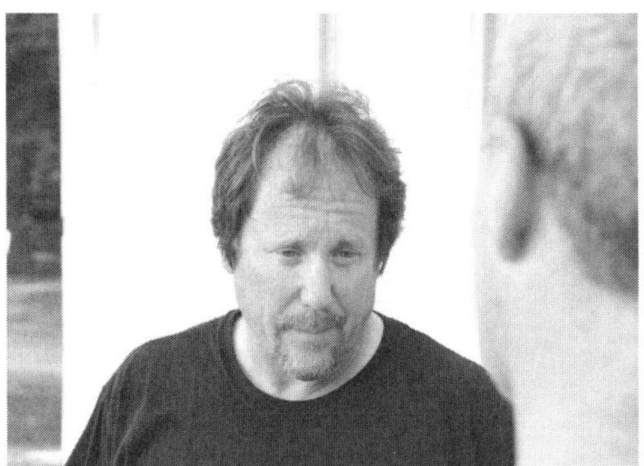

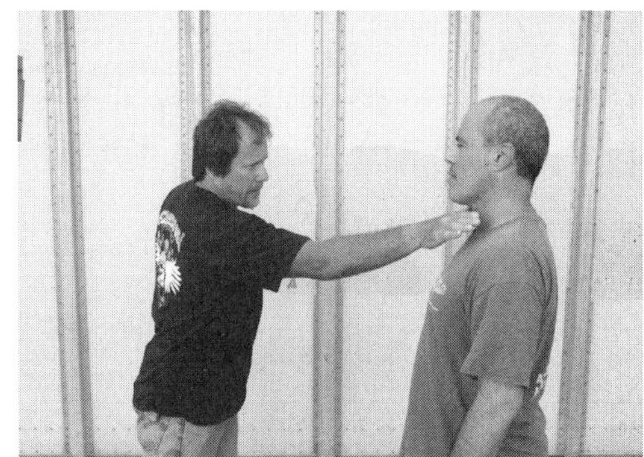

Sighting the throat for a web strike attack.

Disrobing to free the arms (and legs) may also be sign of an adversary preparing to attack.

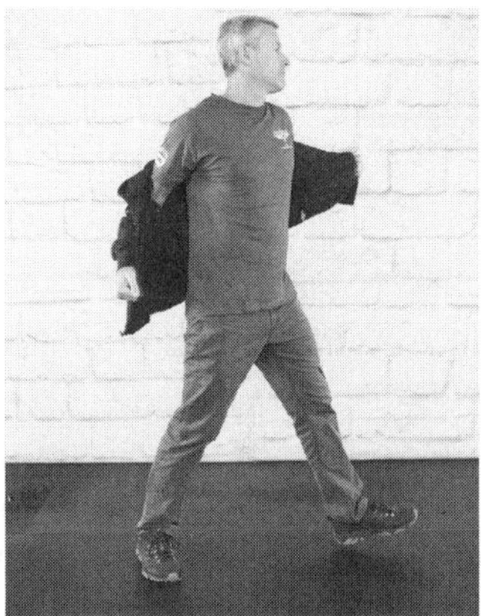

Someone disrobing may indicate forthcoming aggression.

A potential aggressor (or robber) may glance to your left or right or behind you to determine if there are any witnesses or cameras that may see his violent onslaught.

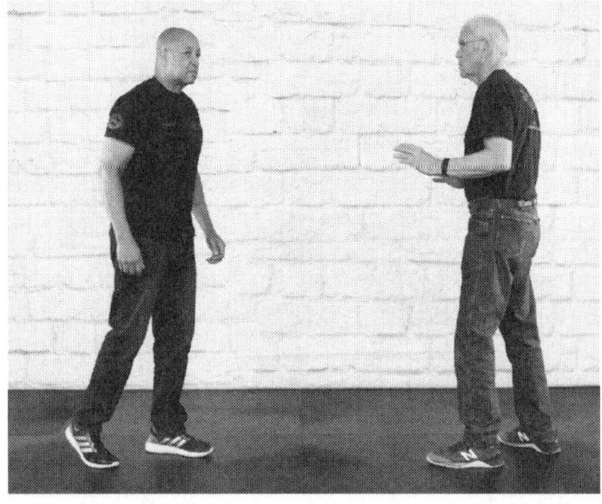

An aggressor looking for witnesses may indicate forthcoming aggression.

Using Reflections, "Selfies," and Other People's Reactions to Detect Rear Threats

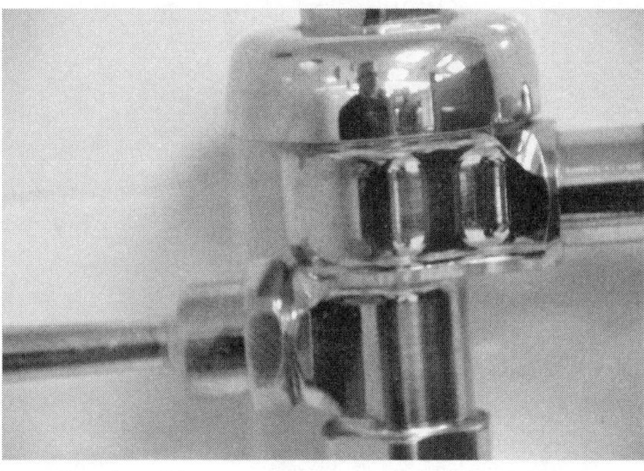

Using the reflective chrome surface of a urinal to detect a rear threat.

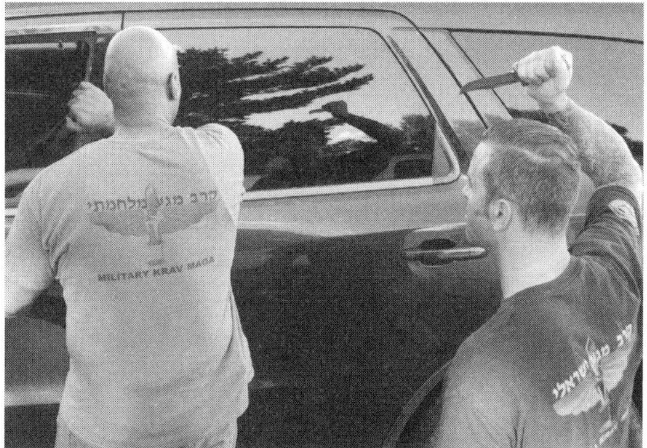

Using the reflection in a car window to detect a rear threat.

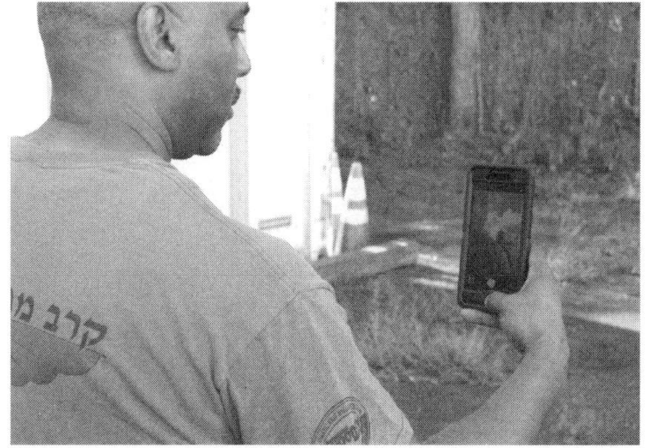

Using a mobile device pretend selfie to detect a rear threat.

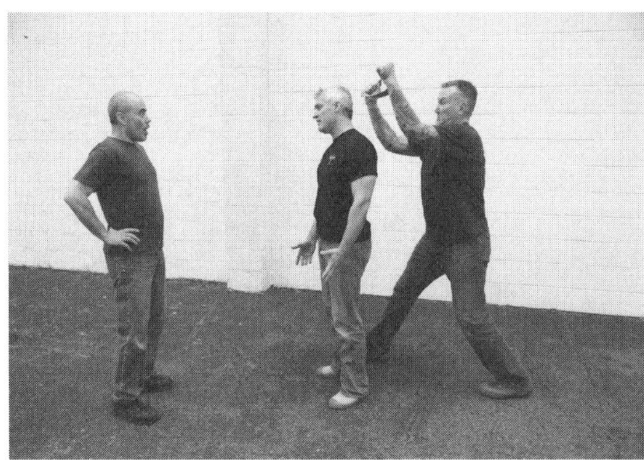

Using other people's reactions to detect a threat.

Reflections from chrome, windows, mirrors, and sunglasses along with an observer's reaction might help you recognize danger. In short, use anything and everything around you to help detect a threat from the rear, including other people's reactions who may be in front of you and see the imminent danger. The advantage is that you can escape, execute a counter-ambush or, possibly, preempt the attack by seizing the initiative. When walking past a corner in an unfamiliar or suspicious environment, it is best to keep a wide distance from it, allowing you to react while surveilling if anyone is standing around the corner. Pretending to use your mobile device to take a "selfie" can also alert you to a threat behind you. To make it less obvious, you could act as if you are "Facetiming" someone, even going to the extreme of having a fictitious conversation as you prepare an escape or counter-ambush.

To scan your rear or "six o'clock," you can feign a trip or stumble to steal a glance behind you to detect a possible threat. Another method is to pat your shoulder and look as though something had fallen on it, but of course, your real intent is to look behind you. Not alerting a possible aggressor that you are aware of his intentions provides an advantage in setting up a counter-ambush.

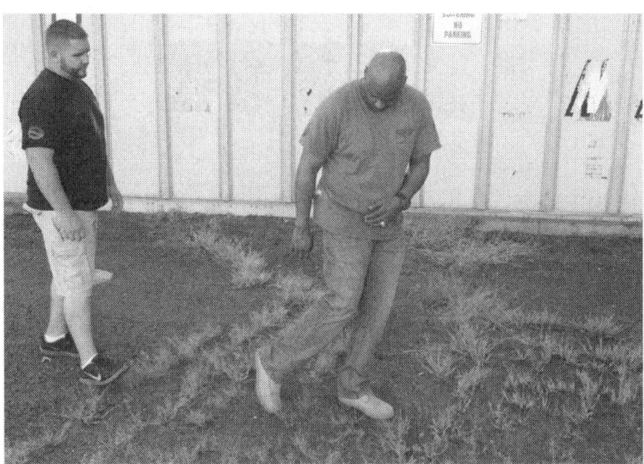

Feigning a trip or stumble to detect a rear threat.

Concealed-Weapon Recognition

Recognition of a bulge on a potential assailant's body—a possible weapon—will allow you to take the initiative to leave or engage him. Threat recognition tips:

1. Most people wear a watch on their non-dominant arm; therefore, the arm without a watch may be the one they prefer to use to initiate an attack.
2. Weapon concealment strategies have one common denominator: accessibility.
3. Look for bulges and loose-hanging clothing to denote a concealed weapon, especially around the midsection or clips in the pockets or waistband.
4. Clothing may hang differently if there is a weapon weighing the garment down asymmetrically.
5. Weapons can be hidden behind a leg, an arm, or the back or secluded under a jacket or newspaper.
6. Would-be assailants often touch a concealed weapon to verify it is in place or to adjust it for a better concealed fit. If an armed assailant is running, he will often put his hand on the weapon to make sure it does not fall out.

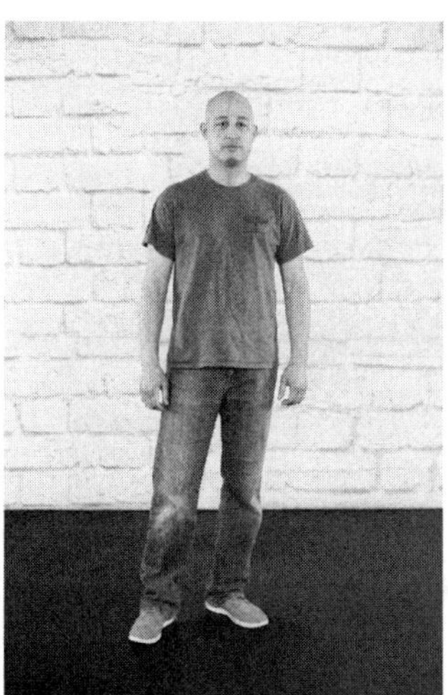

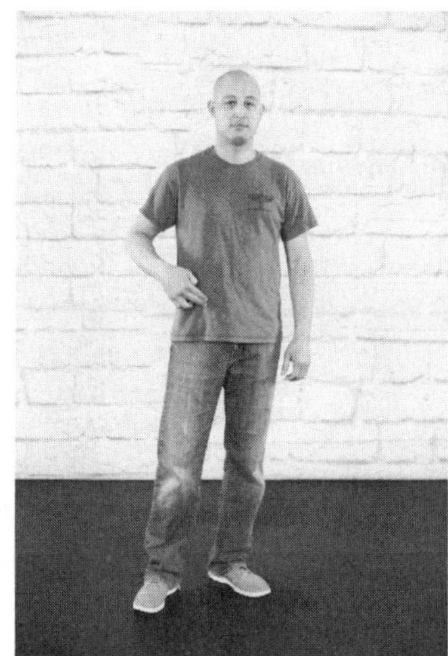

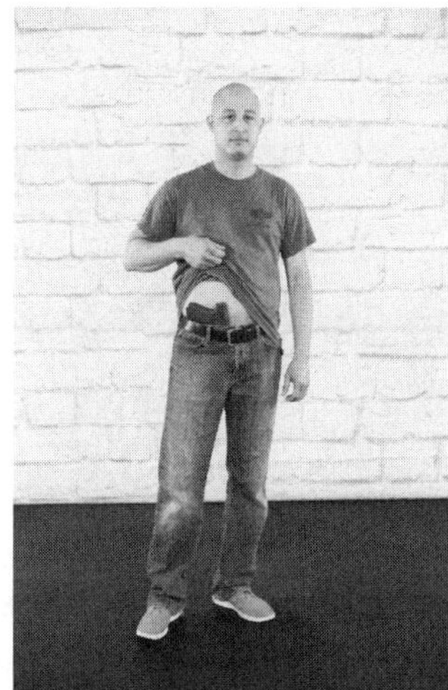

A concealed weapon in the waistband.

A weapon can also be palmed. Note: this may allow you to recognize it as a weapon, as the wielder cannot use his hand for anything else. Another typical method of concealing a blade is to have one's arms crossed in front, hiding the blade behind a forearm.

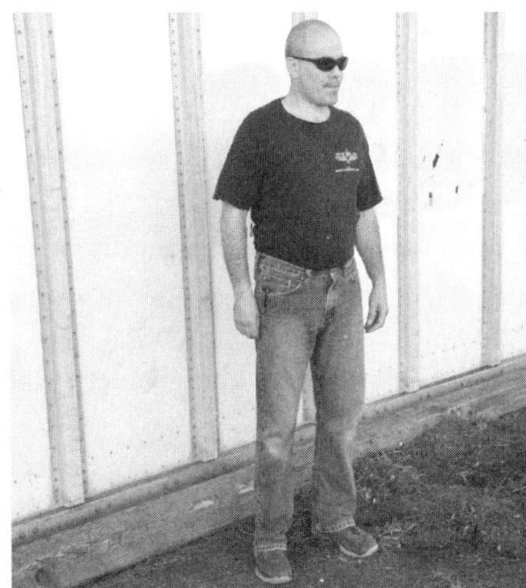

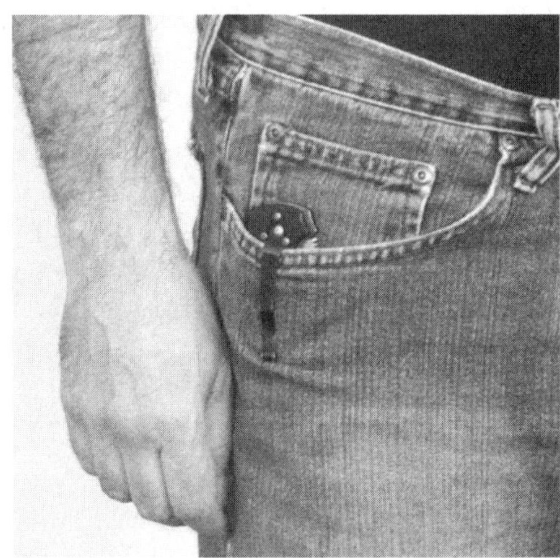

A partially visible weapon.

Watch with ever more vigilance if a suspicious person turns slightly away from you to conceal his hands or his hands drop out of view. Listening for a click or snap, or Velcro detachment can indicate weapon deployment. Be prepared to preempt his attack on you.

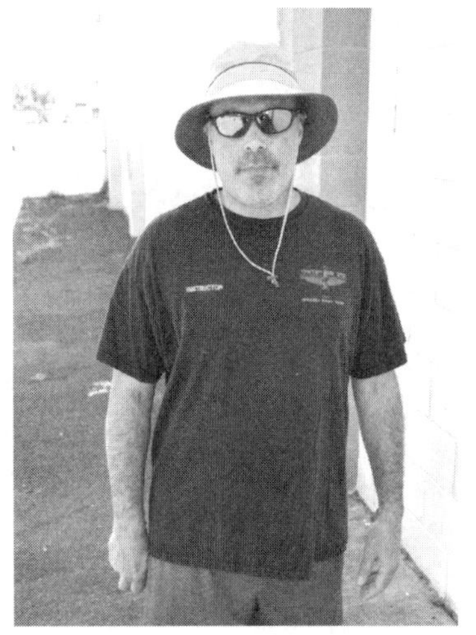

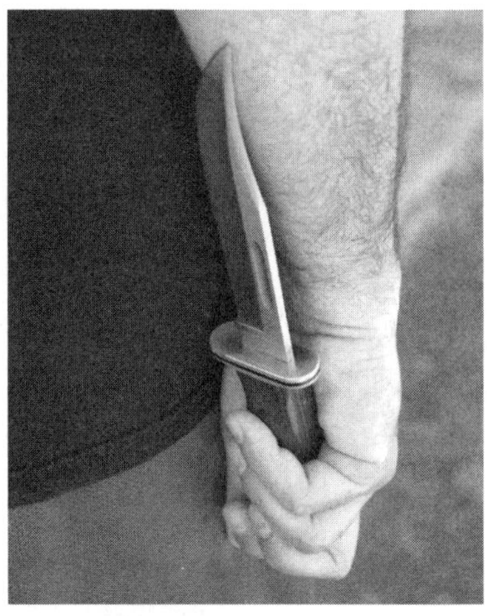

A palmed knife: note the unnatural disposition of the right hand when hiding something.

A preferred method of attack, especially for strong-arm robberies, is for two or more assailants to approach a victim from the front and then veer off to each side of the victim. This enveloping maneuver puts the victim at the disadvantage of facing attack from both the two o'clock and ten o'clock positions. As soon as you recognize two people fanning out in front of you, take the initiative to move and escape or move to the side to line one of the attackers up and debilitate him in short order.

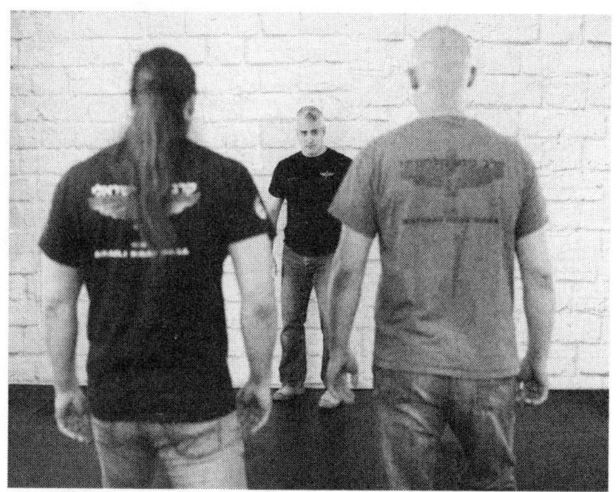

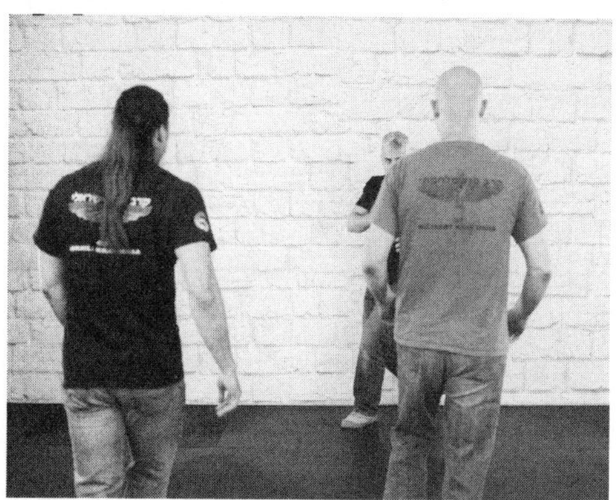

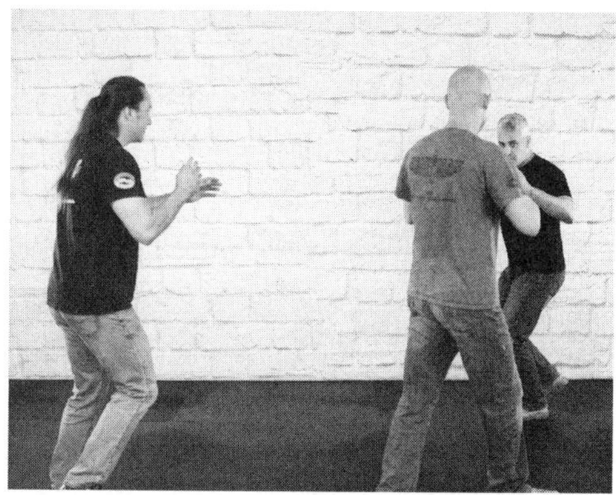

The threat of two assailants fanning out.

Twelve Krav Maga Strategy Principles

When situational avoidance or escape are not possible, Israeli Krav Maga uses the following twelve core principles:

1. Preemption or simultaneous/near-simultaneous defense and attack (violence of action)
2. Defenses and combatives that optimize the body's natural instincts and motions
3. Targeting an attacker's anatomical vulnerabilities; use your closest weapon to attack his closest target, including designated and improvised weapons as well as weapons of opportunity (see section below and accompanying photos)
4. A visceral mind-set devoid of any sporting aspects and rooted in proportional counterforce
5. Economy of motion and tactical simplicity
6. Tactics that work against concerted resistance

7 Tactics that work reasonably well for any size defender
8. Flexible tactics that work against a "family of attacks"
9. Tactics that work against multiple assailants
10. Keeping one's hands properly positioned and not tying both up with the same movement
11. Tactics that allow the defender to decisively and optimally control or secure an adversary and his weapon
12. Tactics that allow a defender to rapidly deploy a weapon of opportunity or designated weapon

Weapons of Opportunity

Remember, whatever object you could use, an opponent could use too. Not only must you be aware of a person's hands, body posture, and any obvious threats, you must also be mindful of potential weapons of convenience he might be able to reach. Anything and everything portable could possibly be used as either a weapon or a distraction. For environmental weapons, the key difference between a danger and an opportunity depends on which combatant recognizes and uses such a weapon first. Here is a partial list of weapons, loosely grouped into six categories:

1. **Blunt objects.** These include impact weapons such as mobile devices, flashlights, stones, chairs, magazines, books, garbage can lids, briefcases, bottles, shoes, wrenches, rings, and mobile devices.

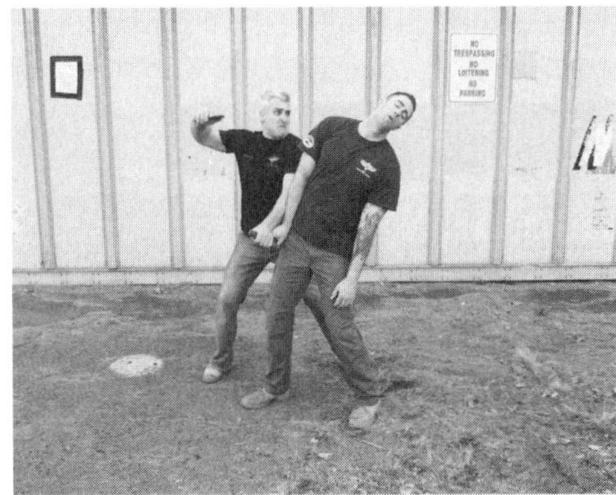

Using a mobile device in defending against a firearm threat.

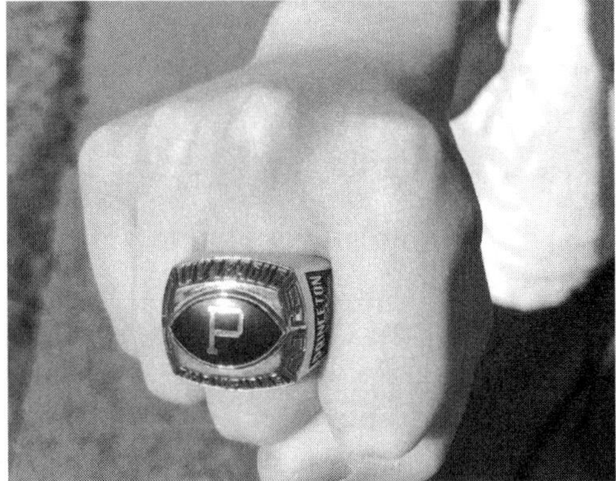

A large ring may be used in combination with a closed fist as a blunt impact weapon."

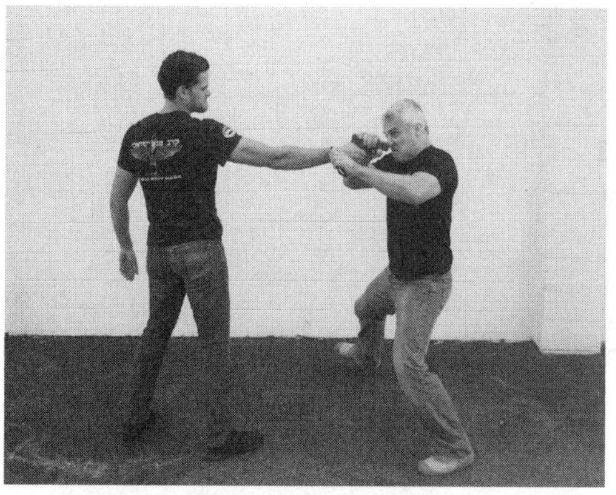

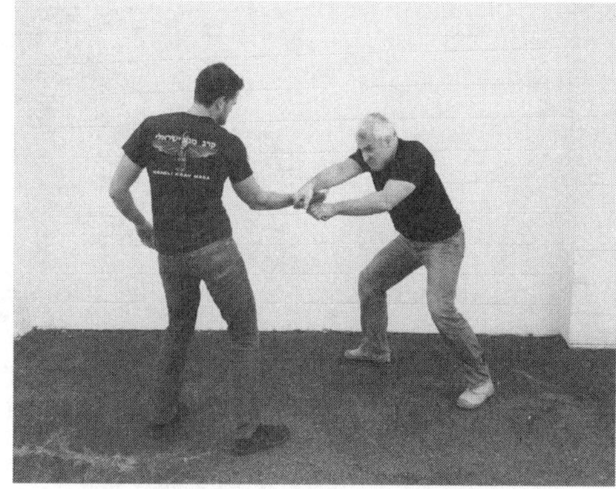

2. **Pointed or edged objects.** These include pens, keys, scissors, forks, cooking thermometers, and broken bottles.

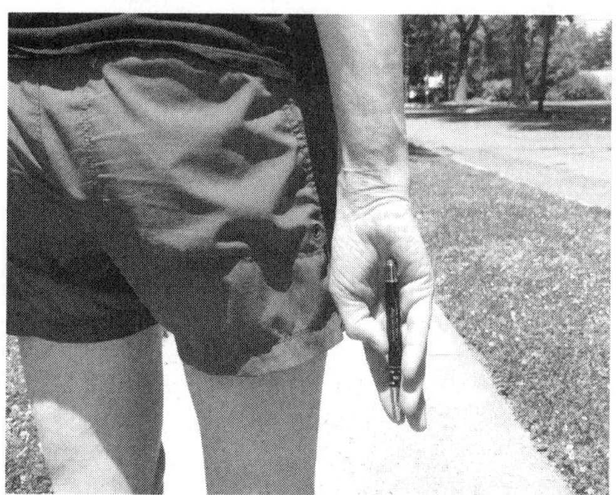

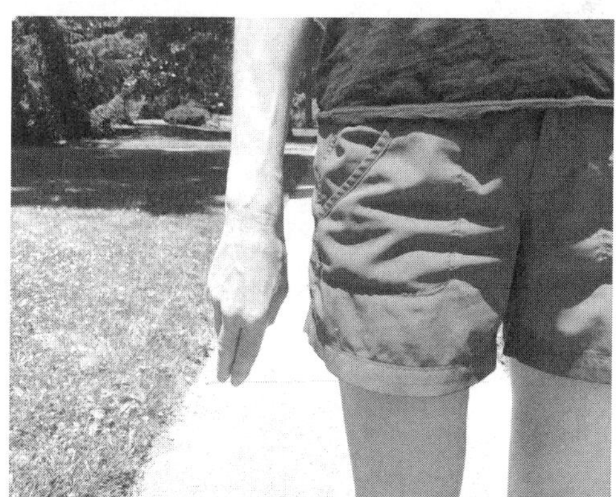

3. **Flexible elongated objects.** These include bags with straps, belts, chains, ropes, jackets, and towels.

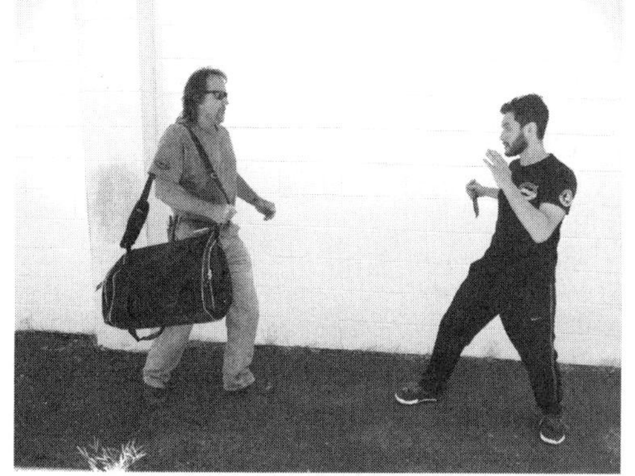

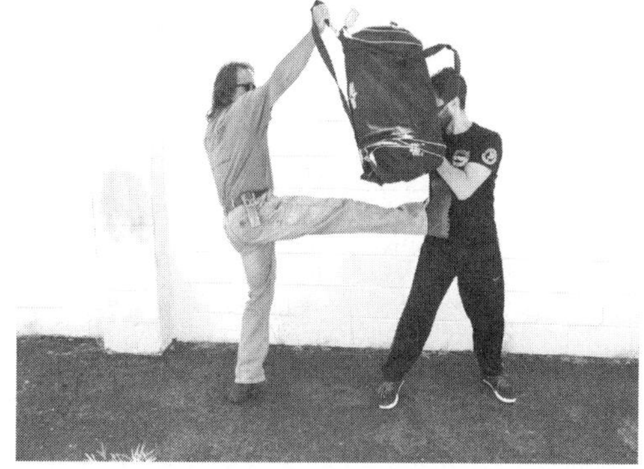

4. **Distraction objects and irritant liquids/sprays.** These include coins keys, watches, loose papers, cellular phones, jewelry, clothing, perfume, spittle, and aerosols. Note that certain liquids or sprays may result in a temporary or even more permanent blinding effect.

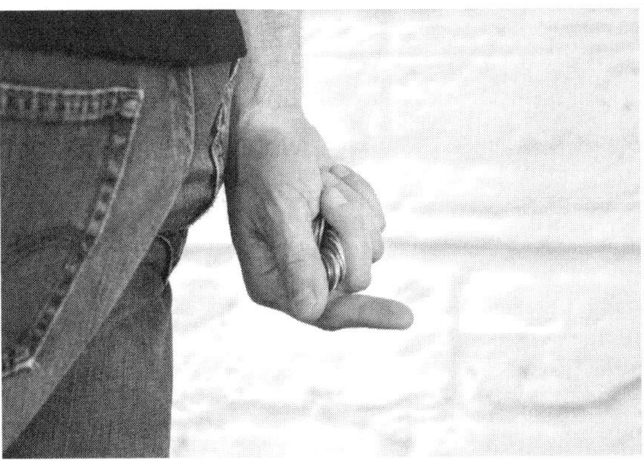

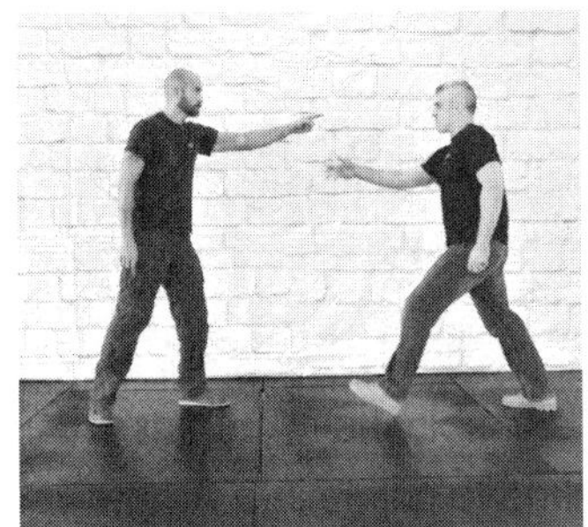

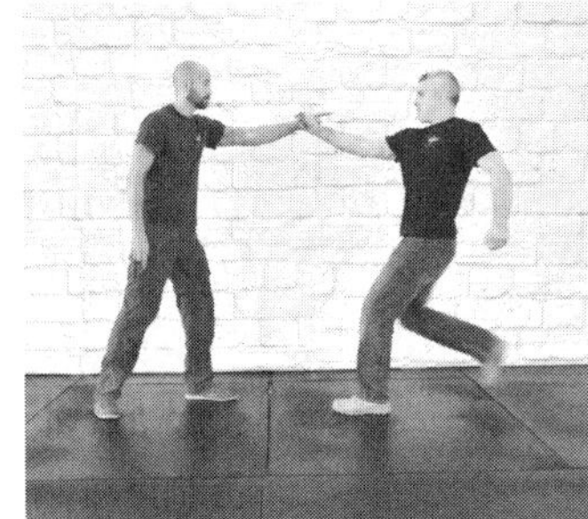

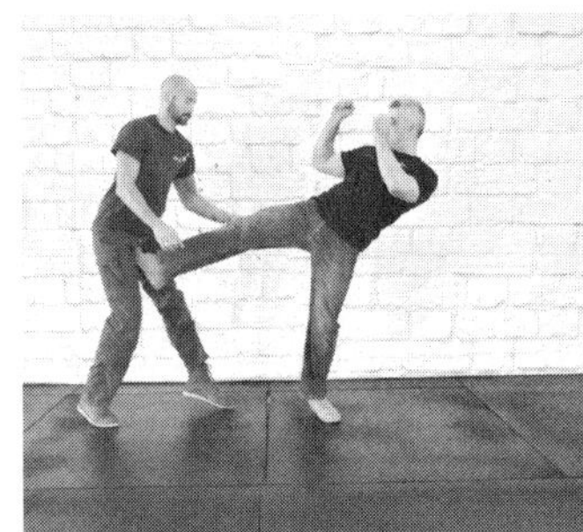

5. **Defensive-shield-type objects.** These include chairs, briefcases, duffle bags, garbage cans and lids, car doors, and other shield-like objects.

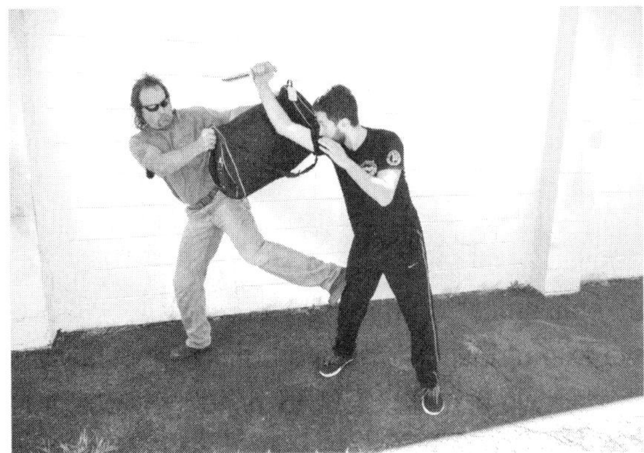

6. **Immovable environmental objects.** These could include such varied things as using a curb to upend an assailant, racing around a parked car when being chased to then turn opportunely on the assailant, or ramming an assailant's head into a wall. Notably, attacking somebody's anatomy when it is pinned against something hard increases your combative's effectiveness since the target anatomy absorbs all the energy and cannot move to disperse it.

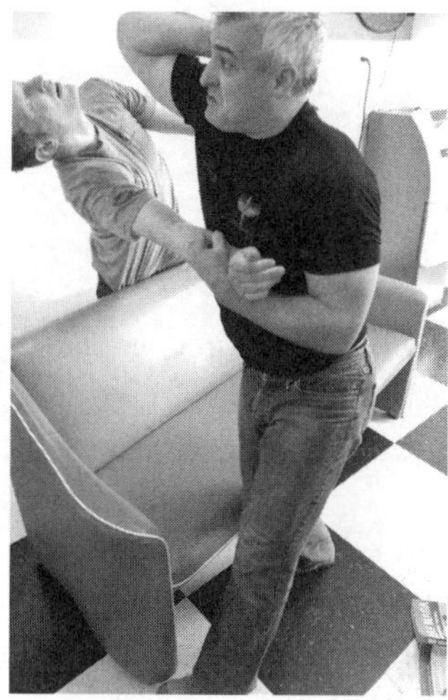

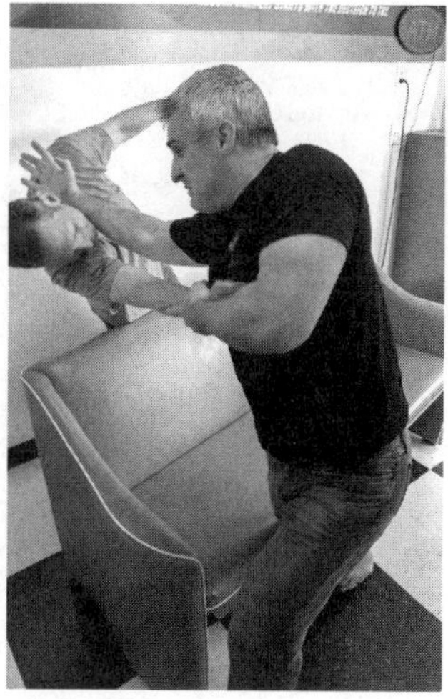

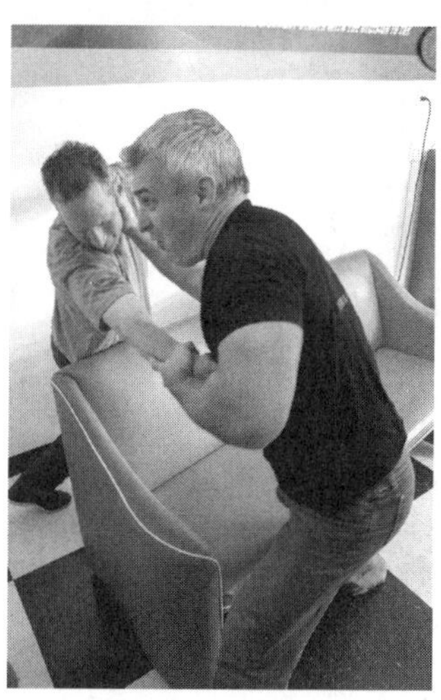

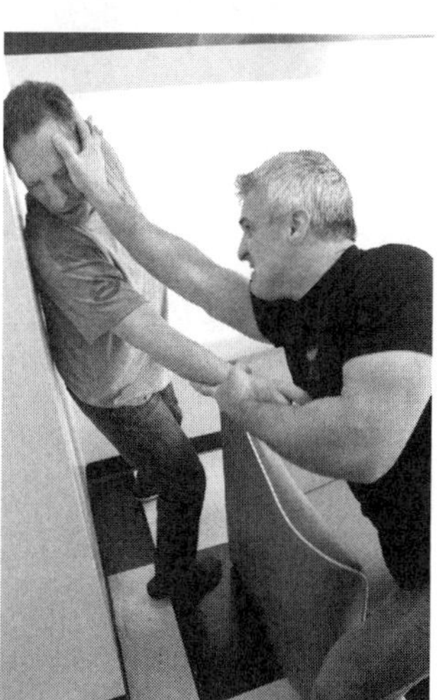

A few more notable points to keep in mind:

- Spitting in someone's face is a weapon of momentary distraction that allows you to attack vulnerable anatomy.
- At close range, screaming into someone's ear can also have a disconcerting affect that can affect the outcome of the fight as you immediately administer debilitating combatives. Jarring, piercing unexpected sounds can immobilize the mind, briefly allowing you an entry to inflict more damage as necessary.
- A flashlight may serve both as an impact weapon as well as a temporarily blinding distraction facilitating escape and an opening to administer debilitating combatives as necessary.
- A car door can be used as a weapon provided your timing and distance are correct.

Key Self-Defense Strategies and Concepts

Here are some additional key self-defense concepts and strategies to keep in mind:

1. In a preemptive self-defense situation, the sooner you neutralize the threat, the less chance the aggressor will have to dominate you. See the preemptive sidekick photo example below.
2. Outside attacks such as hooks and roundhouse kicks are more recognizable because these looping attacks break the attacker's silhouette and must travel a greater distance to reach a target.
3. A competent, well-trained striker will not telegraph his combatives. For example, he will not move his shoulder to initiate a punch. Instead, he will initiate with his hand.
4. One of the most typical mistakes in a fight is not keeping one's eyes on the opponent's whole body. An example would be focusing on his feet. Also, train yourself not to blink. Do not unnecessarily turn away from an attack or close your eyes.

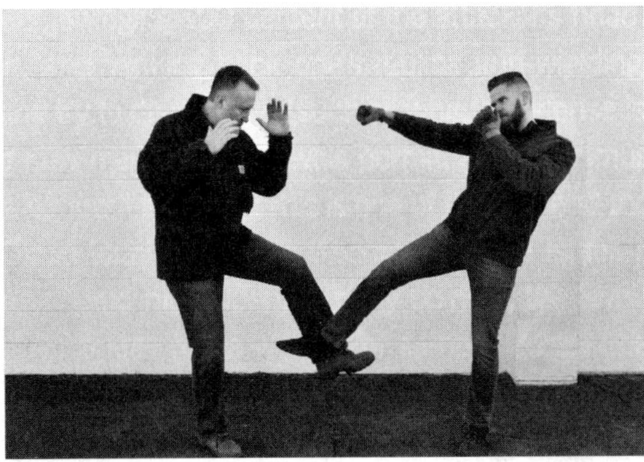

The mistake of looking down and not at an opponent's entire frame.

5. Importantly, a preemptive attack is not launched into an opponent's full attack. This would be incorrect timing (i.e., if the attacker is able to launch his attack, you have not preempted it). A preemptive-timing counterattack is best launched just as the aggressor begins his attack motion, as it is difficult for him to change his attack gears to defend.

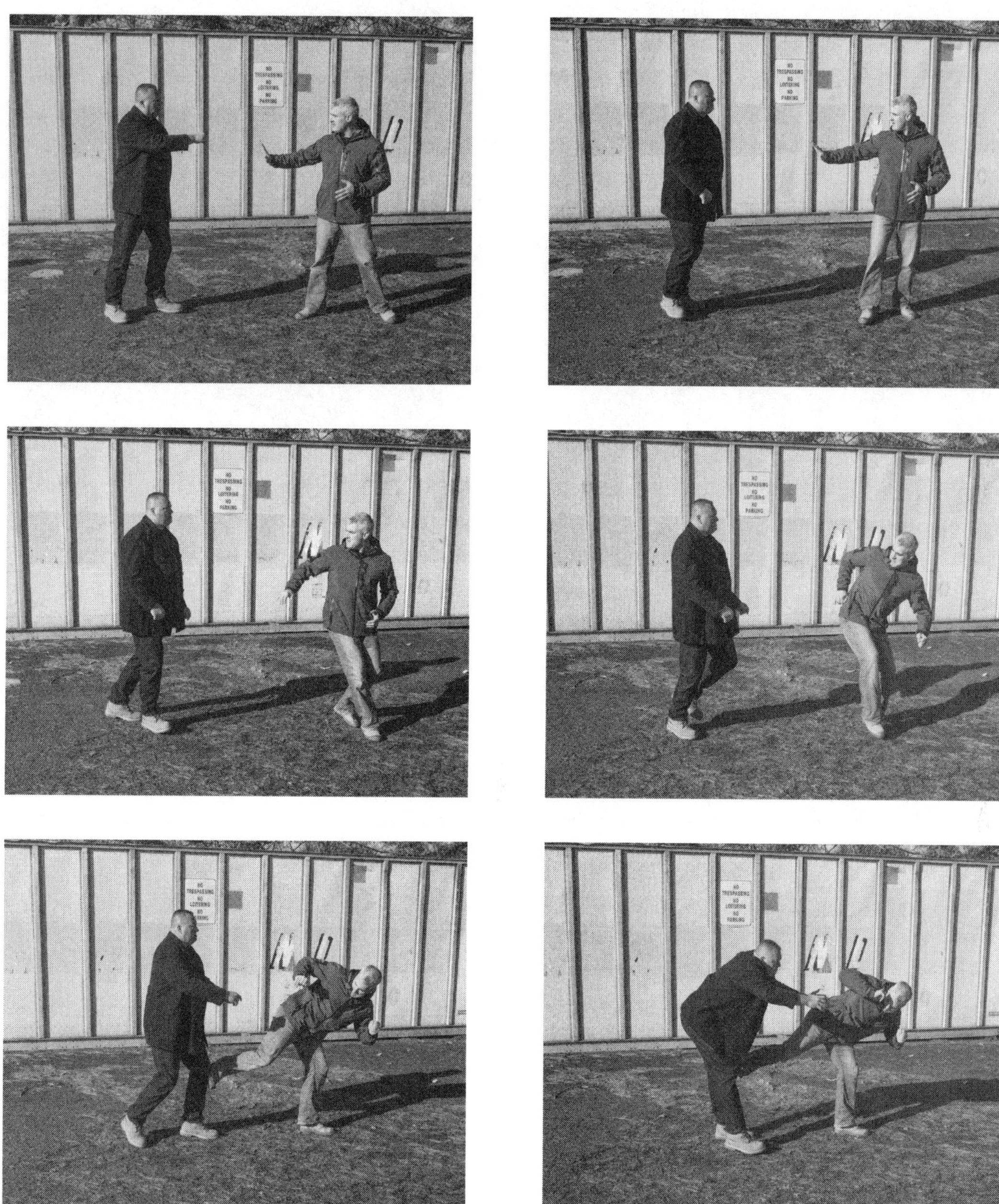

When de-escalation and disengagement do not work, a retreating preemptive side kick targeting the knee can stop the aggression.

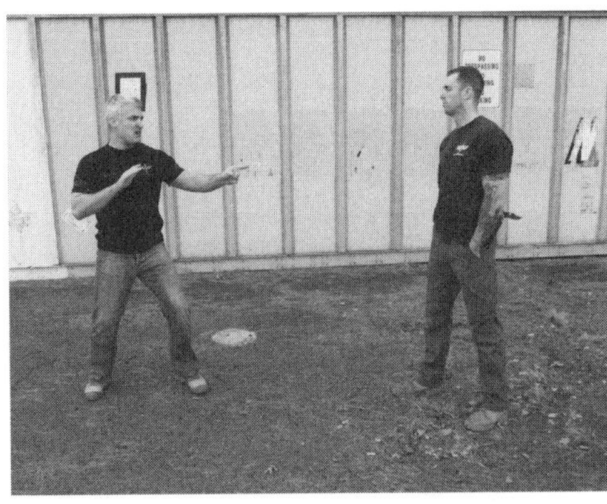

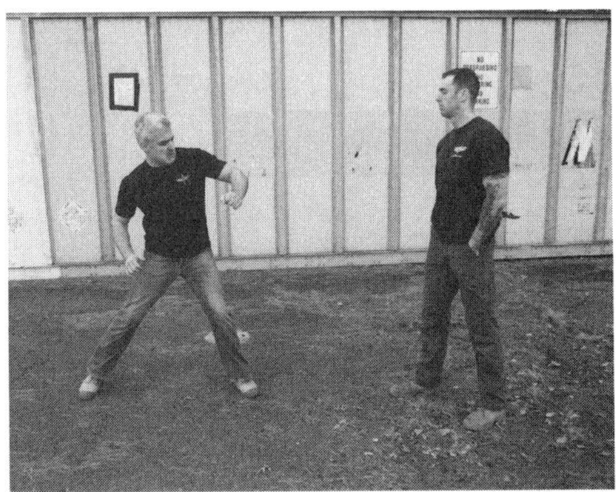

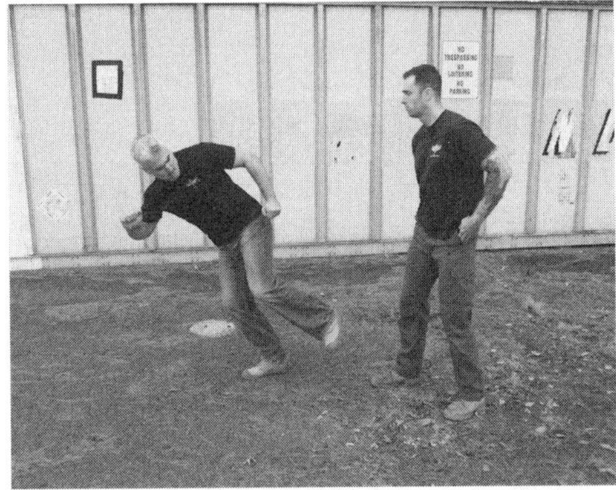

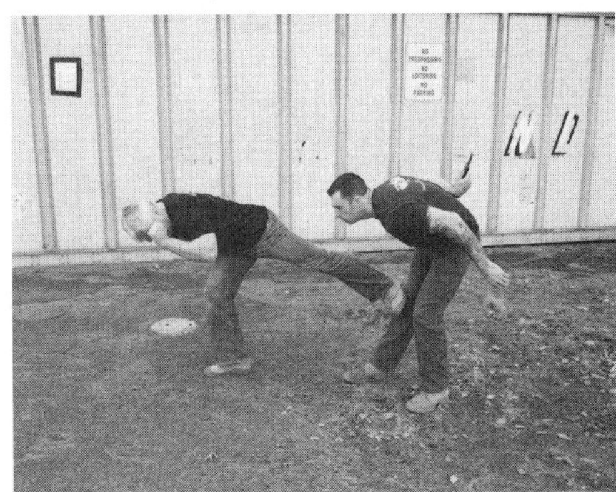

A preemptive side kick against the knee can disable an adversary who is secluding a weapon behind his back.

6. While one cannot always predict how an opponent will move once he is committed, it is difficult for an attacker to change the direction of the attack.

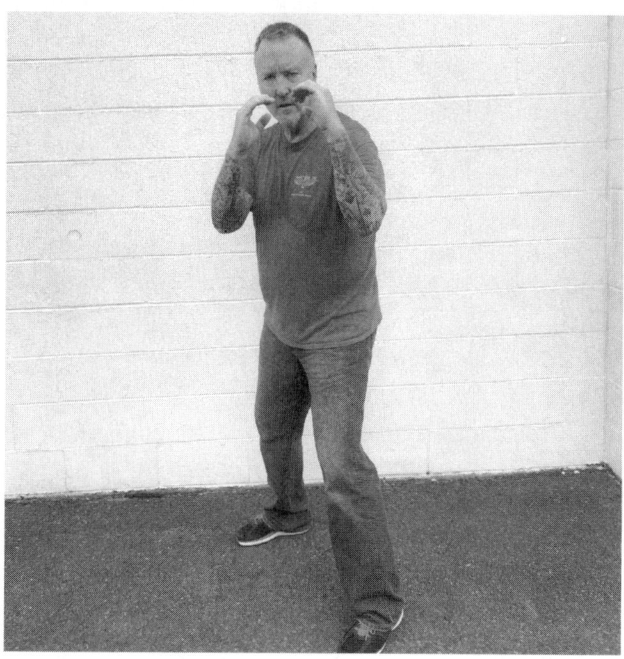

This photo depicts a correct krav maga fighting stance. Note that the defender is bladed to protect his center line. Equally important, this bladed stance immediately lends itself to a front leg side kick to the aggressor's nearest leg—one of krav maga's most devastating preemptive/defensive combatives. Your feet should be roughly parallel and about 55 percent of your weight should be distributed over your front leg. You must subtly be on both balls of your feet to facilitate your movement with your back foot raised ever so slightly off the ground. Raise your arms so that your hands are at about your eyebrow level with your elbows kept close to your torso. Position your arms in front of your face and slightly forward. Extend your arms so your upper arms are parallel to the ground. Bend your elbows to form a 60- to 70-degree angle between your forearms and your upper arms. Hold your hands at eyebrow level, about six inches apart, but do not block your line of sight.

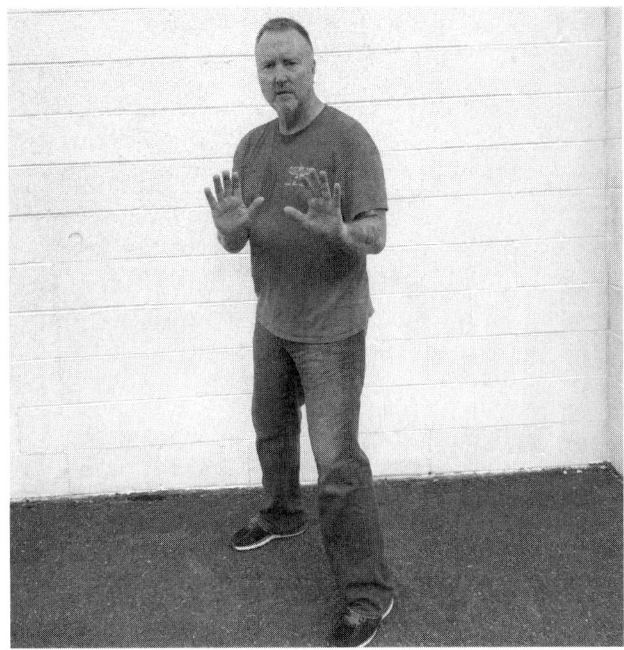

This photo depicts a less aggressive modified outlet stance or low ready position if you are concerned that someone near you may pose a threat. To help you not signal a provocative movement or fighting stance, keep your hands in front of you at sternum level, held in front of you with your palms facing the potential adversary. Only your hand position changes vis-à-vis your fight stance (as depicted above). Your feet are positioned the same as the above fighting stance—be sure to be on both balls of your feet to facilitate movement.

For a de-escalation or an outlet stance, you can choose to stagger your stance with your left or right foot forward. Either side provides an advantage against strikes. Two examples of how a stance can facilitate a defense include:

Left foot forward:

- Against a right straight punch, you can move more quickly to the deadside.
- Against a right straight stab (similar to the right straight punch), you can move to the deadside more quickly to control the knife arm.
- Against a low rear right roundhouse kick, your lead left leg can kick the incoming roundhouse kick or intercept the kick shin-to-foot more easily.

Right foot forward:

- Against a right hook punch, your footwork of stepping away from the incoming punch is easier.
- Against an overhead straight stab (similar to the right hook punch), your footwork of stepping away from the incoming stab is easier.

Against a low rear right roundhouse kick, your lead right leg can preempt the kick by kicking the attacker's torso more easily while your rear left leg is farther away from the strike.

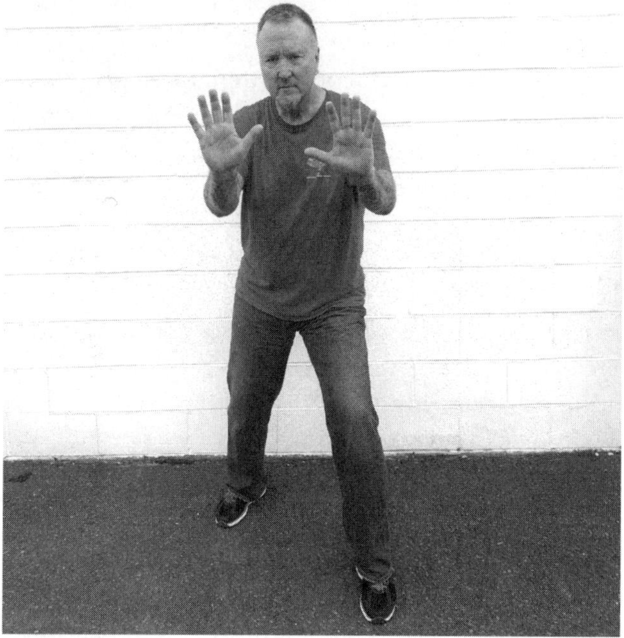

This photo depicts an **incorrect** de-escalation/fighting stance. The defender is squared up to his target exposing his vulnerable centerline. In addition, he cannot readily deliver a low-line sidekick, one of krav maga's greatest weapons.

7. Fighting a novice can be more challenging than fighting a trained opponent, as the novice uses uncoordinated and unorthodox movements to both attack and defend.
8. Learn to recognize an opponent's movements to counter his strengths:
   a) Body lean
   b) Power of strikes
9. Be alert to an opponent's training or preferred tactics, such as:
   a) Boxing/MMA
   b) Jiu-jitsu
   c) Wrestling
   d) Muy Thai
   e) Judo
   f) Taekwondo
   g) Kung fu
   h) Karate

10. Watch for body language, including physical and mental dispositions:
    a) Facial expression
    b) Relaxed or tight body posture
11. Tune in to voice/sound recognition:
    a) "I'm going to kick your . . . " coming from an acquaintance or a stranger
    b) Footsteps
    c) A blade opening
    d) The slide of a gun being cocked
12. Learn to sense danger signs, such as:
    a) Suspicious behavior
    b) Surveillance
    c) Erratic behavior under the influence of alcohol/drugs
    d) Envelopment/flanking movements
    e) Recognizing a shadow either still or moving
    f) A dark, inhospitable environment
    g) Target glancing
    h) Bystanders' reactions to a threat you do not see
    i) Locals' reactions to a threat you do not comprehend
    j) A mob forming

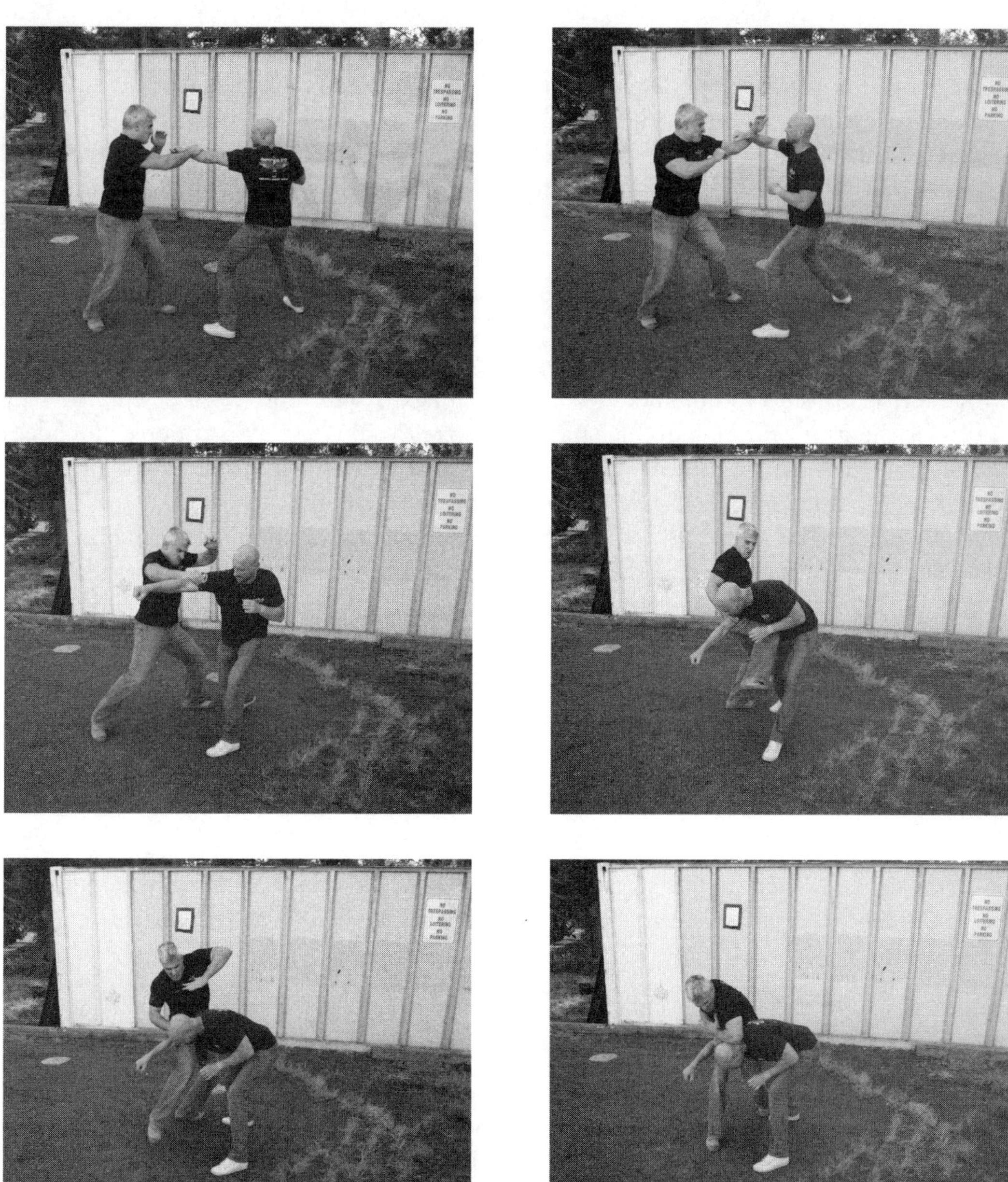

This series shows a the benefits of a correct fighting stance that enables a double parry (should your recognition and timing not allow a preemptive kick) combined with a knee counterattack and switching the hands to trap the opponent against one of the most common trained attacks: a left-jab, right-cross combination. If left unchecked, a trained fighter will unleash a seamless barrage of punches, perhaps up to four every second. Do not let yourself absorb and sustain damage. You must seamlessly defend and counterattack to debilitate your adversary which, when possible, is facilitated by using a solid fighting platform.

An Offensively Defensive Strategy: Attack the Attacker

Because Israel is geographically small with condensed population centers, the Israeli defensive mind-set is to preclude any fight from happening on Israeli soil. In other words, don't absorb an attack. The doctrine of the Israel Defense Force (IDF) is to take the fight to the enemy outside of Israel's borders. Violence in the Middle East has historically been curbed by one inalterable fact: fear of greater counterviolence. The same (un)fortunate logic holds true of street violence: if someone doesn't think he can win, he won't attack.

Accordingly, the IDF's policy is to initiate action against an imminent threat or attacking enemy—on his turf whenever possible. Israeli Krav Maga is an extension of this doctrine: attack the attacker. Avoid absorbing damage and use counterviolence to preempt an attack or, if necessary, utilize a combined defense and attack. A preemptive self-defense strategy (attacking the attacker during his preparation to assault you) is vital. No example in modern warfare is perhaps more illustrative than the 1967 Israeli air assault on the Egyptian, Jordanian, Iraqi, and Syrian airfields. As Egypt continued to mobilize its armed forces against Israel, having blocked the Straits of Tiran to Israeli shipping, this crippling preemptive aerial strike deprived Egypt and its allies from taking the initiative for their planned aggression by destroying approximately 90 percent of their air forces. The maxim "the best defense is a superior offense" applies perfectly here. If you cannot preempt a threat and are caught in an ambush or –5 situation, orchestrate simultaneous defense and attack. Combine your defense and offense into one complete strategy.

American war strategy, as articulated by the renowned historian Russel F. Weigley, also dovetails in part with the aforementioned military logic:

> *[T]he whole history of American strategy since U.S. Grant confirmed that the enemy can be hit with advantage at several places and thus forced to accentuate his weakness through dissipation—as long as the strategy aims at decisive objectives and does not waste itself in sideshows.*[38]

Translated from the macrocosm of war to the microcosm of hand-to-hand combat, the principle of attacking the opponent with all synchronized facets of your combat arsenal (all of your limbs) interchangeably without pause and rules, focusing on deliberate anatomical targeting (not ineffective sideshows against hardened anatomy) is designed to overwhelm an adversary and not give him firm footing to fight back.

Tactically, especially when ambushed, you may not always be able to attack the attacker. In other words, you may not be able to preempt and prevent an initial violent onslaught. Rather, you may have to stop an attack as close as you can to its inception from the position you find yourself in and then overwhelm the attacker with your own superior counterviolence.

38. Russel F. Weigley, *The American Way of War* (Bloomington, IN: Indiana University Press, 1973), 352.

Alternatively, if you recognize an imminent threat such as someone spoiling for a fight, you may wish not to initiate but rather wait strategically in maximum preparedness. If you cannot escape or de-escalate the situation to avoid violence, this strategy allows you to bait him advantageously into committing to an attack. An attacker will always present anatomical vulnerabilities. By waiting for him to initiate the attack, his actual physical committed movement provides you with an opening to administer a devastating counterattack. (Note: once again, this might not be the wisest strategy if you are facing multiple assailants. Rather, preemptive counterattack would stand the best chance of succeeding.) Of course, always bear in mind that defending rather than attacking often has a clear legal advantage: any witnesses are likely to confirm that you were not the aggressor.

In short, if you are caught unaware or recognize the incoming attack late or are simply in a defensive position poised to counterattack, you must capitalize on the advantageous *small window of opportunity that defending any attack affords*. You must understand that delayed recognition and indecisiveness during a physical attack likely equates to you sustaining physical damage you cannot afford. To repeat, this counterattack window is dependent on your recognition and timing as presented by the attacker *as he commits to his attack*—this strategy puts him in a vulnerable position where he cannot easily defend. I believe in addition to possessing the ability to effectively wield preemptive counterviolence, the ability to surgically counterattack using recognition, timing, and distance coupled with optimized counter-combatives distinguishes accomplished professional fighters and warriors. This is certainly what I have watched Grandmaster Gidon and his top instructors implement over the last few decades when challenged. I strive to do the same.

In summary, an attacker, by closing the distance or extending a limb or other movement, will present a vulnerable anatomical target for you to immediately damage. You need to pounce on it. If you must redirect an attack using your limbs, you will fleetingly expose a vulnerable anatomical target. Damage it and continue to damage the original and subsequent anatomical targets as much as objectively necessary.

Regarding anatomical vulnerabilities, both the attacker and defender of course have them. What makes Grandmaster Gidon's krav maga different and superior is that he teaches retzev continuous combat motion. Haim points out that the best MMA fighters and hand-to-hand combat warriors use retzev concepts. Haim's retzev method teaches combat movement that minimizes (and with the best practitioners nearly eliminates) any anatomical vulnerabilities the kravist presents an opponent to counterattack. Analogously, retzev may be further thought of as a sniper rifle capable, after the first precise shot, of fully automatic, aimed fire and operated by a highly trained and skilled professional. In other words, once your first combative reaches its target, the rest of your successive combatives go into full-automatic mode.

Israeli Krav Maga's brutal, highly effective approach to using counterviolence is now legendary. Krav maga's periodic developments are grounded in both street- and battle-proven tactics. Importantly, when taught correctly, krav maga recognizes that the attacker will resist and try to overwhelm you without conceding defeat. Should a tactic fail to be effective in an actual encounter or at full speed and power in simulated training, the system removes or modifies it.

The English translation of krav maga, "contact combat," helps us to understand the required mind-set for any true self-defense situation. Combat is a life-and-death struggle devoid of any rules or fight etiquette. This fact undergirds krav maga's methods and philosophy. Unwaveringly realistic in its approach, krav maga takes into account restrictions that may limit a defender's size, strength, movements, and flexibility. In a street setting, the tactics that a pliable, extensively trained martial-arts fighter may be capable of using are usually markedly different from the average person's capabilities. Nevertheless, krav maga can greatly improve the skills of both the average person and the trained fighter, making it possible to prevail against an ambush or skilled adversary.

The Strategy of Untamed, Targeted Counter-Violence

Knowing how to maim an attacker by counter-assaulting vital points and organs, applying choking pressure to an attacker's neck or breaking pressure to an attacker's joints, or dropping him forcefully to the ground, usually ends the violent encounter—decisively and on your terms. At its core, krav maga does not so much reflect "fighting" prowess or trading combatives so much as the systematic ability to damage the adversary. You must stop the attacker as fast as you can through anatomical targeting. Understand that in a fight involving experienced combatants, specific defensive tactics rarely work or are applied. Rather, it is your offensive capabilities that are paramount. A well-timed, decisive preemptive attack that creates anatomical damage followed by additional combatives usually prevails. Once again, the victor is the fighter who first successfully exploits an opponent's anatomical vulnerability with a well-placed crippling combative and then continues to serially injure the opponent through retzev. Logically, the optimum way to end a violent conflict is to injure the opponent immediately and repeatedly as necessary.

A combatant's superior size strength and speed may translate to little or no advantage in a fight if the more physically imposing or superior athlete does not know how to harness his physical advantages to utilize combatives correctly. The key to delivering optimum strikes is (to borrow a term from ballistics) delivering a form of hydrostatic shock[39] through a target using a well-executed combative with a personal weapon.

There are adversaries you could face who have developed high pain thresholds. Some people simply do not mind absorbing painful combatives and are simply inured or impervious to pain. People with body types of this sort include those who are large framed with fat deposits and lots of muscle. Those who are impervious to pain also include those who are

39. Hydrostatic Shock, https://en.wikipedia.org/wiki/Hydrostatic_shock. Hydrostatic shock is the concept that a penetrating personal weapon can produce a pressure wave that causes remote neural damage, subtle damage in neural tissues, and/or rapid incapacitating effects"in living targets.

intoxicated on drugs, enraged, mentally deranged, and those who simply welcome physical abuse and discomfort. There can be no concrete certainties or conclusions when attempting to disable an opponent, especially when his brain isn't registering pain messages. Fighting an MMA-type fighter is always at the back of my mind when both instructing and training to improve my skills.

When time permits, I watch UFC and other organized MMA fights with considerable interest. I marvel at the tenacity, fortitude, stamina, and skill sets of these sports combatants. I also analyze how the kravist would have to counter such skill and determination. Fortunately, the majority of MMA participants are disciplined, conscientious, law-abiding citizens. But it could happen that you have to face someone using an MMA skill set for illegal or illicit purposes. Your strategy would then be to avoid going up against an adversary's strengths and stand toe to toe, exchanging blows, clinching, throws, and groundwork. Instead, you would have to instantaneously focus on damaging his anatomical weaknesses—and we all have them—notwithstanding those people who can motor on despite sustaining grave physical damage. In other words, you must focus on quickly injuring such an attacker. Notice that I emphasized the word *injure* rather than *hurt*; you must optimize your combatives to deliver the proverbial maximum bang damage for the buck.

When contending with a large or skilled attacker (or someone with both of these attributes) who looks like he may be inured to physical pain, your strategy must be to break down his physical structure so his body cannot function well enough to injure you. One proven strategy for this is to drop him down to the ground while you remain standing and then deliver damage to him. Unbalancing and crashing an adversary to the ground is a highly effective counterattack strategy to disorient him. In addition, a grounded opponent presents anatomical targets that can be attacked with more force because there is no give when a body part is pressed against the ground; all of the combative's kinetic energy is absorbed.

The Strategy of Injuring

It is axiomatic that in violent conflict the party who significantly damages the other party first usually prevails. This is especially true if the defender presses the counterattack home to prostrate the opponent. In other words, strategically inflicting a first-salvo injury against an adversary opens the door for you to unleash subsequent injurious counterattacks. The body's physical reaction to damage is governed by spinal impulses. While physically resilient, your body is still affected by structural injury in a reliably predictable manner. A kravist can consequently often predict how counterattacks will affect the assailant's subsequent movements or continued fighting capabilities. As an example, when an attacker is forcefully kicked in the groin or stomach, he will often lurch over, exposing the back of the neck, spine, and kidneys to further combatives. Use the closest weapon to attack the closest target, and achieve traumatic injury in the shortest time using the most opportune route.

The surest way to prevail in a violent self-defense encounter is to be the one administering overwhelming, debilitating counterviolence. Physical injury inflicted against an adversary compromises his ability both to attack and defend. A unilateral paroxysm of counterviolence must work decisively in your favor. Through controlled but full-speed training that mimics the infliction of terrible, debilitating wounds on an adversary, you learn to shift the balance of power to your side.

Chapter 4

Anatomical Targeting Strategy: Works for Both the Attacker and Defender

To stop an assailant, krav maga primarily targets the body's vital soft tissue, chiefly the groin, neck area, and eyes. The amount of kinetic energy a strike generates to travel through an anatomical target depends on the velocity, the mass of the energy source, and the extent of the kinetic energy transfer. The efficiency of a strike determines the extent and duration of muscle motor disruption.

The human body has seventy exposed anatomical areas, including approximately two hundred targets that cannot be hardened or strengthened through training. These are areas universally vulnerable to damage through anatomical targeting using the most proximate weapon against the most proximate target. Other secondary targets include organs and bones such as the kidneys, solar plexus, knees, liver, joints, fingers, nerve centers, and other smaller fragile bones. Keep in mind that, if an adversary sees his body being dismantled, he will likely suffer emotional trauma that will further sap his will to keep attacking. You, as a defender, must also learn to protect these vulnerabilities on yourself. More will be discussed on this crucial concept shortly. Always keep in mind that whatever tactics you can do to him, he can do to you. To be sure, certain attacks can be lethal, but the body can perform miraculous feats even when severely injured. The body's resilience works for both victim and assailant. Adrenaline is a powerful energizer and allows the body to momentarily insulate itself against pain. Note: an assailant under the influence of drugs acquires yet another layer of pain insulation and artificially increased strength.

Some key concepts for anatomical targeting include:

- Injury breaks down human anatomical structure and function, including both tissue and bones—the aggressor's physical ability to harm you. This, in turn, affords you the chance to impose further strategic injury through retzev.

- Depending on the severity of the aggression or attack, your goal is to produce either superficial or longer-term physical trauma, or both, using the shortest possible path and time to disable the attacker.
- Superior anatomical targeting allows a defender to maximize the use of counterviolence. With correct targeting, a defender can achieve damage regardless of strength, size, physical ability, or professional training. Each successive combative should be more damaging than the previous to prevent the attacker from recovering. Focus on striking vulnerable targets that primarily involve the use of gross motor movements.
- When legally justifiable, administering sequential, injurious, physical trauma epitomizes effective retzev—continuous, opportune, complementary combatives. Target vulnerable anatomy, damage that anatomy, continue to damage it, and move on to the next anatomical target as necessary until the attacker no longer poses a threat to you or others.
- When two fighters are prepared and equal in skill, the fighter who initiates and commits without an overwhelming attack leaves himself anatomically vulnerable to counterattack.

To be an effective fighter you must not telegraph your anatomical targeting intentions. Successful fighting tactics require sound judgment, anticipation, lightning-fast execution, and the ability to instantaneously summon several integrated combatives. Keep in mind that you don't want any type of fighting chess game; instead, the goal is to eliminate any and all of his future counter-movement and counterattack capabilities. In other words, achieve checkmate with your first or second optimized combative as soon as possible. Remember again that whatever *you* can do tactically, the attacker can also do. Human bodies generally move in the same way and have the same defensive and offensive fight capabilities.

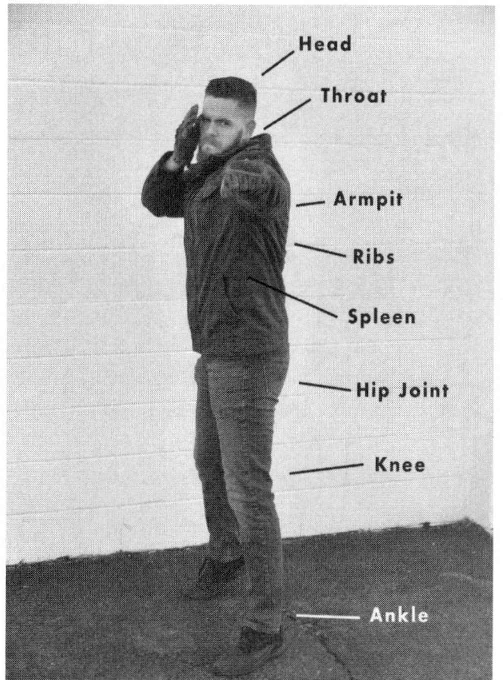

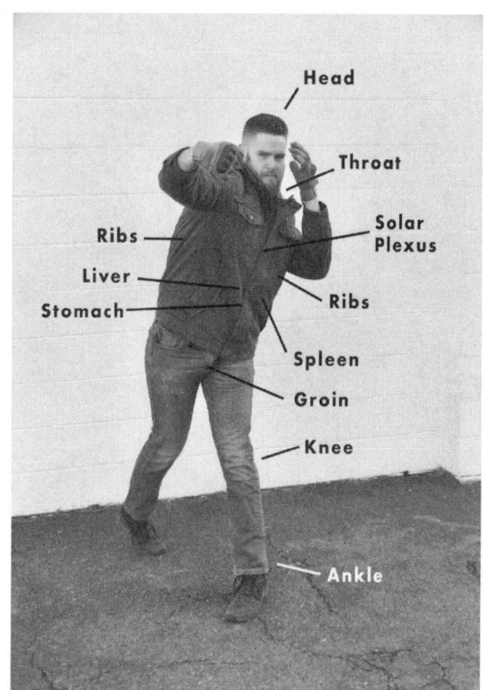

Anatomical targets against a punch attack.

Protecting Your Head

Attackers understand the proven method of debilitating a victim with a blow to the head. The simplest linear type of attack works best when it targets the head. This is usually a straight punch, especially when a victim is unaware. The outcome of an ambush is most often decided in one or two seconds. (This is also true of a fight, although many fights can last longer.) Krav maga, obviously for good reason, places great emphasis on defending attacks against the head. A combative strike to the head transfers kinetic energy from the attacker's impact tool (knuckles, palm heel, elbow, foot, knee, or head) into the victim's skull. The injury types below can result from being struck in the head. Keep in mind that for defensive purposes, this same type of damage as represented in these photo examples can be strategically inflicted on an attacker.

When teaching, I often use the analogy that an attacker's head is the mainframe computer controlling his body (the machine). Disrupt the main circuitry and you disrupt the machine. Attackers fully understand this concept. Take note that an understanding of anatomical damage can be used both for and against you in your legal defense. If you have been attacked, you can explain in your legal defense that you feared the following types of damage if the assailant successfully struck you in the head. Hence your proportional defensive response.

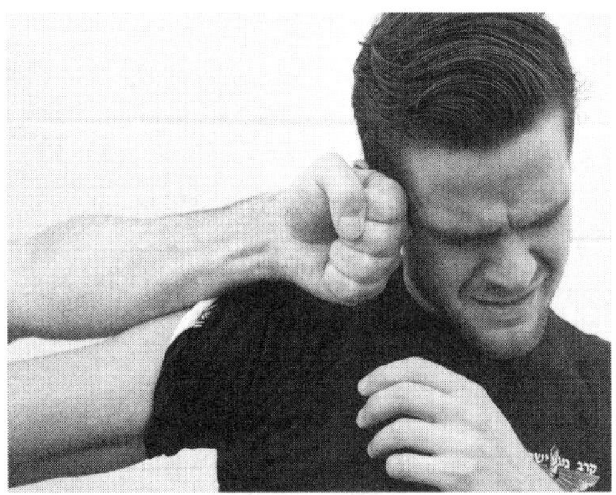
A straight vertical punch to the temple.

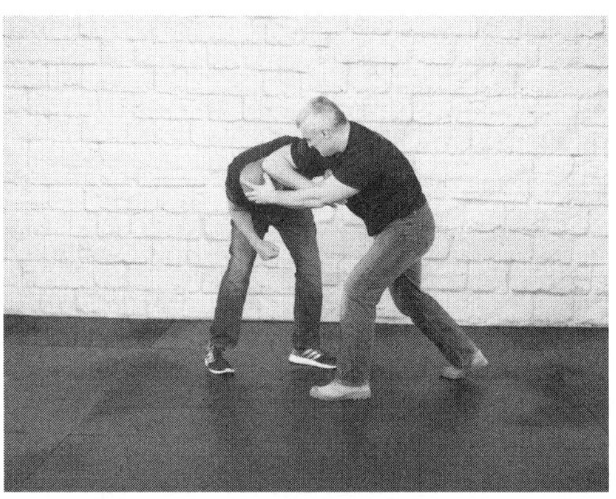
An over-the-top-elbow strike to the skull.

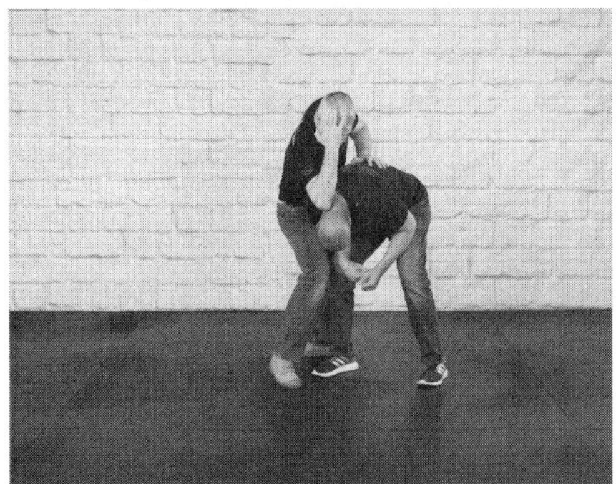
A vertical drop-elbow to the base of the skull.

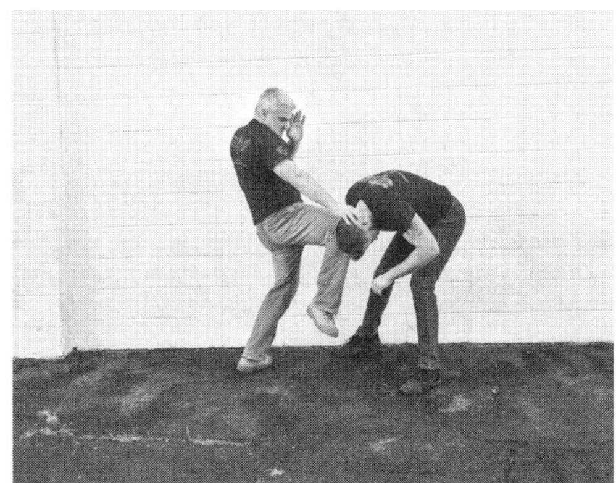
A straight knee to the temple.

Injuries to the Skull and Brain

Globally, there are a significant number of serious injuries and deaths caused by blunt force trauma each year. In the United States, violent assaults account for roughly 10 percent of all traumatic brain injuries.[40] *Skull fractures* account for up to 20 percent for all head trauma.[41] Overall, traumatic head injuries are the most common cause of death among Americans aged forty-five and younger. Up to 75 percent of people with severe head injuries also suffer damage to the neck bones or other parts of the body directly related to the blow to the head. Therefore, deductively, one in five punches to the head could result in a skull fracture.[42]

After age thirty your mortality risk increases after a head injury. Your brain shrinks as you age even though your skull size remains constant. Therefore, there is more room in your skull for the brain to be shaken and, consequently, sustain damage. As noted, blunt force

40. https://www.brainline.org/slideshow/infographic-leading-causes-traumatic-brain-injury.
41. https://bestpractice.bmj.com/topics/en-us/398.
42. https://www.aans.org/Patients/Neurosurgical-Conditions-and-Treatments/Traumatic-Brain-Injury.

injury sustained to one's head in a physical assault can be permanently debilitating or lethal. Since 2007, the British campaign group One Punch Can Kill has recorded more than eighty single-punch fatalities in the U.K.[43] In 2018, a highly publicized tragedy happened when a visiting tourist in Queens, New York, was killed after being punched in the head and subsequently falling backward.[44]

A robust, acute blow to the skull generates a dangerous shock-wave that can disrupt normal brain functions. A violent vibration to the brain can interrupt neurons carrying and intercepting normal signals. This shock could possibly disrupt the nervous system's vital functions, including your heartbeat, breathing, and other life-supporting systems. The cerebellum could effectively switch off, leading to immobility, coma, or death. Of course, from a self-defense standpoint, blunt force trauma attacks to the head are particularly effective in disabling an attacker.

Other serious injuries can result from blunt force head trauma, including internal bleeding when the vessels carrying blood to and from the brain rupture. This causes blood to leak and infiltrate the brain, increasing the chances of death. Traumatic brain injury (TBI) is another serious consequence of a strong blow to the head.[45] When a victim is rendered disoriented or unconscious, his legs give way. This led to the tourist's death in Queens as he smashed his head on the ground. Obviously, a collapsing person could hit his head against any hard object such as the ground, a table, or wall. This secondary impact of the ground, known as a contrecoup injury, often adds to the severity of an injury. The brain is initially smashed against the skull in one direction and then subsequently impacts against the opposite side of the skull, exacerbating the injury. Many military combative programs teach targeting and striking an opponent successively at least three times on opposite sides of the head to generate a maximum contrecoup effect.

An analogy of the effects a punch to the head can have on the brain is a column of jelly on a plate or loosely encased in a jar. If you shake the plate or jar with enough force, the jelly will shake, bounce, and begin to tear.[46] Similarly, when a blow to the head forces the brain to move rapidly inside the skull, the neurons and cells making up the soft brain tissue are readily damaged and torn apart.

Below is a summary of the most common injuries associated with blows to the head:[47]

Concussion—A strong blow to the head may result in loss of consciousness, confusion, memory impairment, ringing in the ears, vomiting, dizziness, coordination problems, confusion, sleepiness, and seizures.

43. https://www.bbc.com/news/uk-38992393.
44. https://nypost.com/2018/08/08/tourist-dies-after-being-punched-in-the-head-in-queens/.
45. https://www.aans.org/Patients/Neurosurgical-Conditions-and-Treatments/Traumatic-Brain-Injury.
46. https://www.health.qld.gov.au/news-events/news/one-punch-medical-effects-can-kill.
47. https://www.health.harvard.edu/a_to_z/head-injury-in-adults-a-to-z.

Simple Skull Fracture—A skull fracture is a crack or break in one of the skull's bones. The skull contains no bone marrow and, consequently, is the human bone structure least capable of absorbing a blow, which often leads to a bruise on the brain's surface.

Pterion ("Temple") Injury—The temple is one of the most vulnerable areas of the skull since the middle meningeal artery sits just beneath it.[48] A blow to the temple can rupture this artery, causing death. Notably, an injured person may initially feel fine. However, as blood accumulates, the victim will develop a headache, become unconscious, and likely die unless a neurosurgeon opens the skull for repair.[49]

Diffuse Axonal Injury (Brain Stem Damage)—The brain is twisted and torn by an acute impact to the skull. Brain cells are damaged without causing bleeding, yet may swell, leading to permanent brain damage or death by disabling the autonomic nervous system.

Epidural Hematoma—A blow tears blood vessels under the skull. Blood collects between the skull and the brain's outermost membranes, causing a hematoma that can expand and become fatal. This severe brain injury typically results in immediate unconsciousness and is fatal about 50 percent of the time.

Intraparenchymal Hemorrhages and Contusions—An intraparenchymal or "in the tissue" hemorrhage pools blood within the brain tissue. An impact on one side of the brain that causes it to bounce within the skull results in bruising. Consequent swelling shuts down arteries and blood vessels that supply fresh blood to the brain, resulting in unconsciousness within eight to ten seconds. Irreparable brain damage and death ensue after four to six minutes of oxygen deprivation without a fresh blood supply.

Injuries to the Eye and Eye Orbit

The eye is perhaps the most vulnerable feature of human anatomy. An intraocular strike to the eye with any type of weapon can damage the eye, eyelids, and muscles or bones that surround the eye. When the eye is subjected to blunt force trauma, it immediately compresses and retracts. Depending on the angle, force, and incident of attack, the eyeball can be damaged, including scratches to the cornea, the lens being knocked loose, or the retina detached. The eyeball can even be split open. Keep in mind that scratches make the eye susceptible to infection from bacteria or fungus that can cause serious harm as soon as twenty-four hours. Trauma from a blow may affect not only the eye, but the surrounding area, including the adjacent tissue and bone structure. In addition, there can be orbital rim and (in)direct orbital-floor fractures.

Note: The most effective type of eye gouge is to attack from the bottom using an upward angle to screw or rotate your finger into the eye to pry the lids open to access the eyeball.

48. http://scienceblogs.com/whitecoatunderground/2009/03/18/a-simple-bump-on-the-head-can/.
49. https://mic.com/articles/117340/this-is-what-happens-to-your-brain-when-you-get-punched-in-the-head.

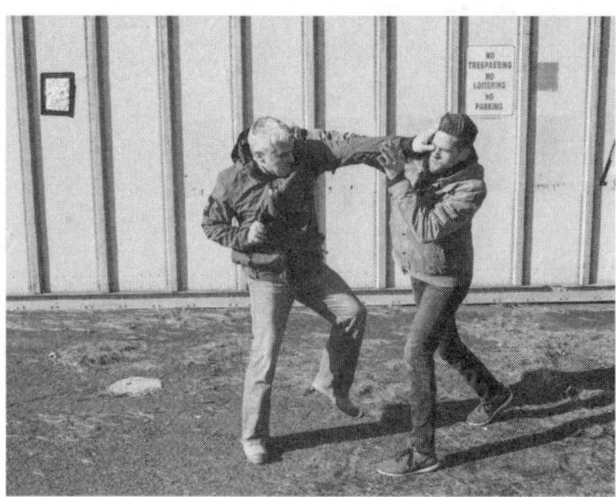

A preemptive thumb gouge to the eye against a hook punch.

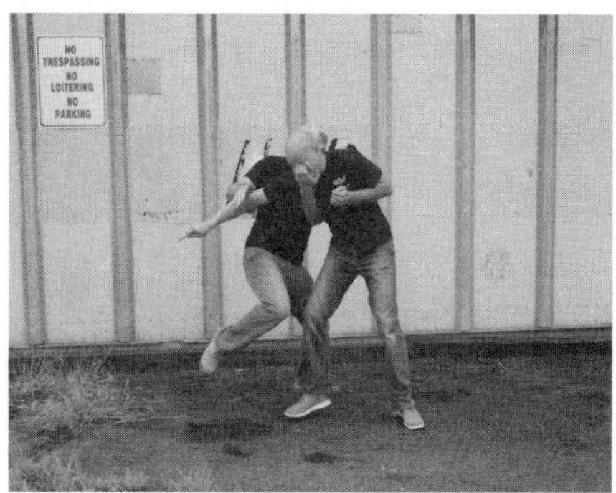

An eye gouge defending an outside slash with an edged weapon.

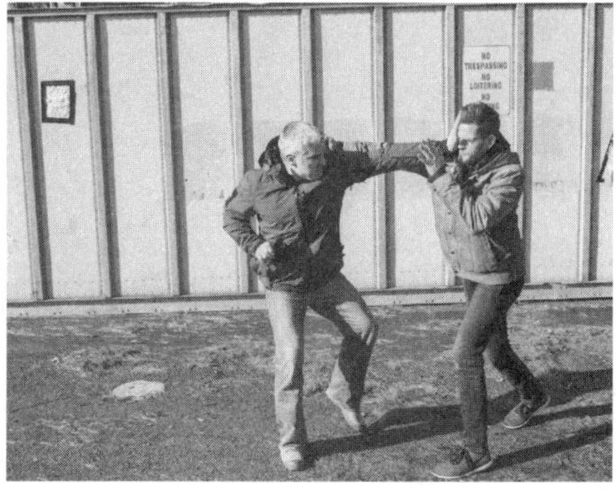

A preemptive straight palm-heel strike to the eye orbit against a hook punch.

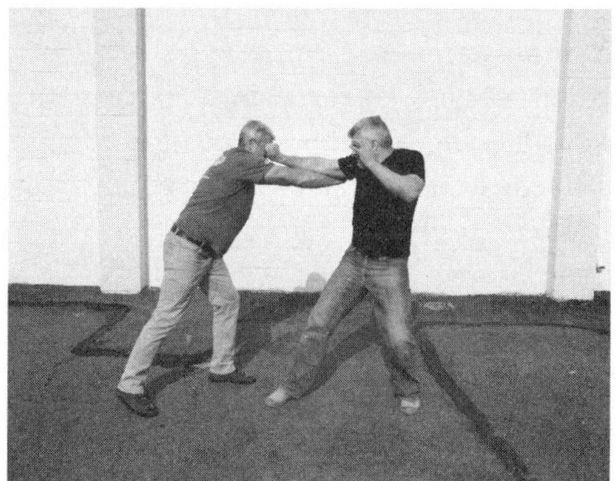

A knuckle eye-rake strike.

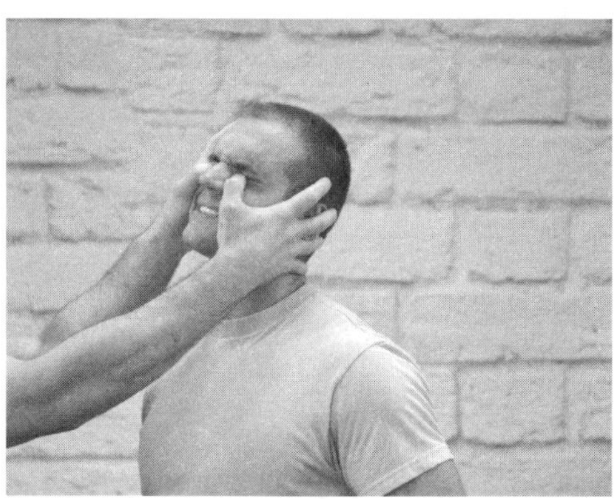

A double-eye thumb gouge.

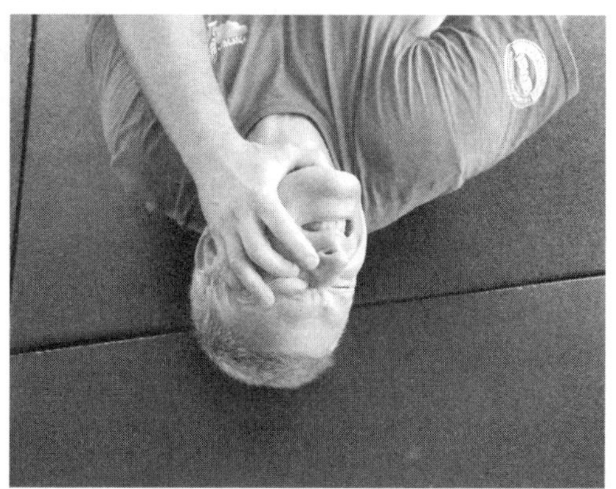

A middle-finger eye gouge.

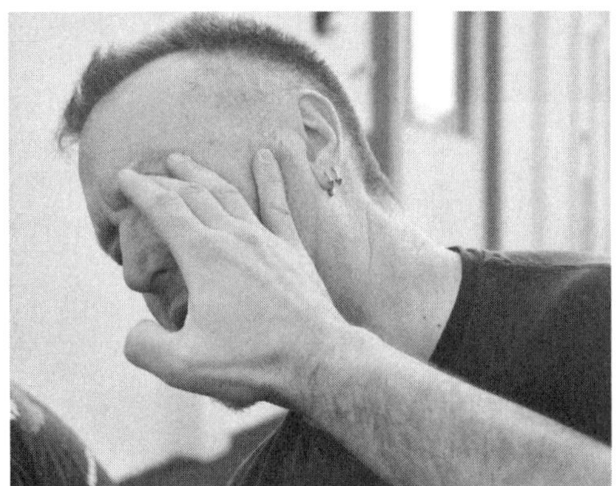
A middle finger eye rake.

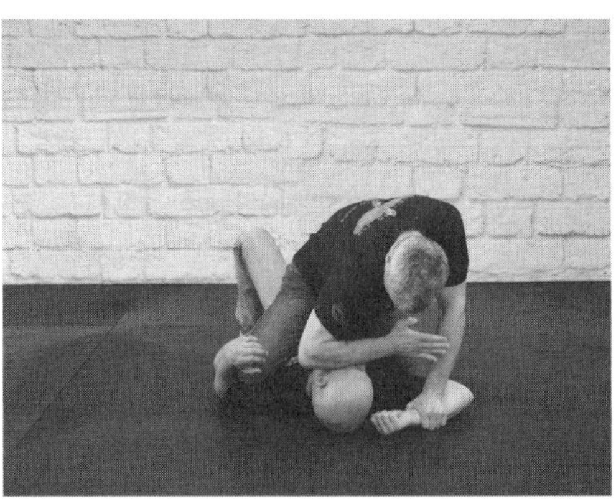
A drop forearm elbow strike to the eye orbit.

Injuries to the Nose

A strong blow to the nose, regardless of whether the cartilage fractures, usually produces reflex tearing, thereby impairing the victim's vision. Such blurred vision can leave the victim vulnerable to further attack. Further, if a blow causes bleeding and gagging, protective responses might be altered.[50]

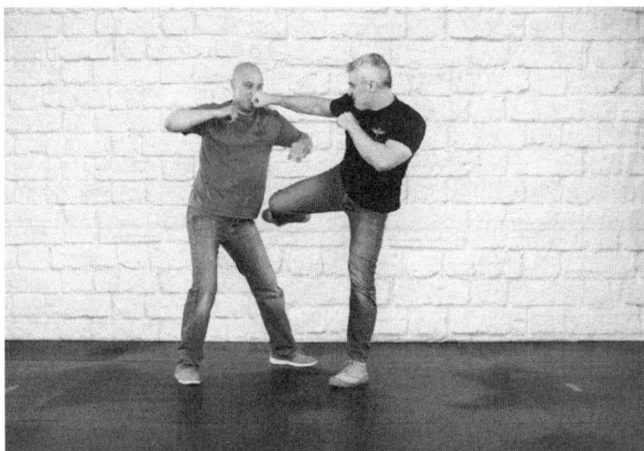
A straight punch to the nose.

Injuries to the Ear

A blow to the ear could not only disorient someone but also be fatal. An ear strike impacts the head above the cervical spine, jolting the head to the opposite side. The spinal cord could be hyperextended or otherwise damaged, causing death.

50. https://haciendapublishing.com/articles/unarmed-assailant percentE2 percent80 percent94-deadly-threat-robert-margulies-md-mph.

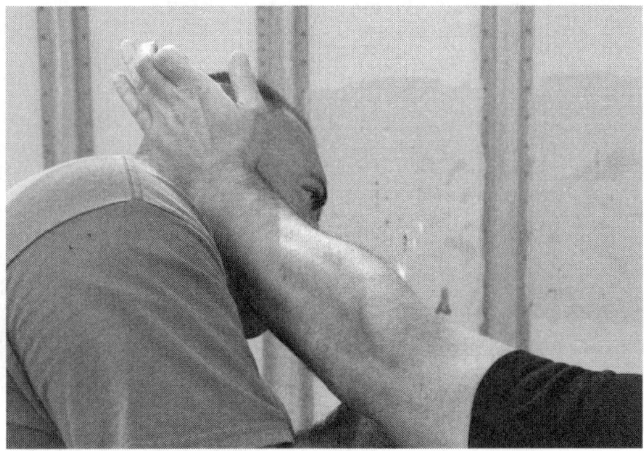

A horizontal palm-heel strike to the ear.

Injuries to the Jaw

The jaw is highly susceptible to injury by direct or indirect forceful contact. The jaw can sustain a fracture anywhere along the jaw bone. Direct impacts to the jaw can result in fractures in the condyles, the area in front of the ear, damaging the bones and muscles controlling the jaw's movement. A posterior dislocation can happen when you are struck hard and precisely on the chin. This type of dislocation forces the jaw back, misaligning the mandibular condyle and mastoid. Also at risk of fracture is the external auditory canal. Superior dislocations often result from being punched on the lower jaw when the mouth is half-open. In summary, posterior, superior, and lateral jaw dislocations can result from a violent high-energy blow to the jaw bone.

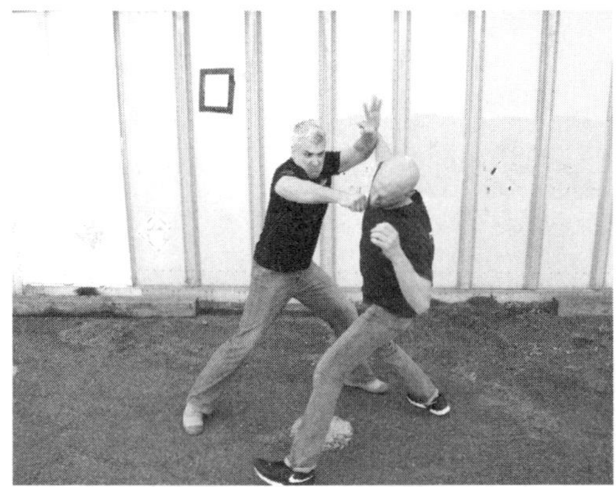

Straight punch to the jaw.

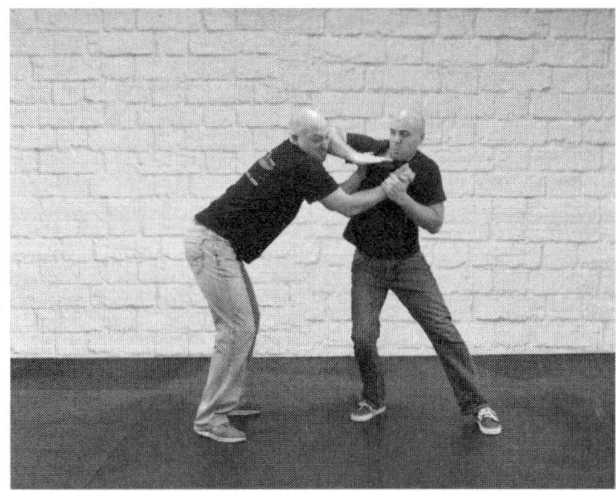

Horizontal elbow strike to the jaw.

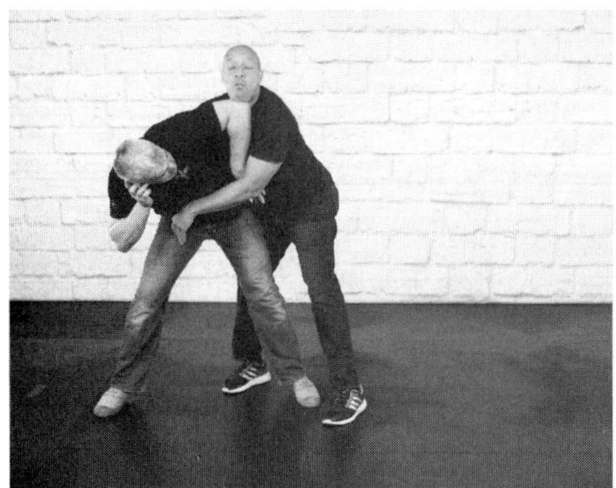

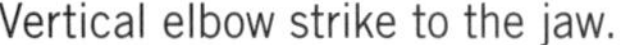

Vertical elbow strike to the jaw.

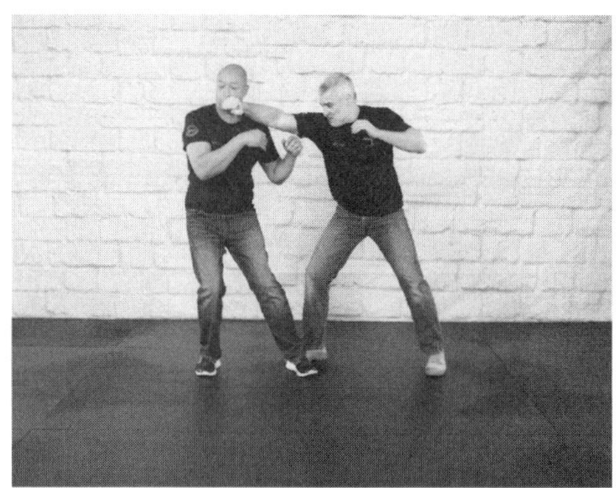

Hammerfist strike to the jaw.

Protecting Your Throat and Neck

A strong blow to the throat can cause laryngeal trauma to the larynx and the upper portion of the airway where the vocal cords are located.[51] Damage can range from minor vocal cord weakness to potentially lethal fractures of the larynx and trachea's cartilage structures. This type of fracture can cause air to escape into the neck and chest, leading to significant respiratory compromise and even death if not diagnosed and treated quickly. A blow to the side of the neck can injure the cervical vertebrae that affect the spinal cord, resulting in paralysis or death.

Accordingly, for self-defense purposes, a throat strike must only be used as a last resort in a deadly force situation.

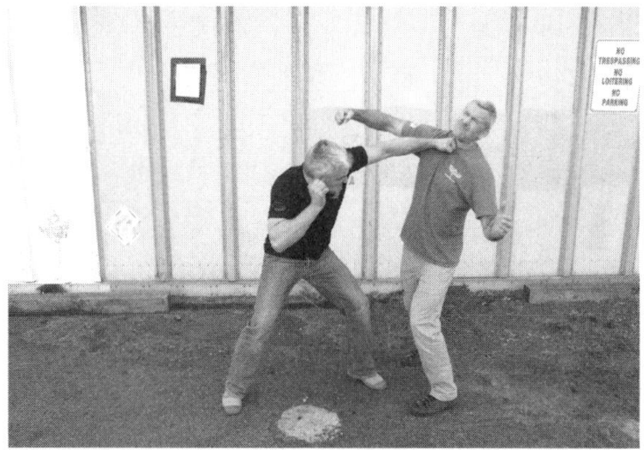

Straight punch to the throat.

51. https://www.chop.edu/conditions-diseases/laryngeal-trauma.

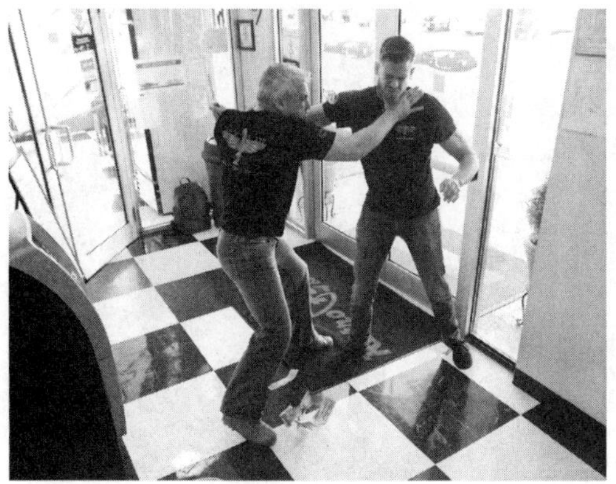
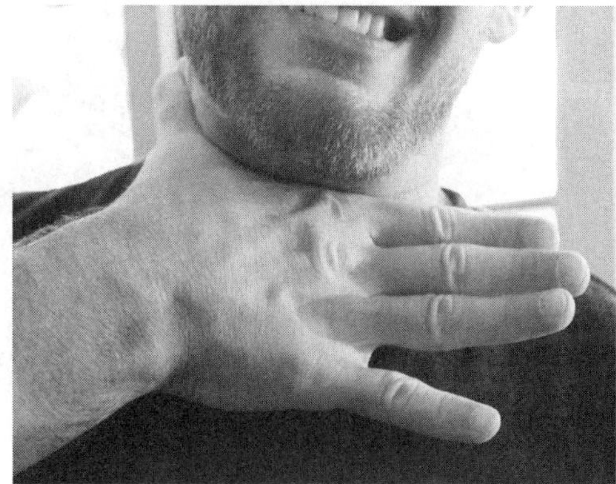

Web strike to the throat.

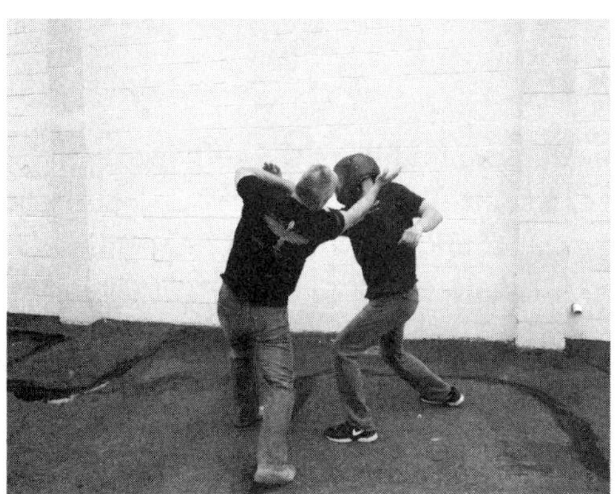

An inside chop to the neck.

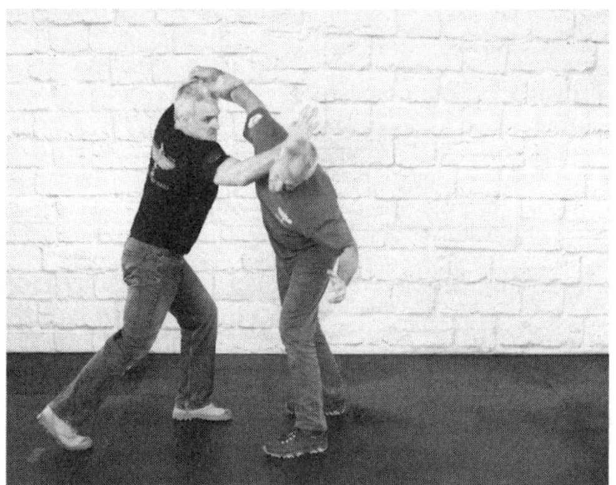

An outside chop to the neck.

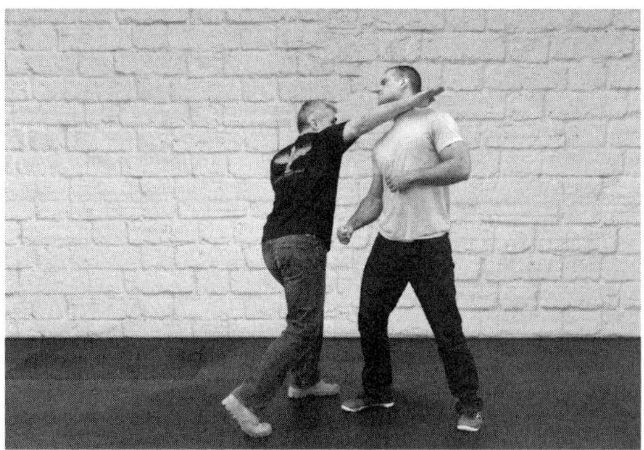

An *arimi* forearm strike to the neck.

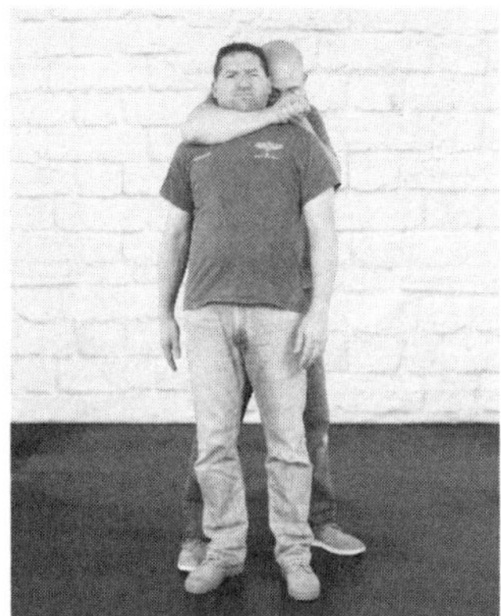

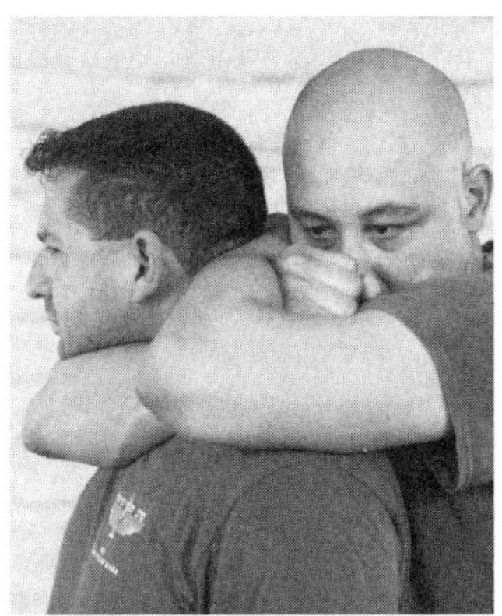

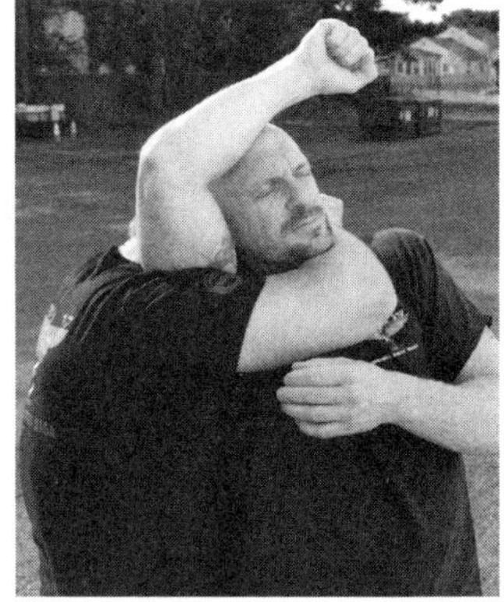

Air and blood chokes.

Protecting Your Torso

A strike to the solar plexus, a nerve bundle positioned in the middle of the abdomen, can be highly debilitating. The solar plexus is considered the control center between the abdomen and the brain. Comprised of two large conjoining nerve bundles or ganglia, it lies behind the stomach and below the diaphragm, close to major arteries and the abdomen's essential organs and glands—the adrenals, stomach, liver, kidneys, and intestines. A blow here creates a momentary paralysis of the diaphragm and the sensation of having the wind knocked out of you. While this type of injury is generally not permanent, it can cause significant physical distress through acute pain and shortness of breath, which often induces a feeling of panic.

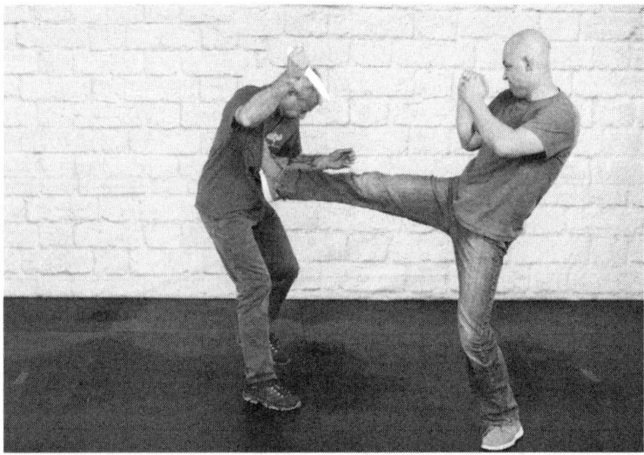

A straight kick to the solar plexus.

The abdomen is a relatively unprotected area and, therefore, susceptible to blunt trauma, including contusions and lacerations along with puncture wounds. For protection, the abdomen relies solely on the soft tissue of the abdominal wall, fascial layers, and skin. The abdominal cavity houses many vital organ systems that could be injured during a fight. Blows rarely cause severe contusions to the abdominal musculature, as the muscle and abdominal contents are soft and dissipate the majority of most blunt trauma. Organ damage is the most dangerous abdominal injury resulting from blunt trauma. A strike to the spleen can cause a splenic rupture, which can result in symptoms as serious as internal bleeding, a dangerous condition and common cause in athletics of death by abdominal trauma.

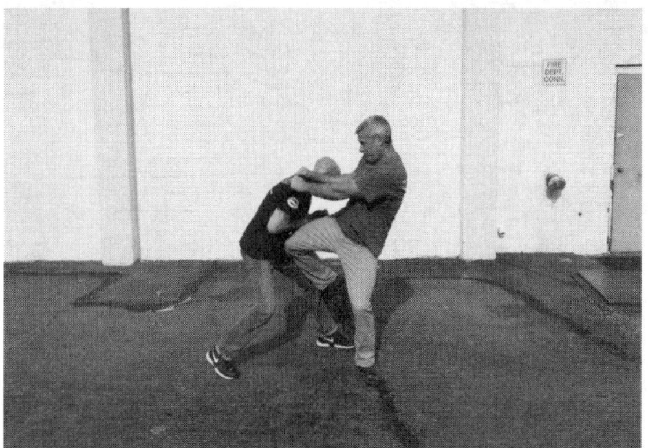

A straight knee strike to the abdomen.

The liver is located on the right side of the body, partially under the ninth and tenth (floating) ribs. Of all combative body shots, perhaps a blow to the liver is the most effective and damaging. Liver trauma can be potentially fatal through hemorrhage. Surrounded by nerves, the liver directly connects to your autonomic nervous system. When these nerves are overstimulated from a blow, your body goes into a sort of shut-down mode. A liver shot is often a punch, palm heel, chop, kick, or knee strike under the right side of the ribcage, orchestrated at a slight upward angle. A sudden blow creates internal pressure changes, stretching the organ. Such reconfiguration causes a complex chain of physical manifestations, including a sudden dilation of blood vessels everywhere in your body (except your brain), while also decreasing your heart rate. This combination of dilated blood vessels and heart-rate drop causes a sudden drop in blood pressure, causing you to collapse. A strong enough liver strike can render you unconscious. Simply put, you cannot control your body's reaction. Blunt force to the liver is usually excruciatingly painful and an especially effective combative to incapacitate someone.

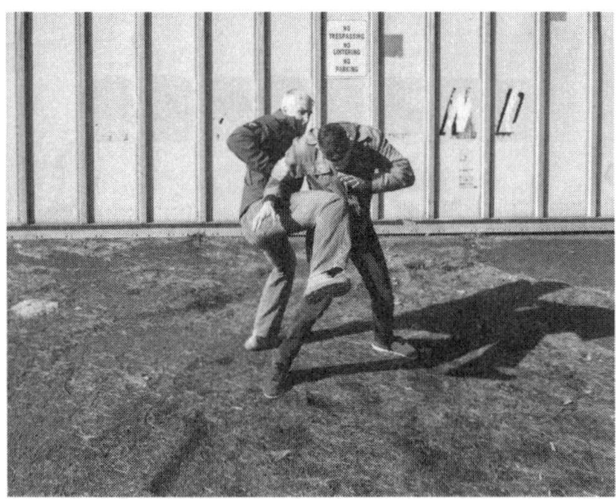

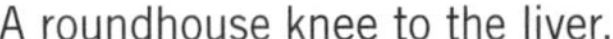
A roundhouse knee to the liver.

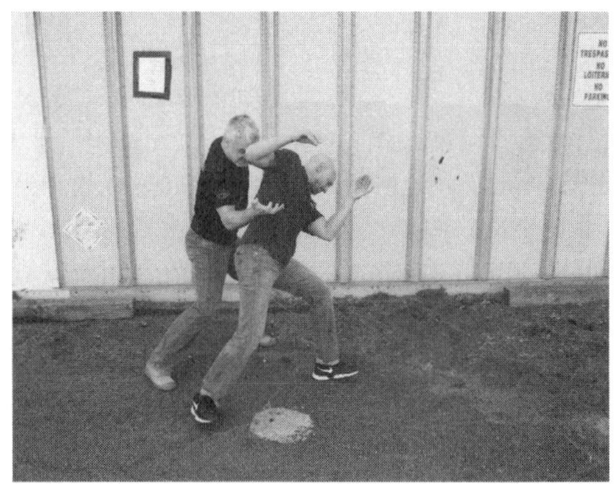
An inside chop to the liver.

The kidneys, located on both sides of your mid-back just below your ribcage, are protected only by soft tissue. The kidneys serve as your body's filter, removing waste and excess fluid. The most common combatives to the kidneys are body punches, palm heel strikes, chops, knees, and kicks. Fighters targeting a kidney often aim for the area on the torso just behind the opponent's same-side elbow. Since they are on the back of your body, the kidneys are especially difficult to protect. A blow to the lower back can result in a contused or ruptured kidney. Back and flank pain, nausea, vomiting, and even shock are possible with significant trauma to the kidneys. An acute direct blow to the full bladder can rupture the organ, resulting in hematuria.

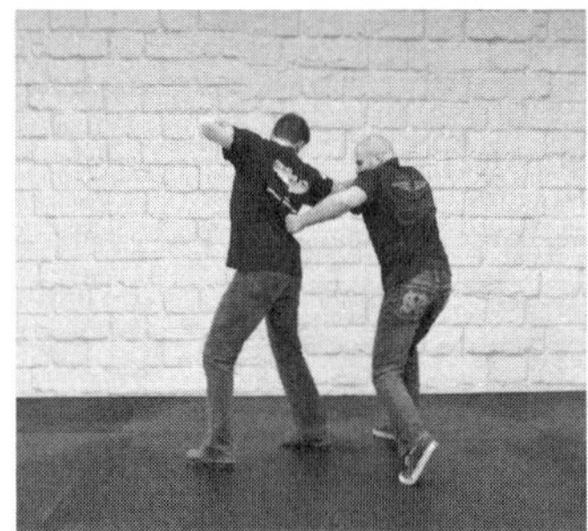
A body-hook punch to the kidney.

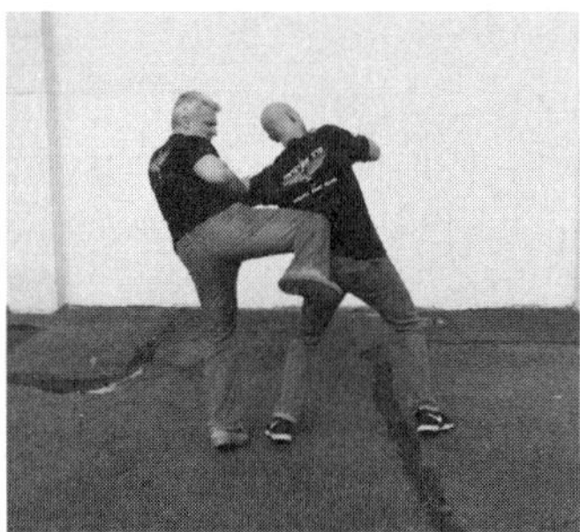
Roundhouse knee to the kidney.

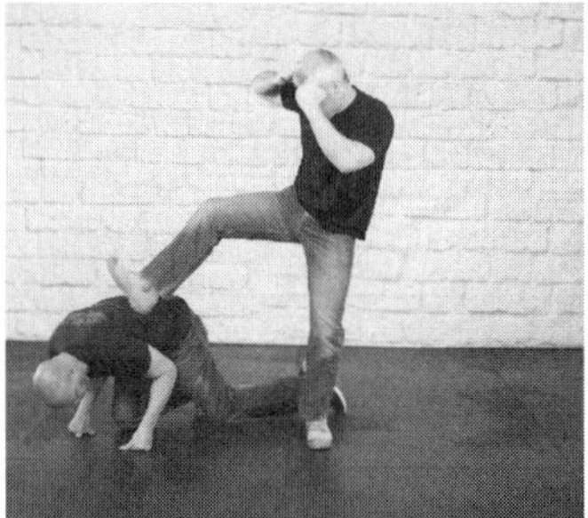
Heel kick to the kidney.

Protecting Your Groin

A swift combative administered to the groin is one of the most widely heralded and emphasized self-defense tactics. In most cases, blunt trauma to the groin, especially through a kick or knee strike, can instantly debilitate an opponent, though do bear in mind that an adversary could be wearing loose pants or tactical pants that provide a barrier against a shin kick reaching the testicles. (Only a minority of opponents can withstand such an acute blow and continue to attack you.)[52] A groin strike's effectiveness results from the testicles' vulnerability. The scrotum affords the testicles little protection from a blow. The sole protection is a layer of fibrous tissue called the tunica albuginea. While resilient enough to withstand some pressure, this tissue can only absorb limited trauma. Because of the high concentration of pain nociceptors surrounding the testicles and the myriad interconnections between testicular nerves and organs throughout your body, when physically assaulted, the testicles hijack the vagus nerve to send the body into disarray. Examples of the debilitating pain a groin strike causes may readily be seen in MMA fights gone awry. Fighters debilitated from a strike to the groin lie on the mat for several minutes. The nausea, tears, dizziness, and collapse that usually accompany a groin strike are your body's mechanisms for coping with the pain through the brain's cervical sympathetic ganglia. Groin trauma signals are launched up to your brain at about 265 mph, along with a neurotransmitter, Substance P, which is released by the testicles to induce pain relief.[53] Pain relieving endorphins drop your oxygen level, often resulting in an acute headache and nausea. Moreover, the brain is contemporaneously launching signals to your groin and abdominal area, keeping you convulsed in additional pain. Your heart rate increases, accompanied by a higher body temperature that induces sweating. While the pain, medically termed "blunt scrotal trauma," typically subsides without long-term damage, permanent injury can occur.

The most common short-term result from a groin strike is a bruise or testicular contusion, though testicular ruptures can occur. Testicular bruises result when the arteries and veins in the scrotum are injured and broken open. Blunt trauma may cause a hematoma, ecchymosis of the scrotum, or injuries to the testicle, epididymis, or spermatic cord. Traumatically induced testicular torsion is another well-documented injury that occurs when a testicle twists, cutting off its blood supply. Testicular torsion can result in the loss of a testicle if not treated soon after sustaining such an injury. Testicular rupture occurs when the testicle receives a forceful direct blow or when it is crushed against the pubic bone. Testicular rupture, similar to testicular torsion and other serious injuries to the testicles, causes extreme pain, swelling in the scrotum, nausea, and vomiting. Infertility can also result. A less common injury is a testicular dislocation when a testicle is forced into the abdominal cavity. Other trauma could include a lacerated urethra or a penile fracture. In conclusion, while groin strikes may lead to serious complications, most urologists agree this type of combative is generally not lethal.

---

52. Four examples of why someone might not be instantly debilitated by a groin strike include someone who: (1) has "testicular immunity" or immunity to being struck in the groin; (2) is under the influence of pain-numbing alcohol or drugs; (3) is wearing baggy pants or strong jeans that prevent the strike from full contact; (4) is wearing groin protection.

53. Taylor Kubuta, "Here's What Happens to Your Body When You Get Kicked in the Groin," *Men's Journal,* n.d., https://www.mensjournal.com/health-fitness/what-really-happens-after-a-kick-to-the-groin-20140528/.

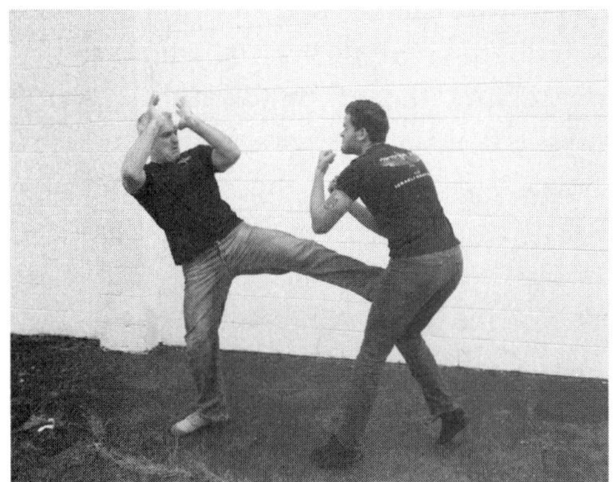
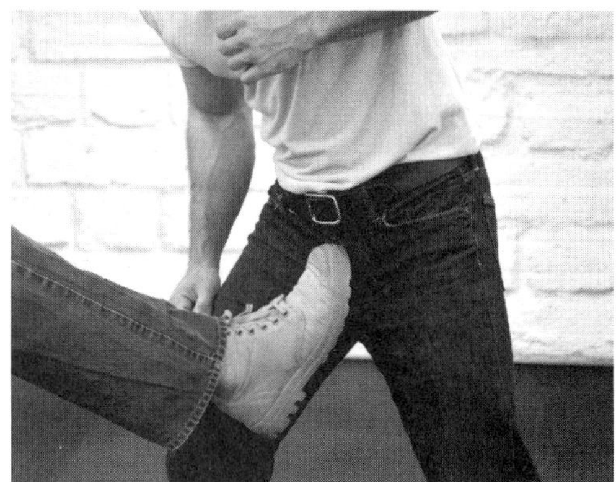
A straight kick with the ball of the foot targeting the groin.

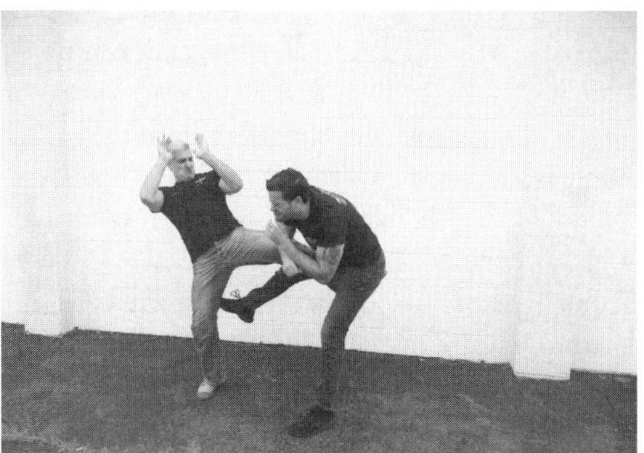
A straight kick with the shin targeting the groin.

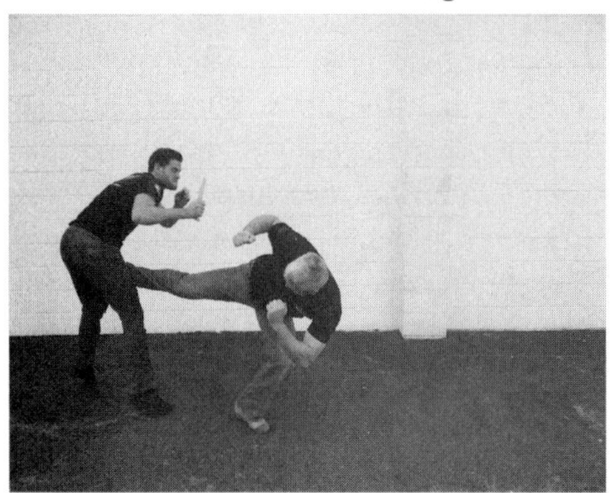
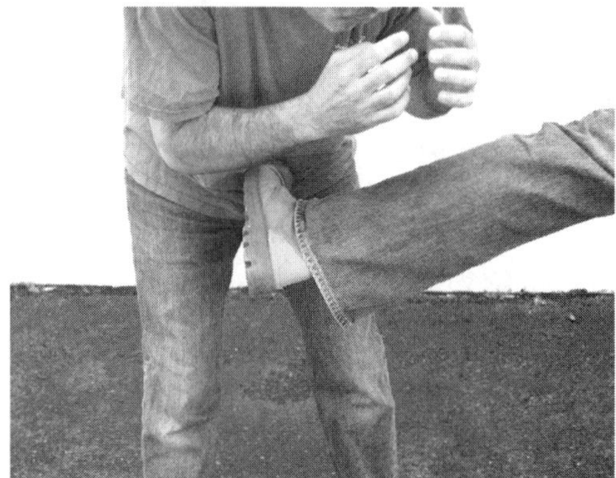
A roundhouse kick targeting the groin with the ball of the foot.

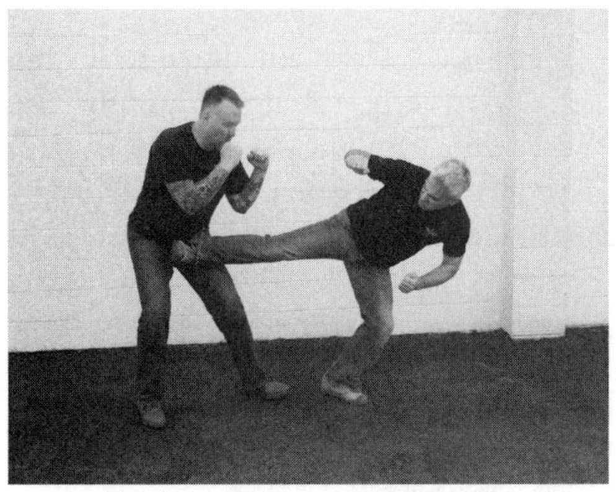

A reverse roundhouse kick targeting the groin with the heel.

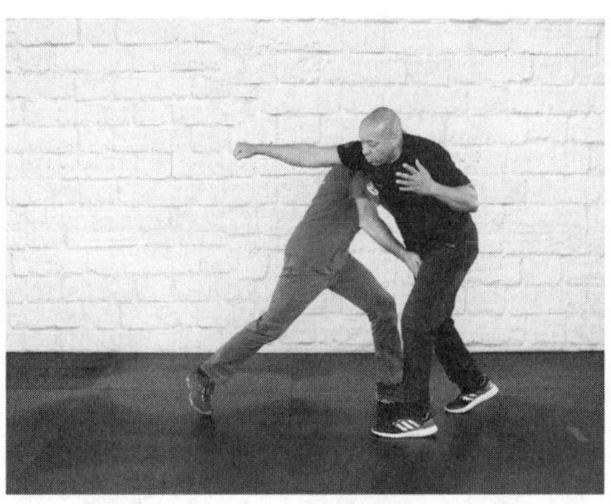

A palm-heel strike targeting the groin.

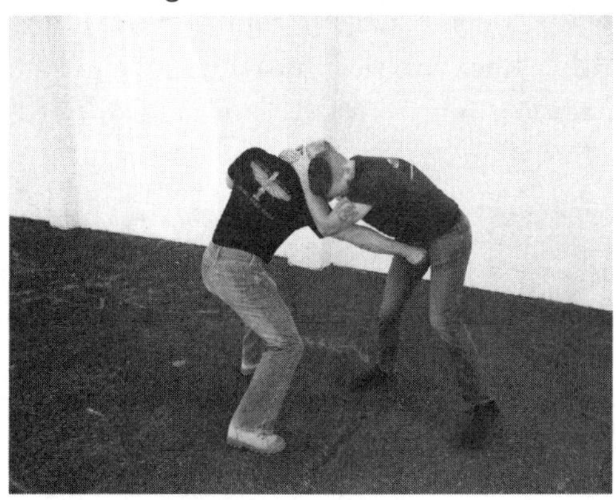

A hammerfist strike targeting the groin.

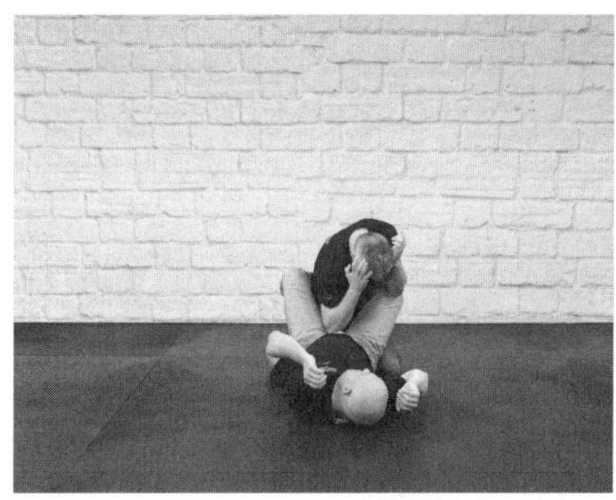

A drop-elbow strike targeting the groin.

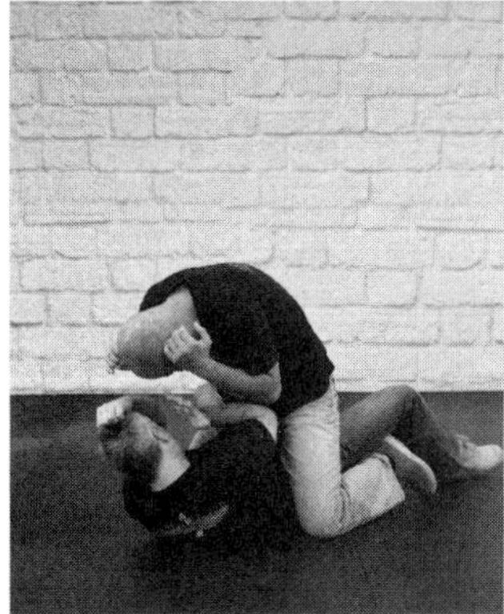

A drop-elbow strike targeting the groin.

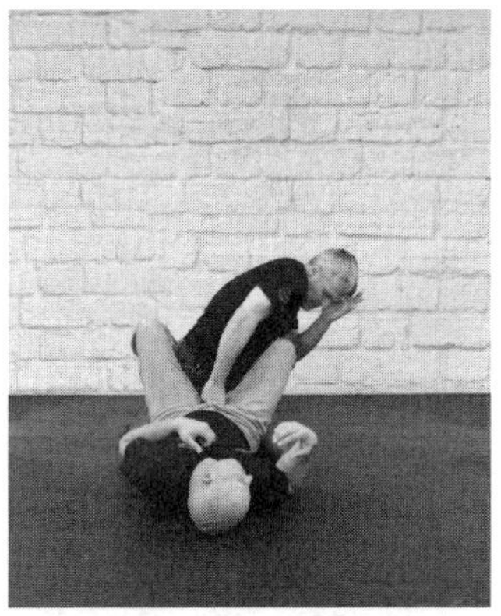

A straight punch targeting the groin.

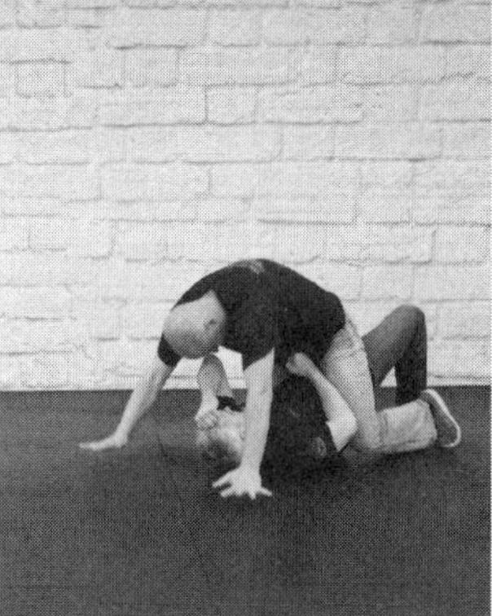

A hammerfist targeting the groin.

Protecting Your Knees

In my opinion, a forceful kick to a standing attacker's knee is the best method to disable him. A precise, strong side kick or stomp using the heel or, alternatively, a straight kick using the ball of the foot against the front or side of an opponent's knee, can cause significant damage that will drop him immediately. The knee is a hinge joint fastened together by four ligaments. A ligament is found on each side of the knee (the collateral ligaments) with two additional ligaments that cross, the ACL and PCL, deep inside the knee. Both ligaments attach on one side to the end of the thighbone (femur) and on the other to the top of the shinbone (tibia).[54] During movement the ACL regulates how far forward the tibia can move with the femur. When the knee is attacked from the outside-in or inside-out, it is forced in an unnatural direction. Blunt force trauma from a kick can damage the PCL and ACL ligaments on both the outside and inside of the knee depending on the relative position of the kick. A targeted kick could collectively damage these ligaments, along with the patellar tendon. Damage may vary from a small crack in one of the small ligaments to a total rupture of the exterior or interior collateral ligament, or both. Other knee injuries caused by a deliberate kick could be hyperextension, hyperflexion, or rotational injuries with associated valgum/varum stress, while other knee structures are also often damaged.

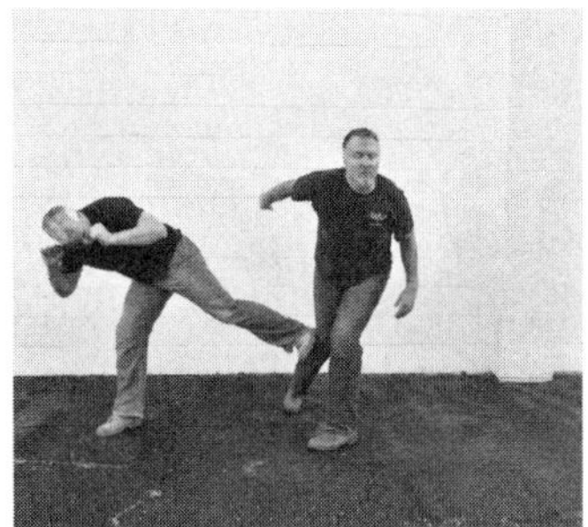
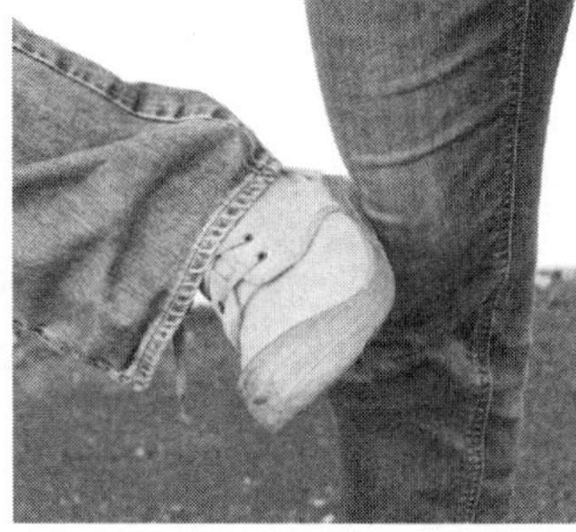
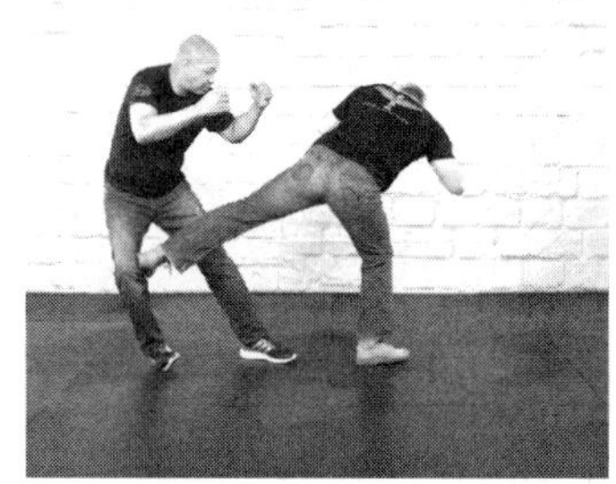

A side kick targeting the knee.

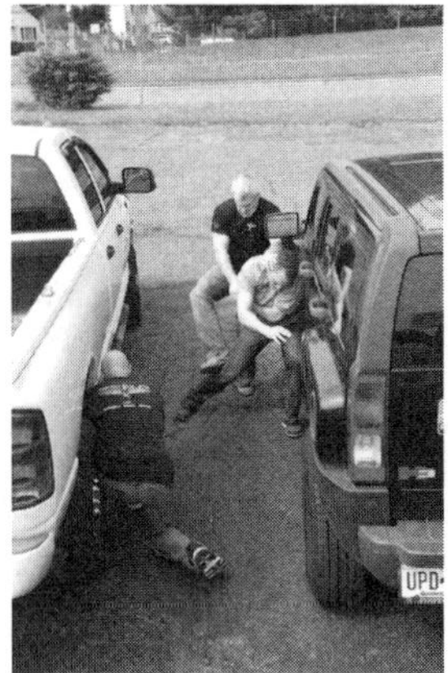

A stomp targeting the knee.

54. https://www.hopkinsmedicine.org/health/conditions-and-diseases/acl-injury-or-tear.

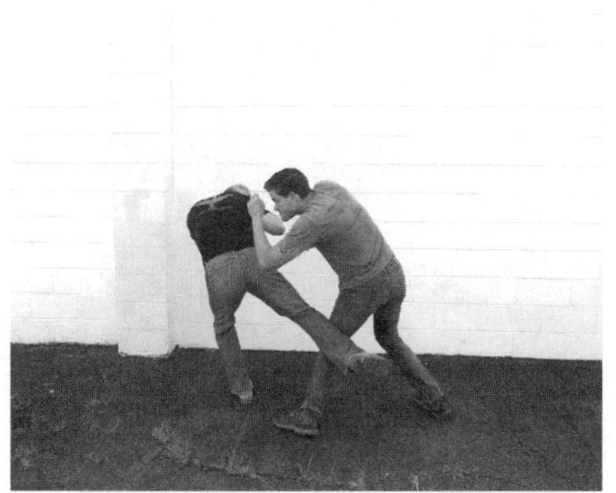

A roundhouse kick with the shin targeting the knee.

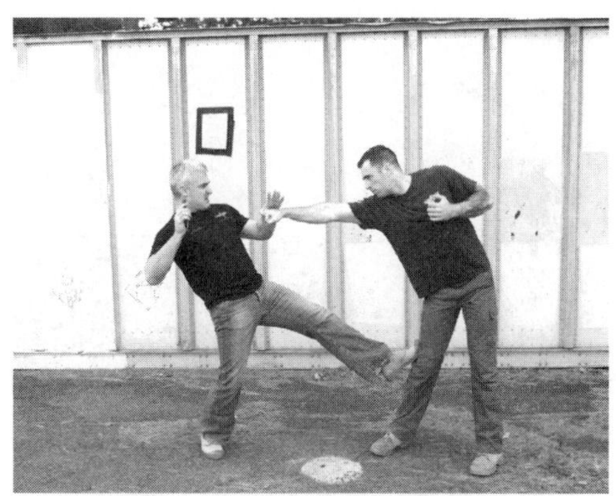

A straight kick targeting the knee.

Protecting Your Achilles

Your Achilles tendon or heel is highly vulnerable to attack. It is most readily attacked from the rear or deadside. Therefore, along with the many other targets made available by deadside movement, don't allow an opponent to position himself where you cannot see an attack being launched. (If your head is stunned, the rest of your body—including your deadside—can become vulnerable, so you must protect your "computer.")

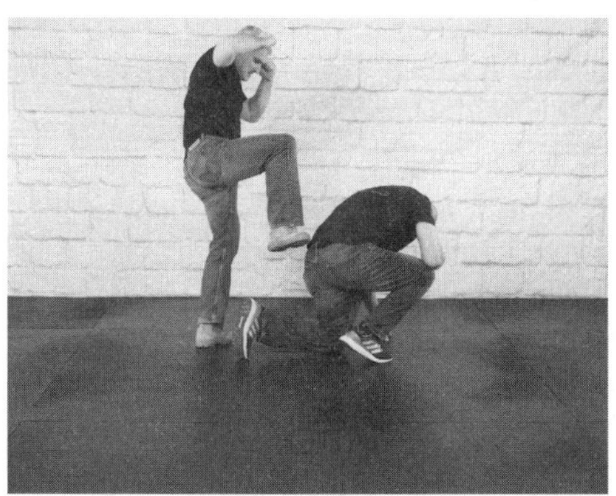

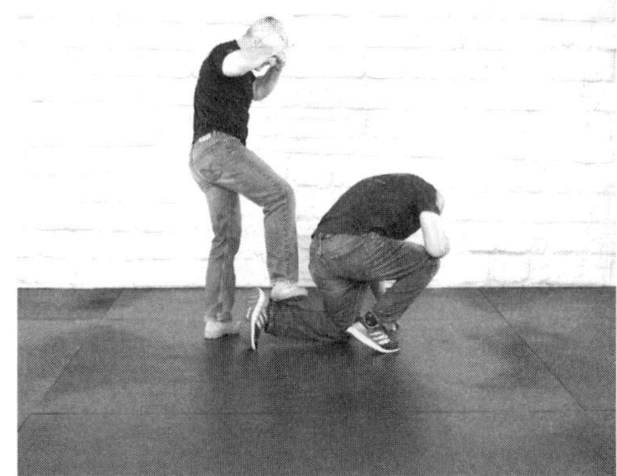

A stomp targeting the exposed Achilles tendon.

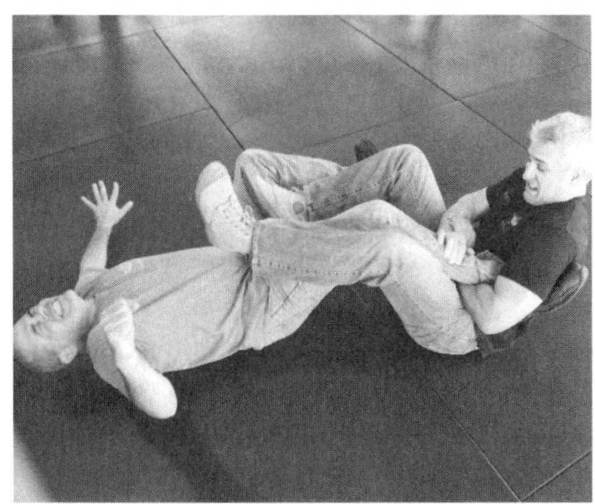

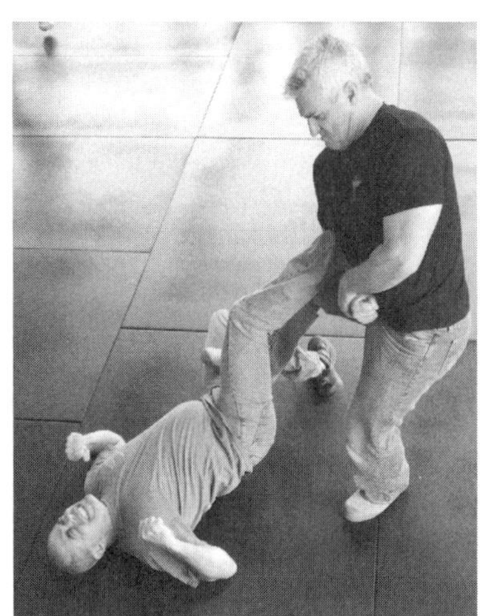

Blade of the forearm Achilles tendon lock variations.

Defending against Martial Arts Kicks

Any self-defense strategy is to defeat an attack and, obviously, not all attacks are the same. If you must contend against a trained fighter, his arsenal is probably both greater and more refined than an average street brawler. Most commonly, a trained martial artist can deliver strong kicks.

The ability to defend against and withstand kicks (and launch them), especially low-line ones, often separates a trained, reality-based fighter from a tough, capable street brawler. While most aggressors favor upper-body attacks, a trained fighter can launch a devasting kick from three heights: low, medium, and high. If you don't keep your hands up, a high kick to the head, usually a roundhouse kick, can cause serious damage—often a knockout. Therefore, keep these tactics in mind as part of your strategy to protect your entire body.

Preferably, you should not drop your hands against low kicks. Krav maga's strategy, when possible, is to defend using "legs against legs." Using your own legs to intercept and deflect an incoming low- to medium-height kick provides two advantages: (1) your lower body is stronger and more capable of deflecting or absorbing the power of an opponent's kicks and (2) an opponent may also launch a near-simultaneous upper-body attack (similar to krav maga's emphasis on combined lower and upper-body attacks optimized by retzev). The following examples highlight krav maga's approach to defending against kick attacks at different heights. You'll note the following defensive strategies combined with immediate counterattacks:

1. When possible, as noted, krav maga uses your legs to deflect and intercept along with counter kicking or closing to deliver an upper-body counterattack. Note: for low roundhouse kicks, krav maga focuses on intercepting the kick with a counter-modified straight kick either against the attacker's leg or at the attacker's vulnerable foot with your shin, not in a shin-to-shin crash.
2. When possible, krav maga emphasizes getting off the line of attack from a kick. If you cannot get off the line, retreat or move away from the power of the incoming kick. If you must absorb a low kick, strengthen your body while exhaling when possible and counterattack immediately.
3. If a high kick must be defended with your hands, it is best to use a rotating deflection where you make your arm strong by flexing it, either tensing the hand or making a fist to redirect the kick away. If you must intercept a kick with your arms, it is best to use the inside fleshy part of your forearm or your palm. If you must absorb a high roundhouse kick with your arms, try to use both of them, keeping your elbows bent beyond 90 degrees and using the inside fleshy part of your forearms.

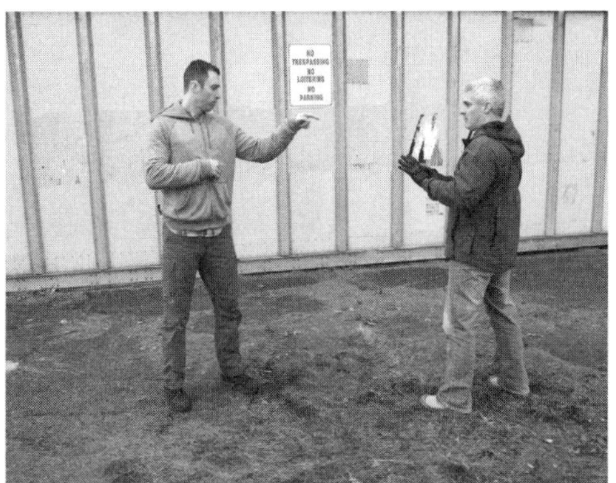

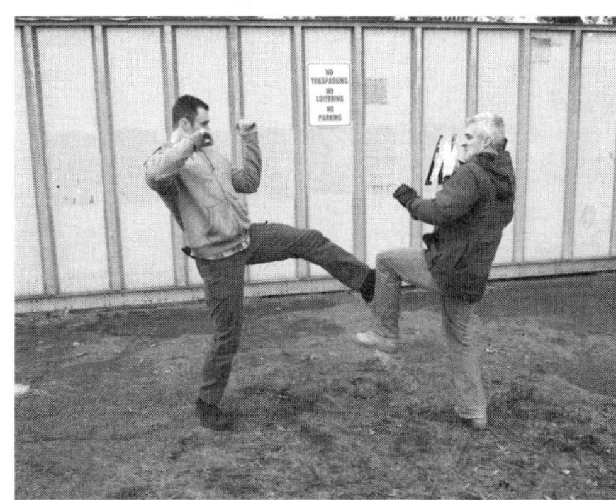

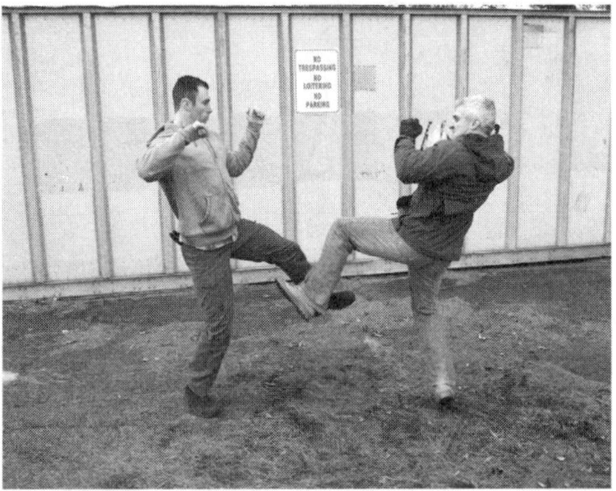

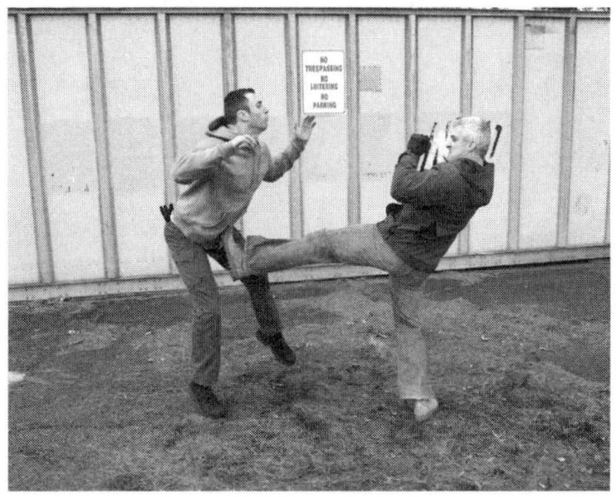

This series depicts a lead-leg low-straight kick defense that uses a shin deflection and straight counter kick. This harnesses the deflecting leg's momentum to target the attacker's groin.

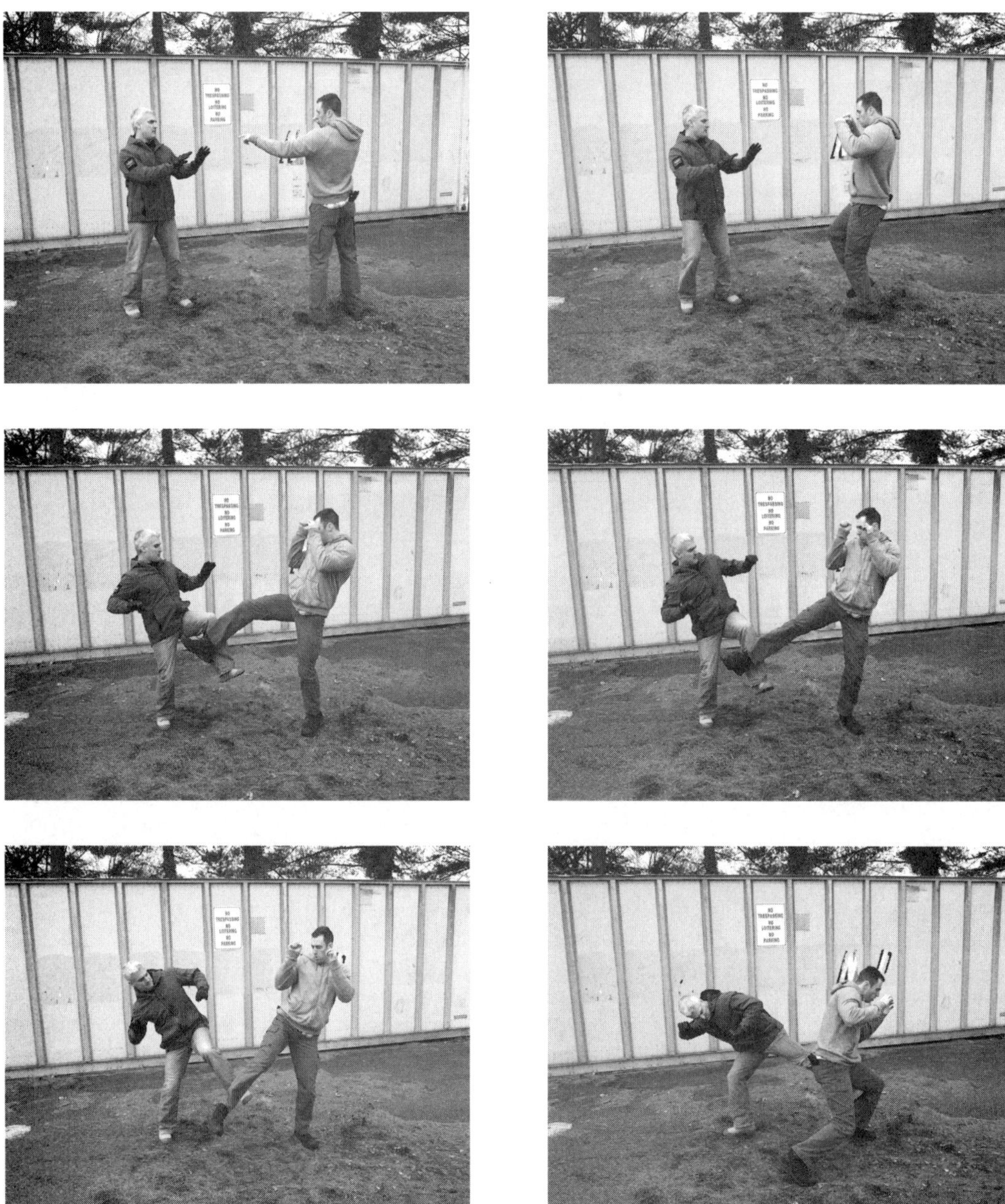

This series depicts a lead-leg low-straight kick defense that uses a shin deflection and side kick counterattack. This harnesses the deflecting leg's momentum to target the attacker's non-kicking base leg.

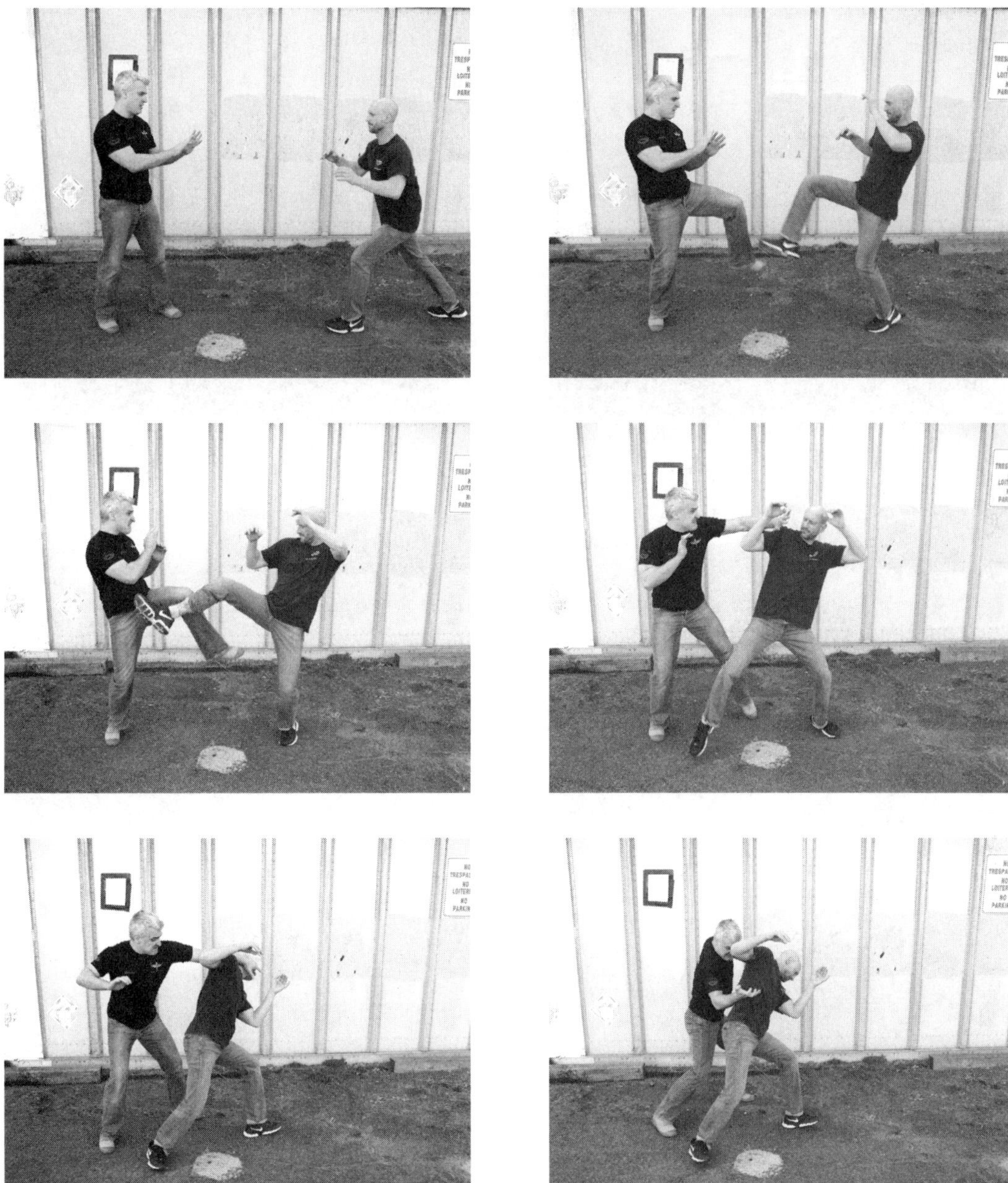

This series depicts a low-straight kick defense using a shin deflection that sends the attacker's leg inward. This deflection places you advantageously to the attacker's deadside. Counterattack with your preferred combatives, strategically using the closest weapon against the closest target.

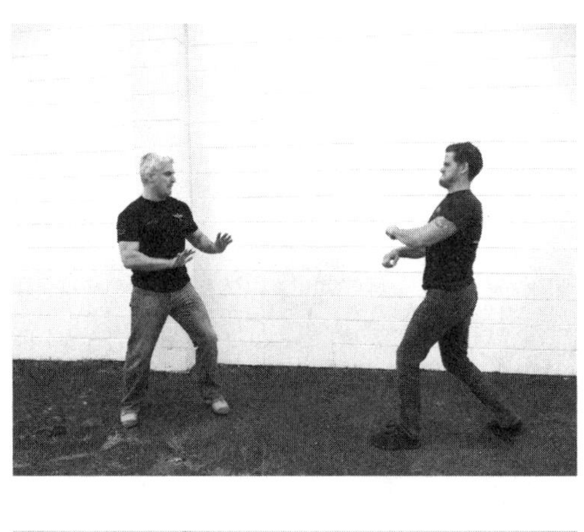
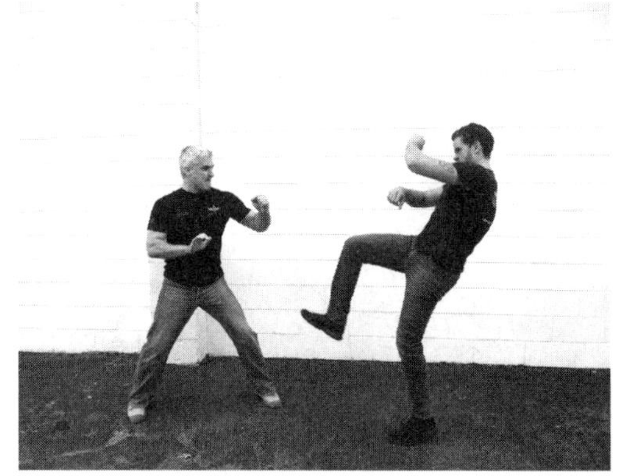
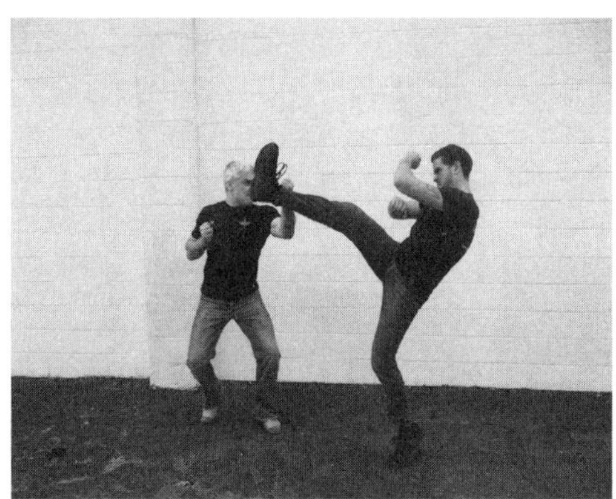
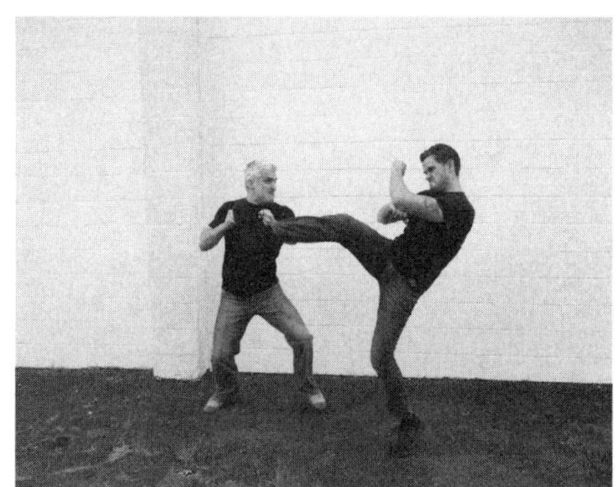
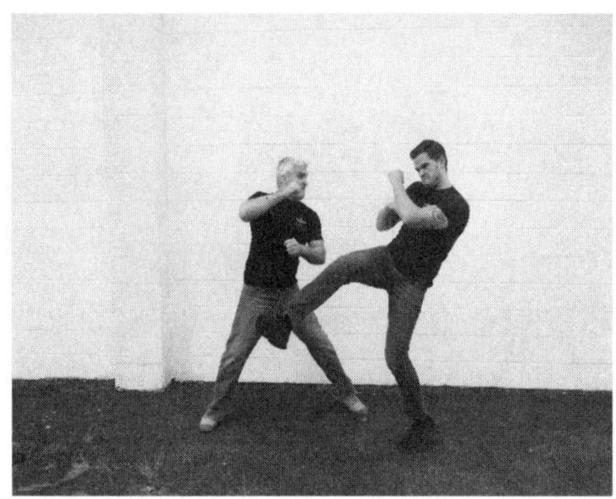
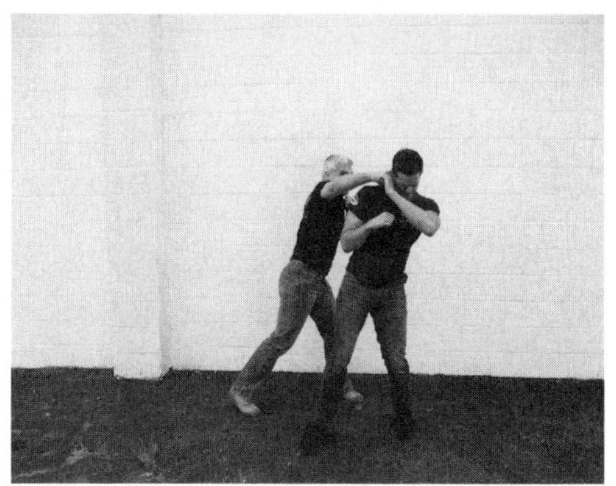

This series depicts a high-straight kick L-parry parry (with closed fist) defense with sidestep and counter punch that sends the attacker's leg inward, taking you advantageously to the attacker's deadside. Strategically counterattack with your preferred combatives using the closest weapon against the closest target.

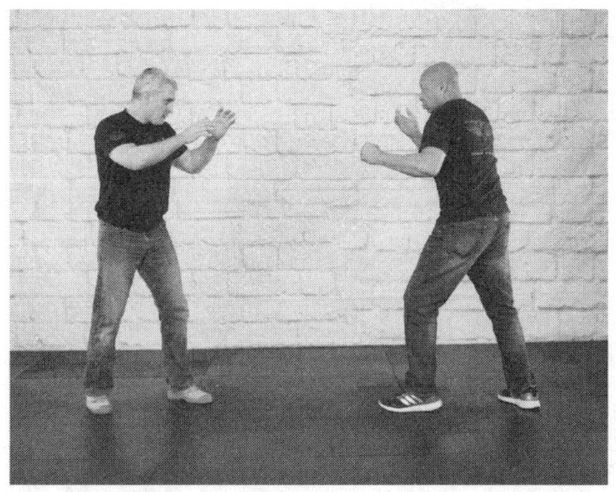

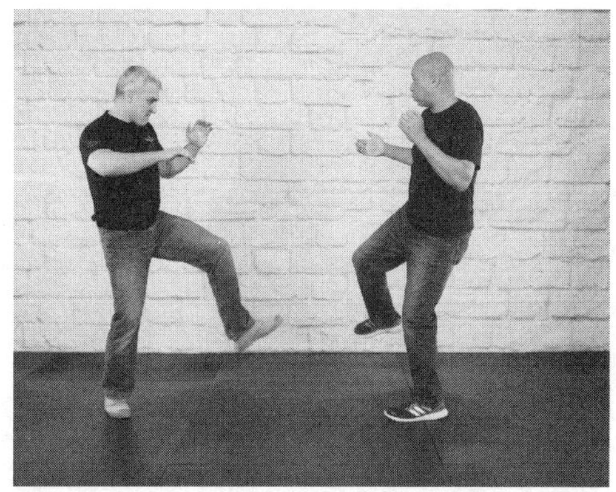

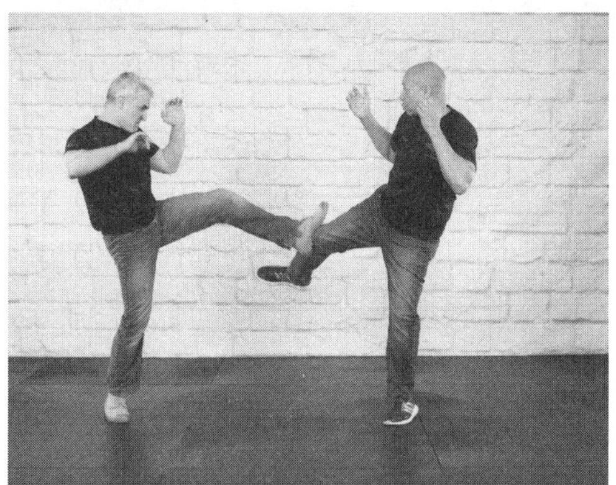

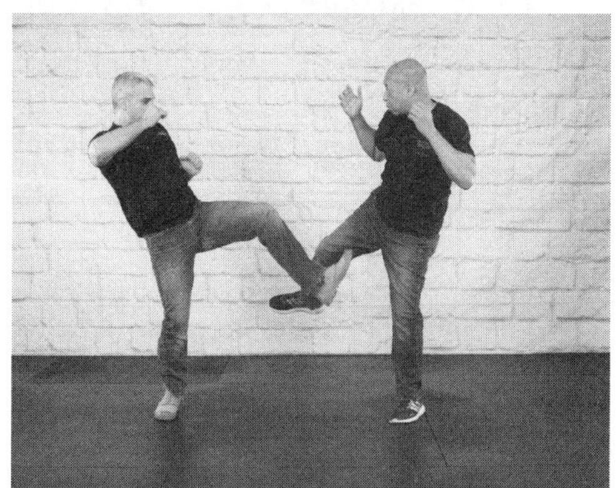

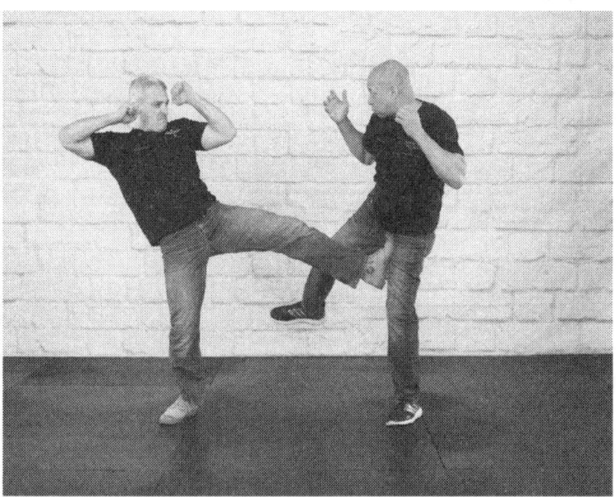

This series depicts a low-roundhouse-kick interception defense combined with a same-leg counter straight kick emphasizing the bedrock principle of attacking the attacker. Alternatively, you could also touch your left leg down and use your right leg to deliver a counter straight kick. The tactic harnesses your interception leg's momentum to target the attacker's groin.

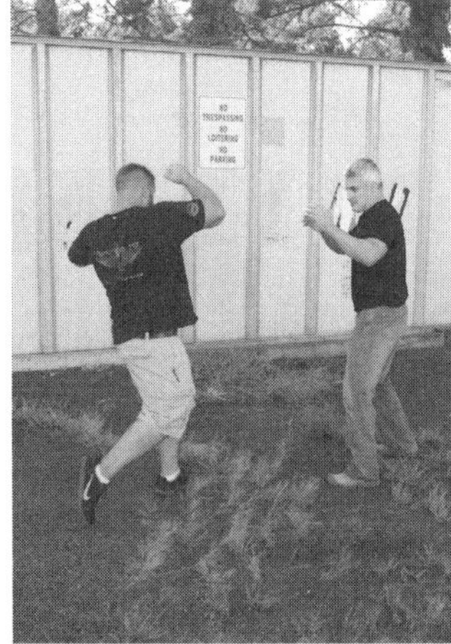
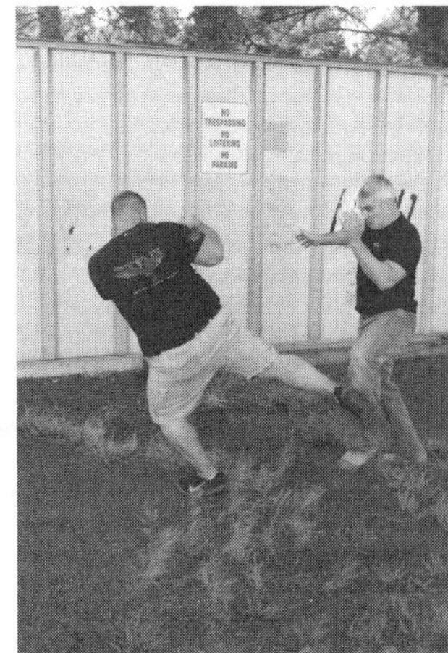
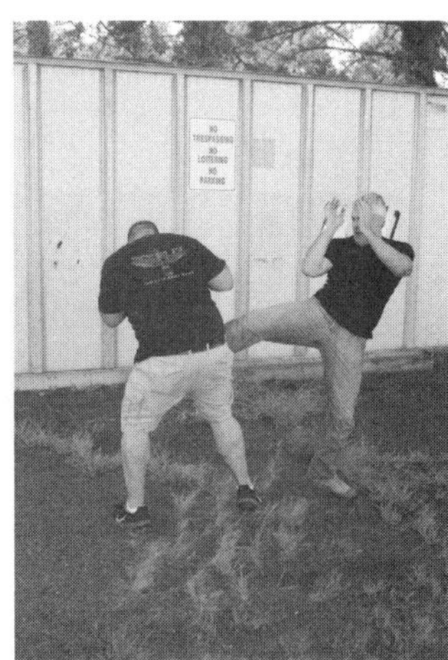

This series depicts a low-roundhouse-kick interception using your shin to intercept (and possibly damage) the attacker's vulnerable foot. Launch an immediate counterattack straight kick.

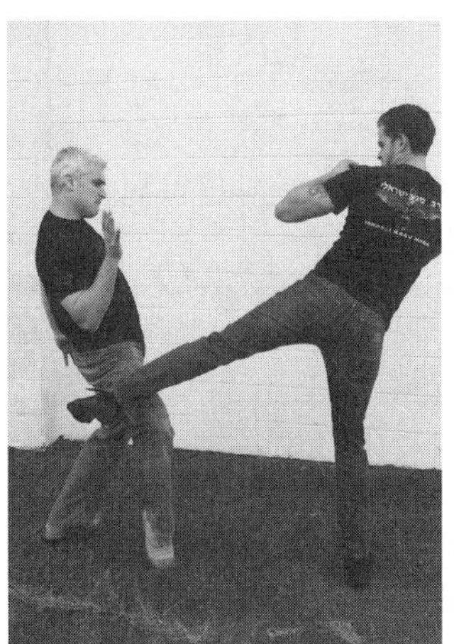
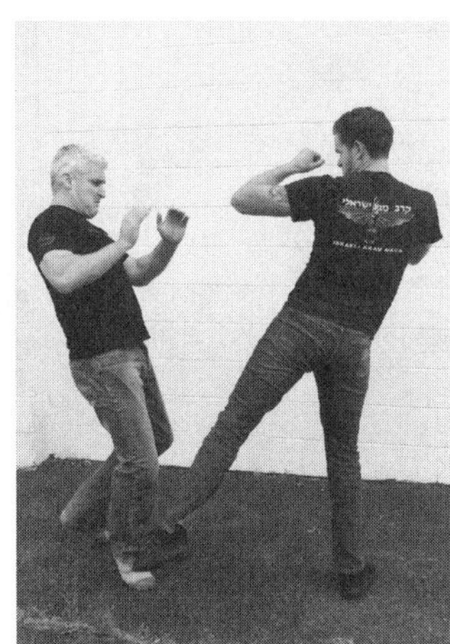
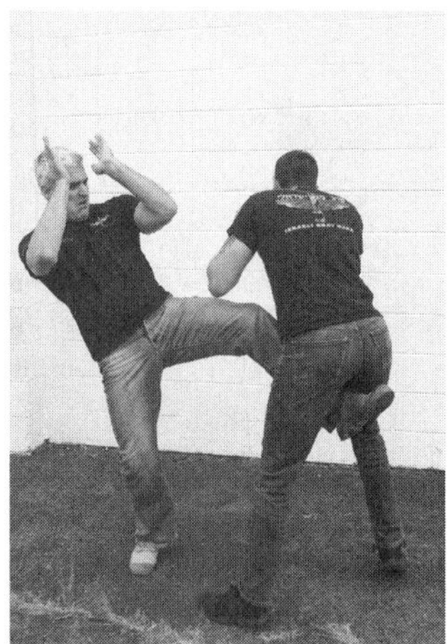

This series depicts a low front roundhouse kick (late, suboptimal) absorption defense that allows you to deliver an opposite-leg counter straight shin kick.

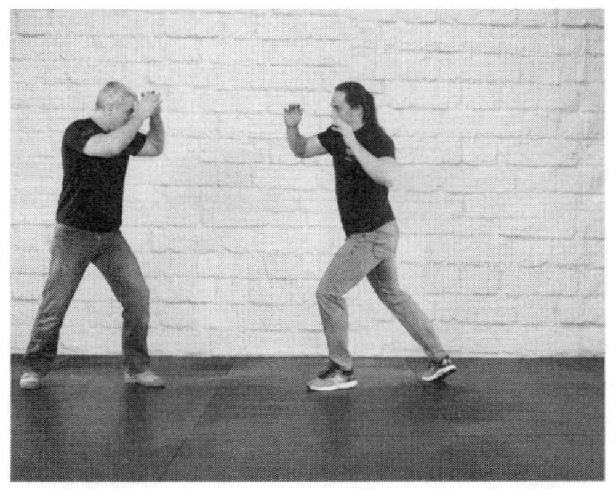

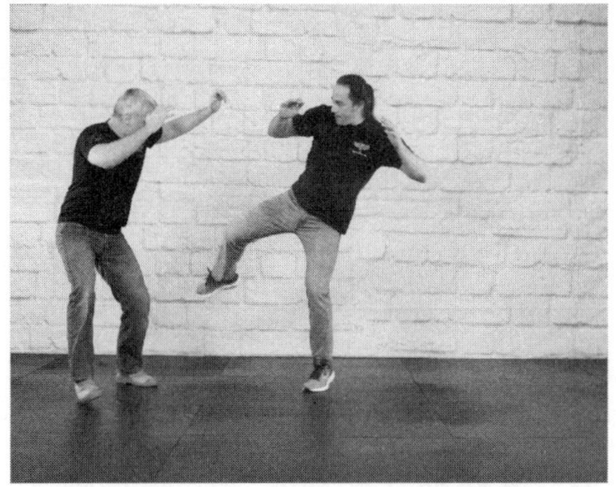

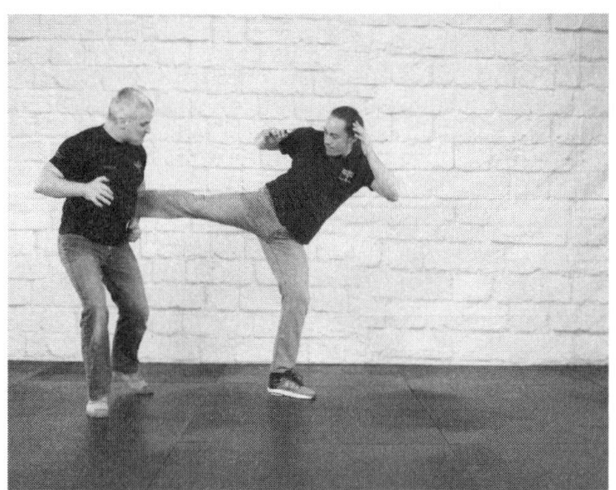

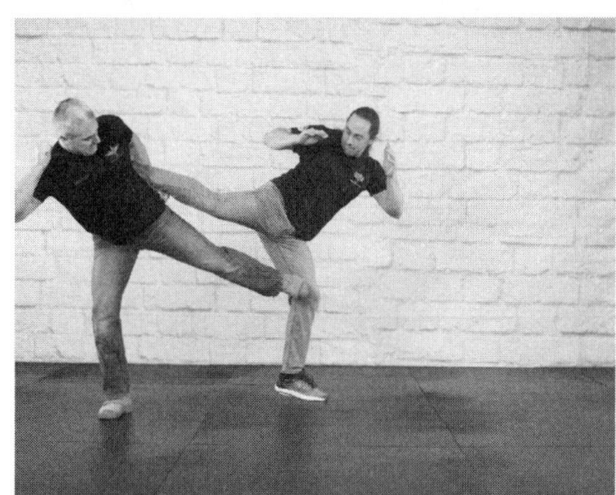

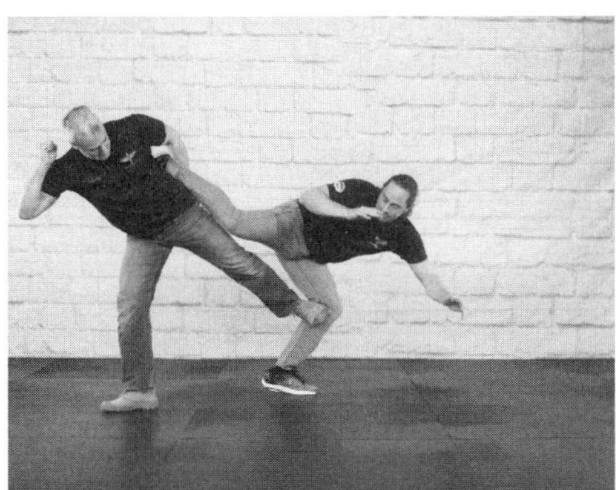

This series depicts a medium roundhouse kick defense accomplished by stepping off the line, enabling you to absorb the kick (only one third of the kick's power) against your lateral muscle and catch the attacker in a compromised position. You may counter with a side kick to the attacker's knee or use other counterattacks such as wrenching the attacker's caught knee.

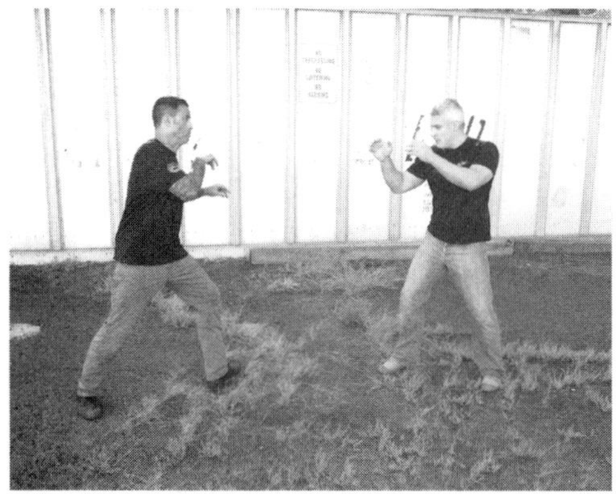

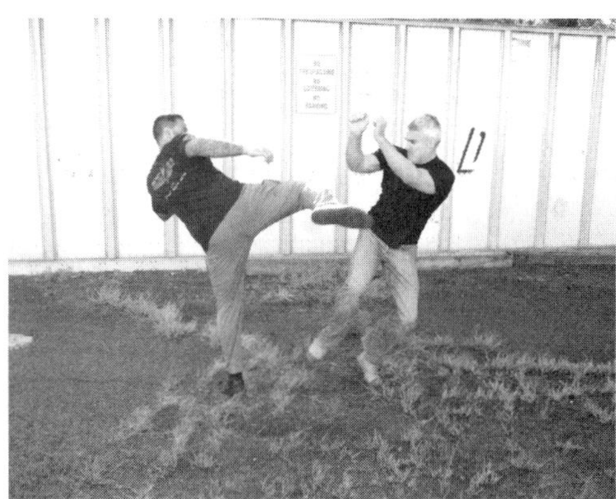

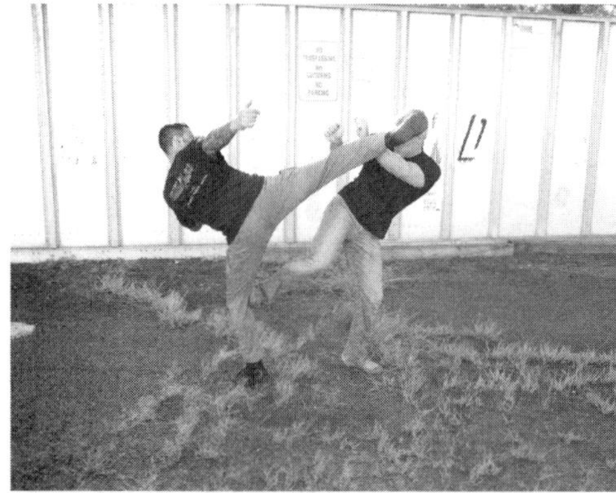

This series depicts a high-roundhouse-kick double forearm block defense combined with a side kick to the attacker's vulnerable base-leg knee.

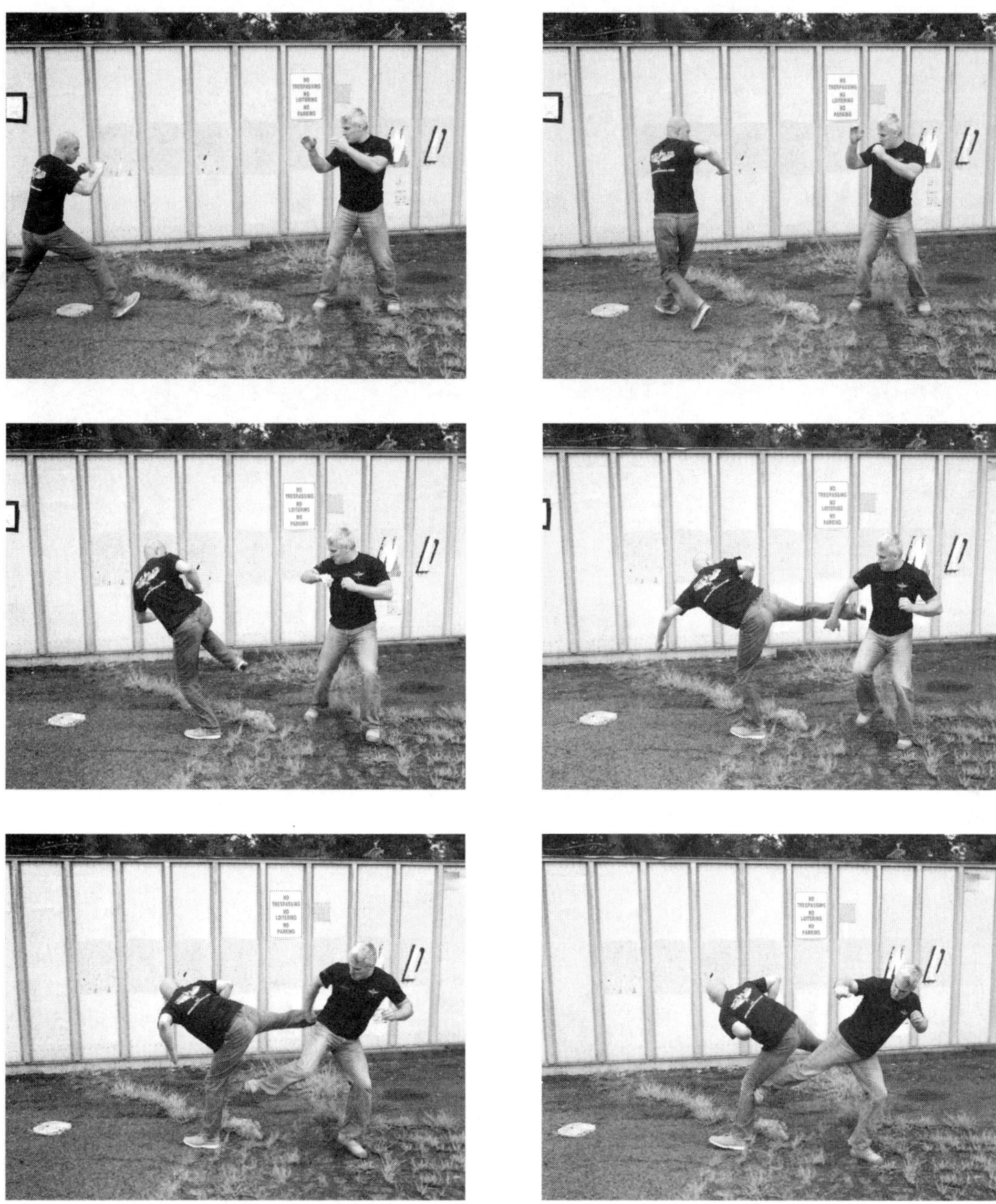

This series depicts a low-side-kick leg defense using a hand scoop while simultaneously stepping off the line of attack. Combine this integrated body defense and hand deflection with a counter side kick to the attacker's vulnerable base-leg knee.

Chapter 5

Representative Decision-Making Strategies

Krav maga training emphasizes that you practice both disciplined and legally justified mental and physical responses in handling confrontational situations. Here are some crucial krav maga situational analyses and self-recognition concepts:

1. Counterviolence must only be used as a last resort tool.
2. Until you are physically assaulted, you still have the options of avoidance, de-escalation, and escape.
3. Understand your own triggers: what you will accept and what you won't accept. It is best to remove all triggers prompted by social violence (when you can walk away).
4. Indecision and inaction can get you killed. The person committed to winning a violent confrontation unfailingly raises the stakes. He can often win regardless of tactics.

A few road-rage examples facing an assailant armed with an impact weapon serve as examples of:

5. Decision #1: Staying put in your vehicle and calling the police.
6. Decision #2: Exiting your vehicle while summoning help and using it as a barrier between you and an assailant.
7. Decision #3: Engaging an assailant who is destroying your property to stop him.

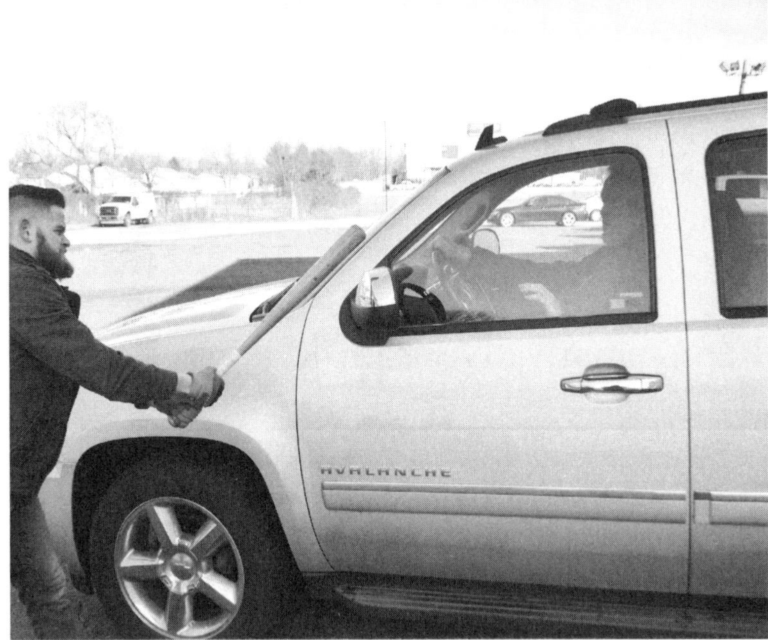

The decision to stay put in your vehicle and weather a storm of violence to your personal property may be natural and the best course of action. Most people are likely to be incredulous or bewildered by the onslaught of such violence and consequently freeze in place. Try not to freeze, and then immediately move away from the attack to another part of your vehicle to better avoid the danger of an object penetrating your windows. Of course, call the police immediately when facing an irate person. Note that most people do not practice dialing their phones under pressure and will fail in their initial attempt(s).

Exiting Your Vehicle to Escape an Assailant Coming at You

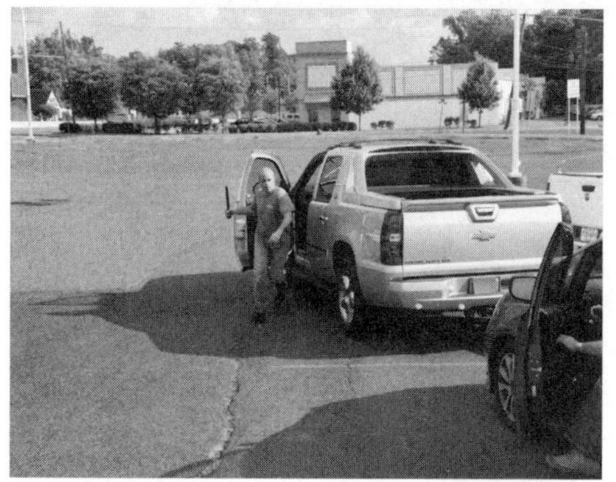

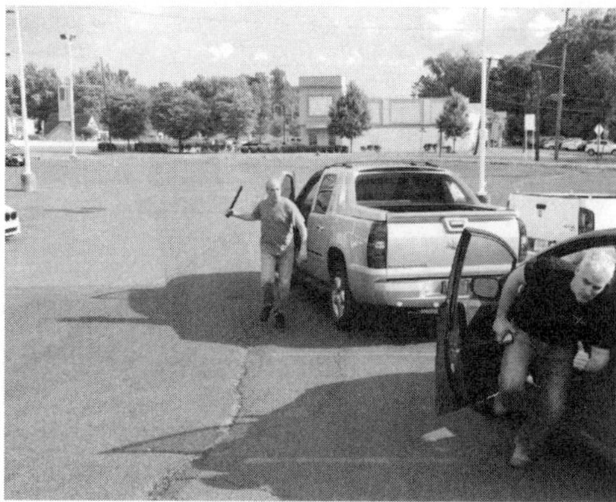

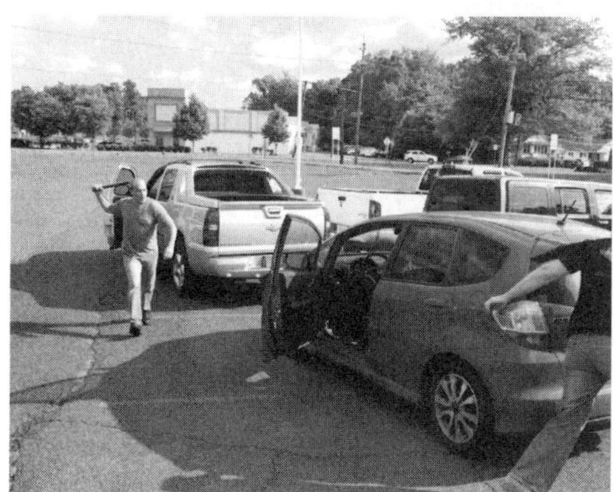

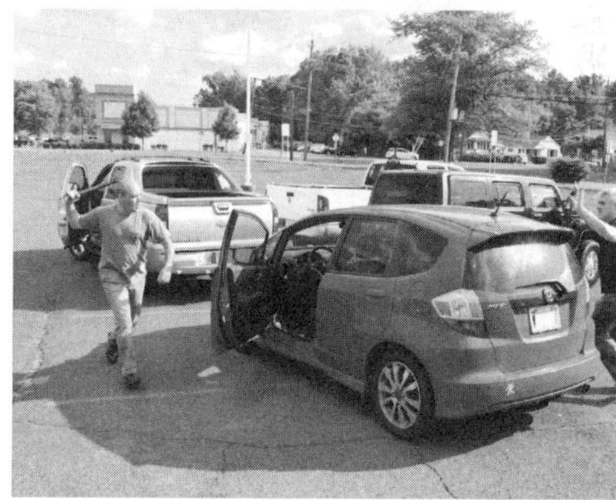

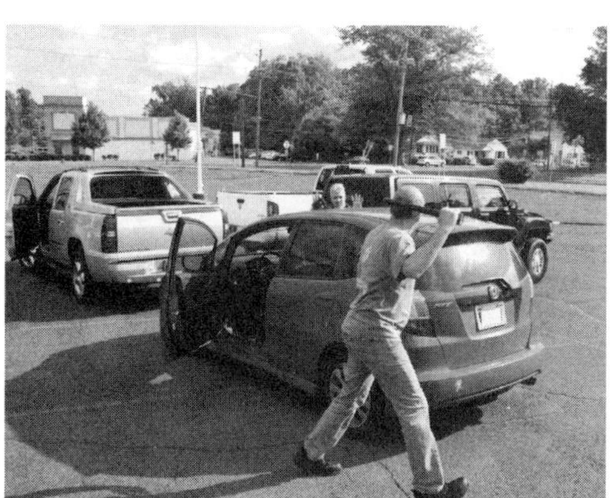

In this example, you can exit your vehicle (provided you are alone in the vehicle and do not have other passengers to worry about) and run around it, using it as a barrier between you and the assailant. Hopefully, you or a witness can immediately summon police help. You could also, of course, run away by simply leaving your vehicle and the scene.

A Strategic Choice: To Defend One's Property or Solely Rely on Legal Remedies

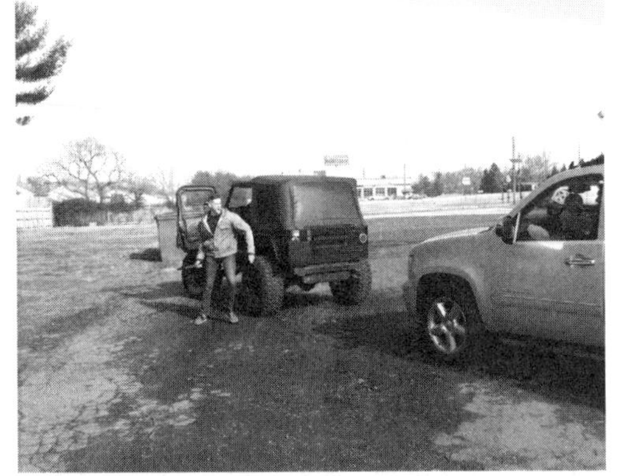

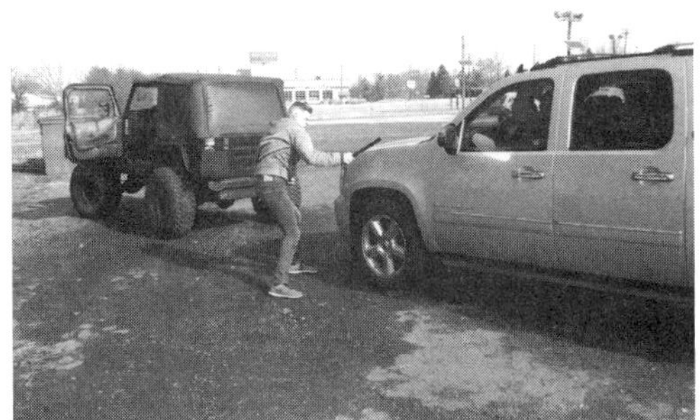

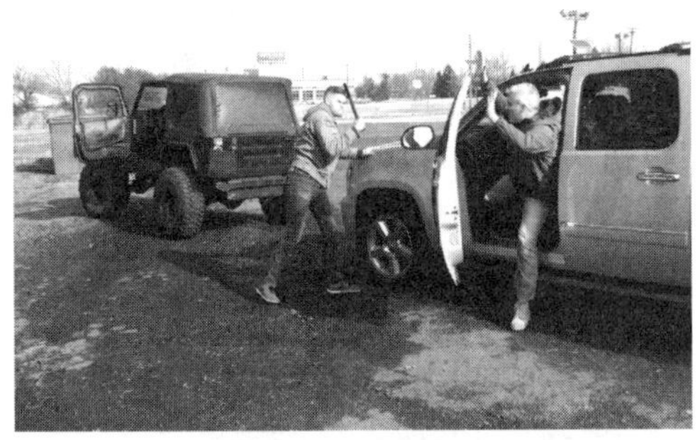

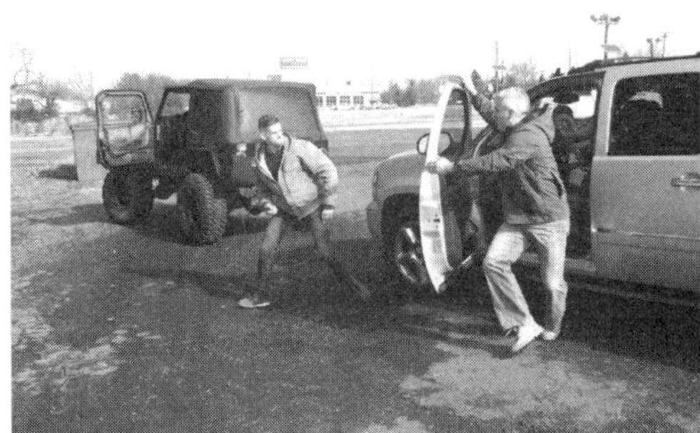

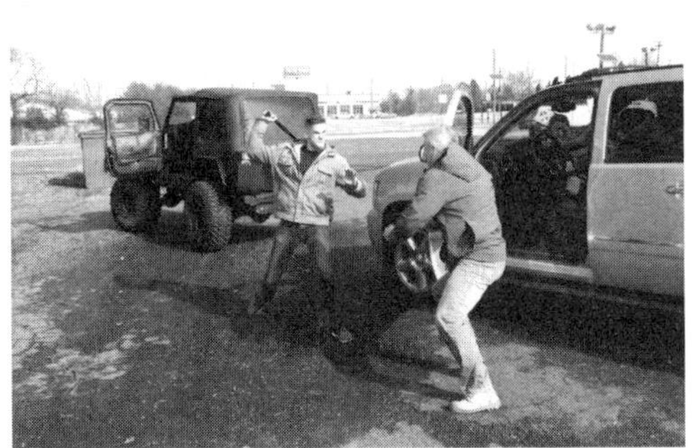

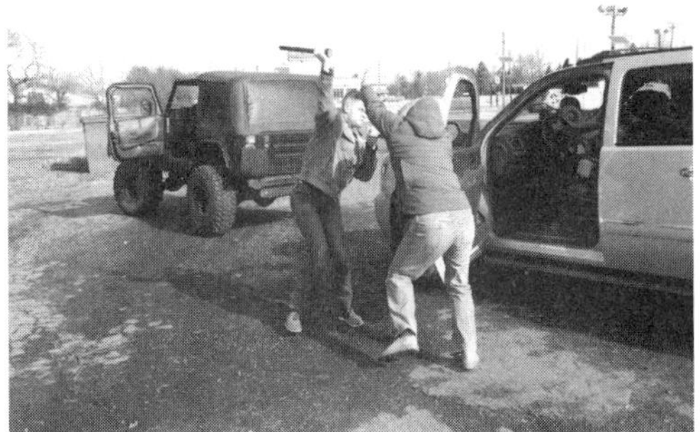

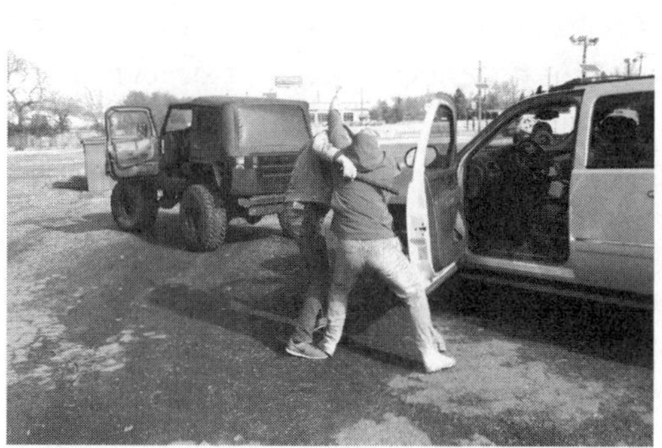

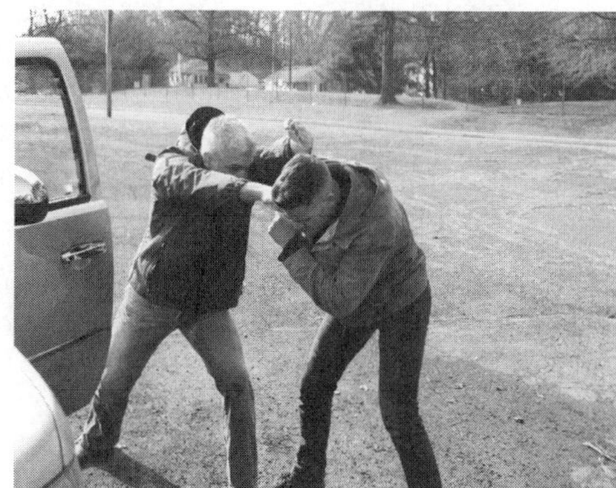

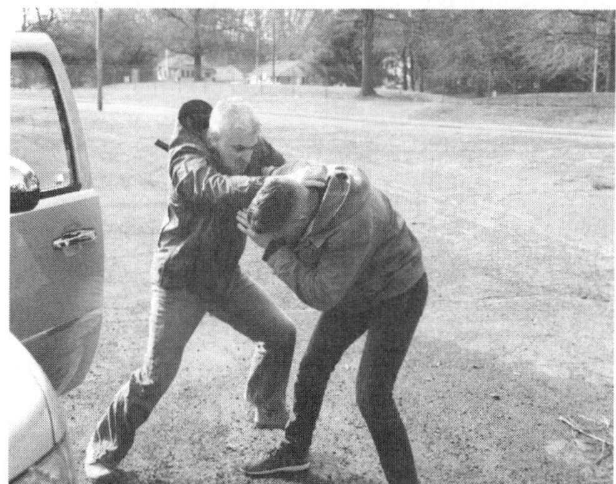

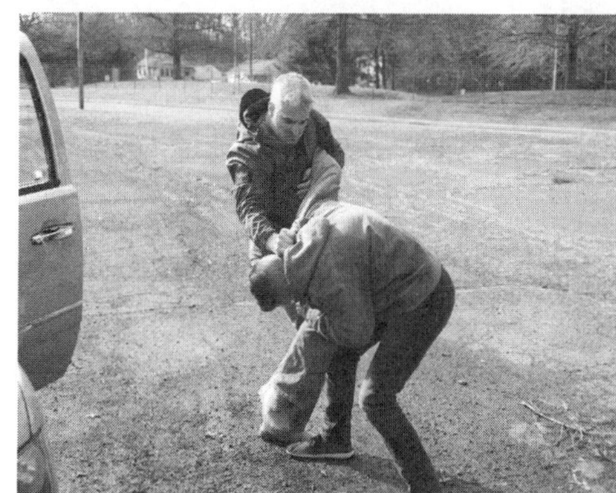

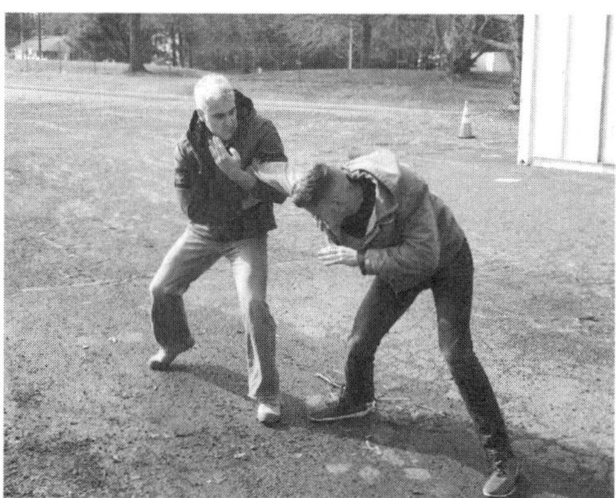

This series represents defending your vehicle from an *ongoing* attack by closing on the aggressor to deflect and redirect the overhead impact-weapon attack and remove it. Of course, in this type of direct confrontation you risk being injured or incurring liability should you use unreasonable force to defend your property. Accordingly, you must obviously weigh your response. Think about this now so you have a plan of action were this type of scenario to arise.

In the United States, you generally have a right to defend your personal property, including your automobile. The law allows a citizen to defend his property using objectively reasonable force, but not deadly force. However, as compelling as it may be to defend your property and stop an aggressor, your exercise of this right may not be the right strategic decision. Depending on the outcome, you could end up injured or have used excessive force in the eyes of a court. Historically, the law has always valued human health and life over the preservation of property. So, you should think ahead of a strategic planned course of action if you find yourself in this situation. If you do not plan ahead and visualize this type of unavoidable encounter, you may freeze or overreact at your peril.

I will use my home state of New Jersey's NJ Rev Stat § 2C:3-6 as an example of the rights afforded a citizen in protecting his personal (and real) property. In a case like the one in the photo example, you must be in control of the automobile you are driving, including being licensed and privileged in its use. You must rationally believe that the reasonable force you use is necessary to prevent or terminate the commission or attempted commission of a criminal trespass and battery against your vehicle.

Prior to using reasonable force, you must "request" that the aggressor not damage your property unless that request is useless or dangerous to yourself or another, or if substantial harm would be done to the property before your request can effectively be made. Once again, deadly force may *not* be employed to repel a battery upon one's personal (or real) property. In other words, you may physically intervene with objectively reasonable non-deadly force to prevent active damage and harm to your vehicle. However, if the aggressor damages your vehicle and then walks away, thereby disengaging or breaking the continuum, you are not legally justified in using force to avenge yourself or settle the score. If the aggressor damages your vehicle and then attacks you, self-defense rules of engagement of course immediately apply.

NJ Rev Stat § 2C:3-6 (2014) Statutory Example

2C:3-6. Use of force in defense of premises or personal property

c. Use of force in defense of personal property. Subject to the provisions of subsection d. of this section and of section 2C:3-9, the use of force upon or toward the person of another is justifiable when the actor reasonably believes it necessary to prevent what he reasonably believes to be an attempt by such other person to commit theft, criminal mischief, or other criminal interference with personal property in his possession or in the possession of another for whose protection he acts.

Krav Maga Strategy and Methodology

What a defender does instinctively he does faster. A few instinctive defensive tactics will enable you to survive the most common violent onslaughts. In other words, developing a minimum selection of preferred, broadly applicable techniques that you can summon immediately will allow you to prevail. If the situation requires, krav maga teaches you to hone your instincts to maximize the damage you can inflict. Overcoming the threat is solely dependent on your intent and determination, combined with correct anatomical targeting. True self-defense focuses not simply on survival but rather on how to optimally injure, cripple, maim, and—in extreme life-and-death situations—kill a murderous adversary. You will have to debilitate an attacker both physically and mentally to end the confrontation decisively on your terms. Be sure to keep in mind that if you are engaged against a sport-oriented fighter and you up the ante by using eye gouges, biting, or groin strikes, your adversary may do the same. Therefore, when you rely on "dirty" fighting—a krav maga mainstay—you had better damage your opponent immediately and convincingly to prevent his adopting the same strategy.

Krav maga may be thought of as defensive offense. If an aggressor has violent intent, you must have superior unwavering counter-violent intent. Rely on injuring the aggressor—not simply hurting him—to stop the assault. You must short-circuit his physical capability and will to continue. While you cannot underestimate an attacker's ability, the paradox is that the attacker's skills, in the end, are irrelevant—provided you seize the decisive counter-initiative.

Krav Maga's Four-Pillar Strategy

Krav maga's four pillars of self-defense are:

1. Awareness
2. Avoidance
3. De-escalation/escape
4. Last resort preemptive combatives or simultaneous defense and attack

Retzev Key Points

1. Retzev may be compared to a professional law enforcement or military assault, which uses overwhelming violence of action and a preponderance of firepower.
2. Retzev teaches instinctive combat motion that does not require you to think about the next logical move. If attacked, the kravist must, within the boundaries of the law, become the most violent person present, capable of defeating any threat.
3. Defensive movements transition automatically and seamlessly into offensive movements to neutralize the attack, leaving an adversary little or no time to react.
4. Retzev allows you to switch tactics immediately if one of your combatives does not succeed at reaching its target, thereby providing for a seamless flow into the next available combative. Keep in mind that optimized combative combinations require sound footwork and target prioritization.
5. Retzev merges all aspects of one's krav maga training.

Krav Maga Training Strategies and Emphases

There is one key difference between hand-to-hand combat and sport-oriented fighting. Hand-to-hand combat avails itself of all of the fouls and prohibited moves (biting, gouging, kicks to the knees, throat strikes) sport-oriented fighting bans because these tactics cause injury. For both hand-to-hand combat and a lesser, restricted extent sport fighting there is a correct natural and practical temptation to use a just few core combatives against vital anatomy. Yet, in a sporting context, "legal" combatives against a tough, trained adversary may not always work. Hence, the need to incorporate "illegal," specifically designed injurious combatives. You must comfortably use all limbs and other personal weapons from all angles and opportune distances. Each combative sets you up for a complementary combative (principle of retzev). Keep in mind that the average person has about a dozen seconds or so of maximum fighting effort or "burn time" until they will be overcome with fatigue, according to Bruce Siddle's research.

Learn a few preferred core combatives to optimize whatever individual martial-arts capability you have. When training, many people are detrimentally lulled into a false sense of their tactical effectiveness because a training partner does not resist as a real assailant would. You must train against full-speed and full-force attacks to equip your body and to understand how to handle a real-life violent encounter. The caveat is that you and a partner must develop complementary and reciprocal skill that precludes injuring one another when counterattacking. Lastly, use the internet to watch actual street violence to a gain a better understanding of the engagement speed, viciousness, and circumstances where people (often needlessly) go after one another.

Essential Defensive Strategies and Fighting Prowess

The old adage singularly applies: the best defense is a superior offense. The IDF relies on quality of military prowess instead of quantity (though, of course, quantity is always welcome). This is especially true when facing multiple adversaries at the same time—another difficult scenario to which the IDF is accustomed. A similar analogy may be made for Israeli Krav Maga as well. A select group of optimized, instinctive, superior combative tactics, adaptable to many situations, that bring overwhelming firepower to bear in a time of need, is krav maga's essence. It is crucial to remember krav maga's historical roots. Jewish defenders were usually outnumbered by attackers and prevailed by using superior tactics. Keep in mind that attackers may think only about winning—not about a fair fight. There are dangerous people who are professionally trained or have acquired enough "no rules" fighting experience to be considered experts. They will methodically assault and maim you. Recognize they exist, but fortunately they are not the ones who usually escalate matters or display bravado.

Most importantly, adopt an unbeatable mind-set. No matter who you might have to face, under desperate circumstances you will physically prevail, using no-quarter anatomical targeting. Krav maga and like-minded training will provide you with an effective tactical solution.

Communicate nonverbally with a potential attacker, if possible, to nip the potential assault in the bud. Use body language and positioning to unequivocally indicate you are confident you will win a physical confrontation. The following are nine key defensive strategies to prioritize:

1. Become an expert on core combatives along with basic evasive deflection movements. Each core combative involves two interrelated, yet unique phases:
   - Why and how it should be done.
   - When it should be done.
   - Example: A rear straight kick versus a front straight kick.
2. While concepts may be considered more important than specific techniques, optimized krav maga self-defense relies on sound, proven tactics—for both tactical and legal reasons.
3. Your mind-set is not if but how you will incapacitate an attacker. Successfully recognizing vulnerable anatomical targets is achieved by instantly identifying what tactic will work best. Instant analysis may include an opponent's poor foot positioning or open stance that makes the groin susceptible or exposes his throat.
4. Preemptive strikes work best, provided pre-attack recognition allows them.
5. If discipline and fortitude allow, when facing a threat or impending attack, non-physical reaction can be used to feign initial acquiescence or compliance for an optimum counter-ambush. In other words, the aggressor does not expect you to physically disable him.
6. The difference between a kravist and a less experienced fighter is this: the kravist avails himself of each vulnerable opening and opportunity, while immediately creating more of the same. A kravist also protects himself against strikes targeting vulnerable anatomy, including joint locks and chokes.
7. Try at all times to be on balance and in control for both enhanced offensive and defensive capabilities.
8. The fastest route between two points is a straight line; hence the effectiveness of linear combatives.
9. A low-line kick is delivered under the radar and is more difficult to defend. In addition, straight-line attacks are more difficult to recognize and, therefore, to defend. If an opponent lowers his hands to defend a kick, you are in an advantageous position to then target his neck and head with seamless upper-body combatives.

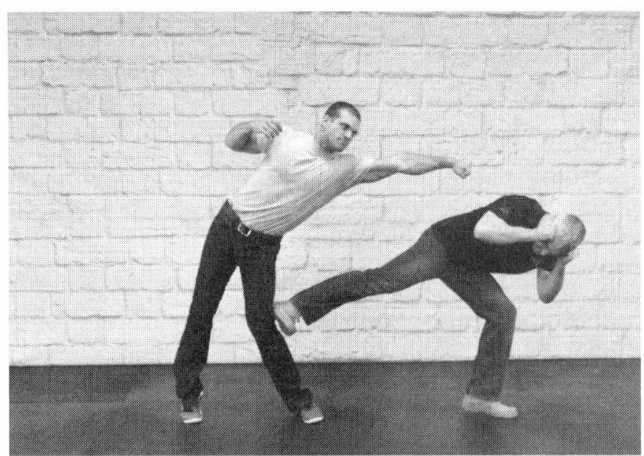

A low-line side kick against a straight punch, combined with a body defense.

Lower and upper-body combatives must be combined seamlessly, harnessing the momentum and weight transfer from each previous combative.

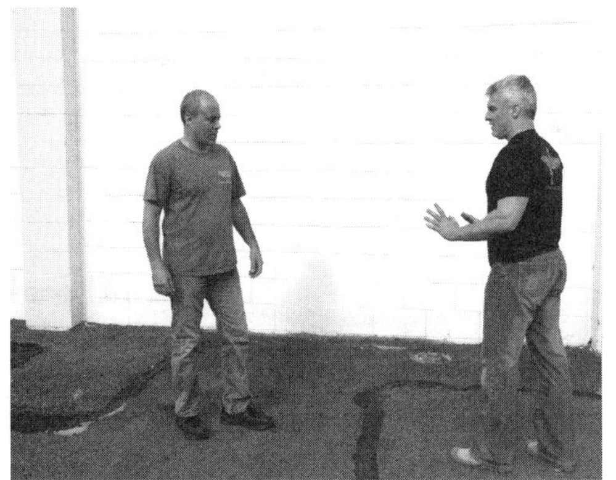

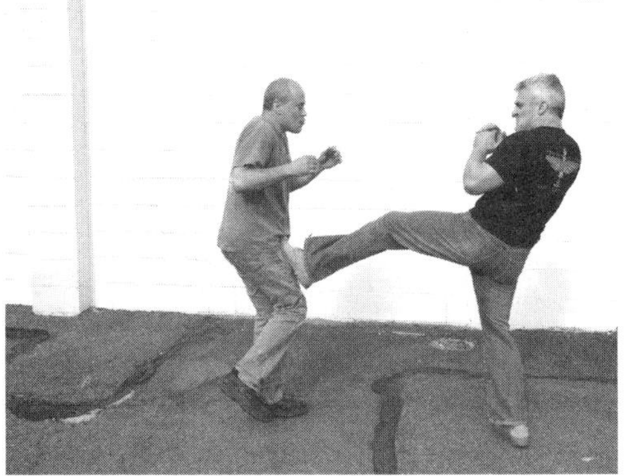

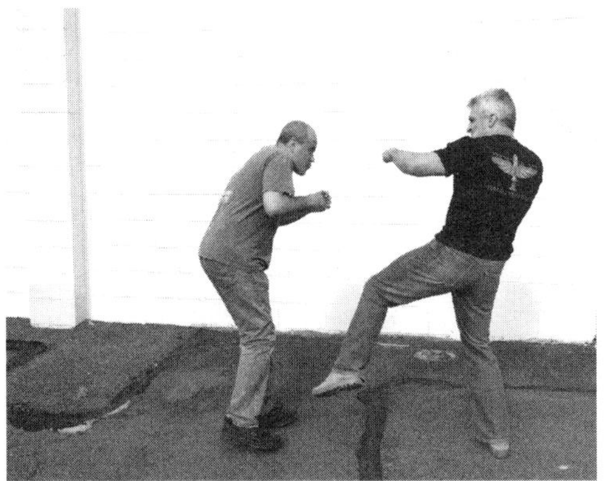

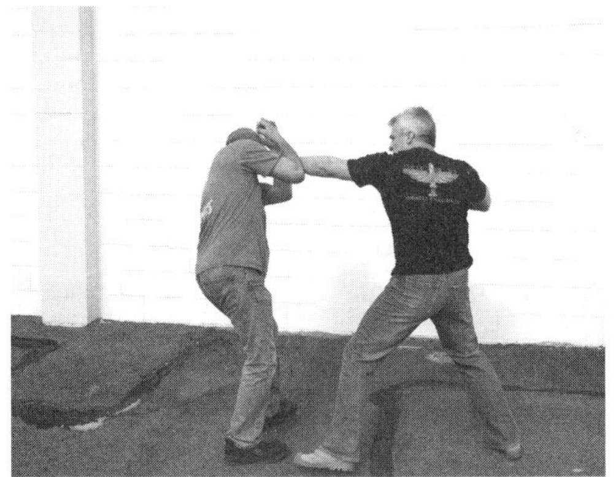

This series depicts a lower- and upper-body straight kick and straight punch combination.

Compound Kick: Economy of Motion Strategy

Economy of motion is one of the strategic pillars of krav maga. Compound kicks using the same kicking leg epitomize economy of motion by harnessing the momentum from one kick and using it instantaneously to launch another kick. Compound kicks require both balance and strength. The key is to avoid touching your kicking leg to the ground.

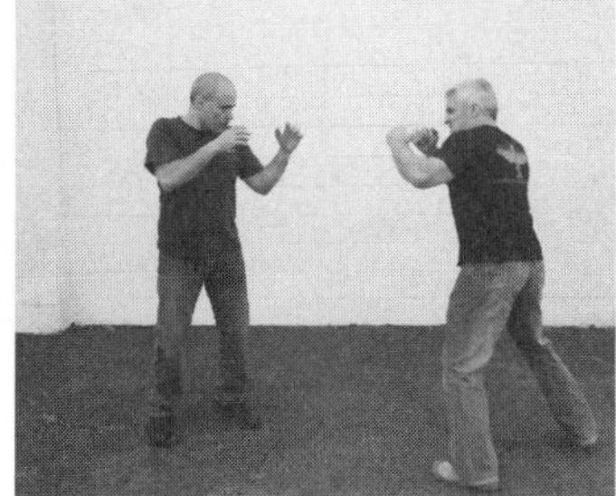

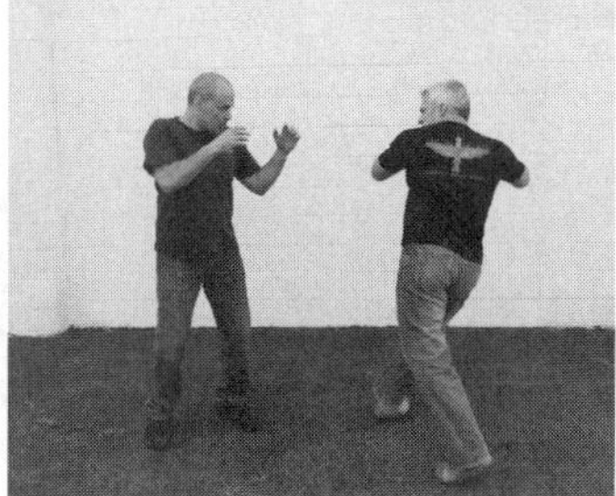

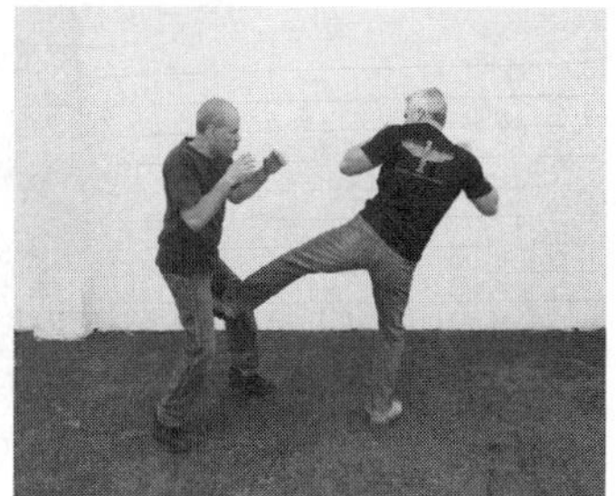

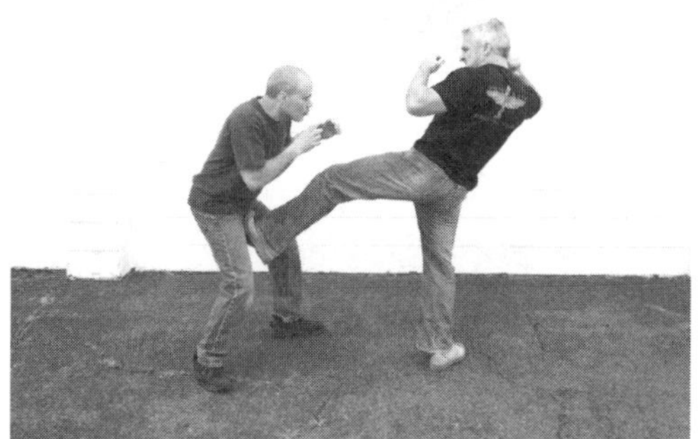

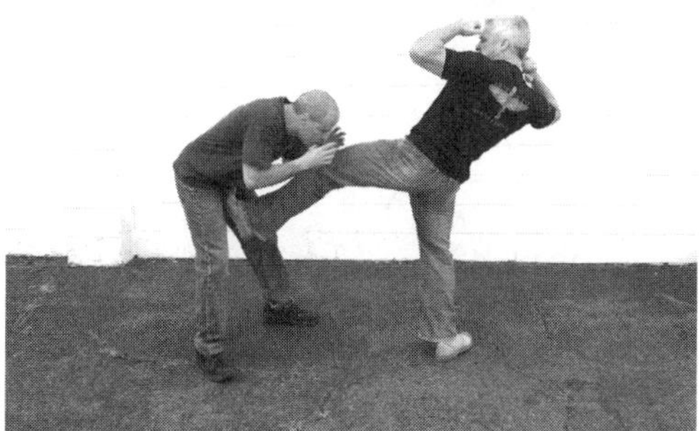

This compound kick example depicts a roundhouse shin kick to an opponent's inside knee followed by a seamless transition into a straight ball-of-the-foot groin kick. Using an economy of motion strategy, a compound kick uses the same kicking leg to harness the momentum of one kick and then to instantaneously launch a second kick. A skilled opponent will defend his groin. Therefore, you need to create access, and this kick does it.

Trapping

Trapping is pinning the opponent's arm(s). Traps are used

- when having successfully angled for advantageous position or countering;
- to control an edged weapon;
- to prevent an opponent from initiating combatives.

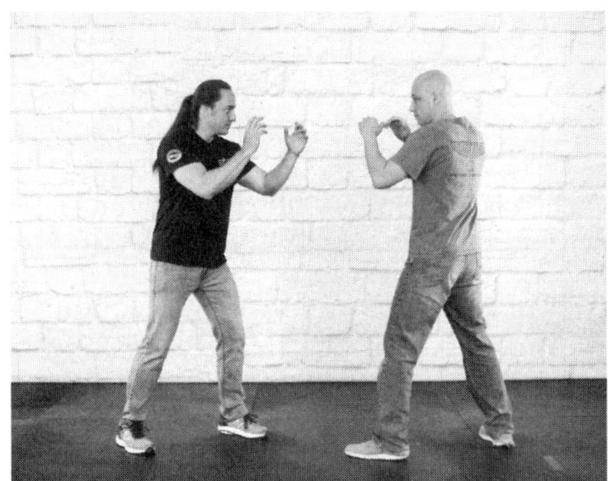
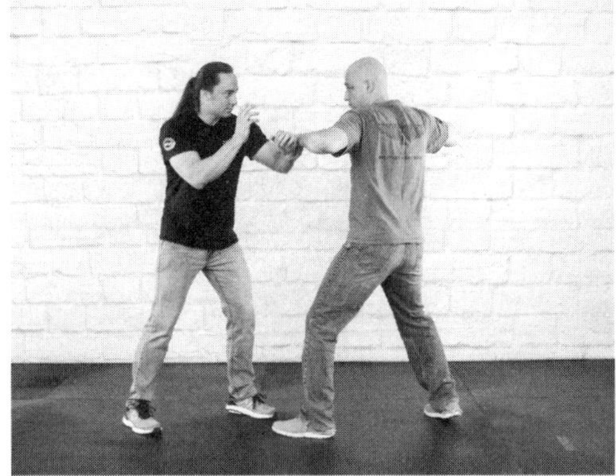
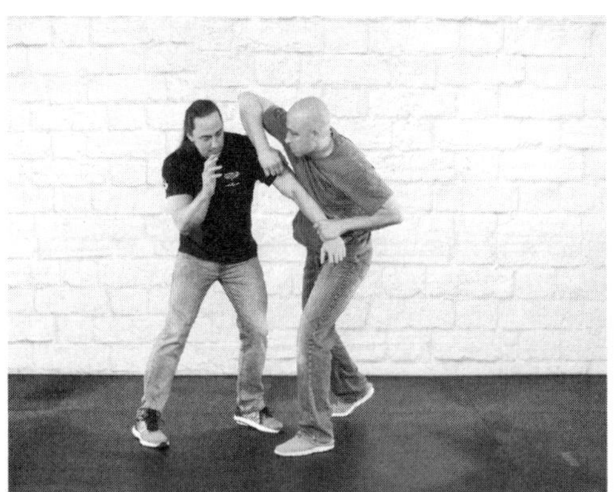
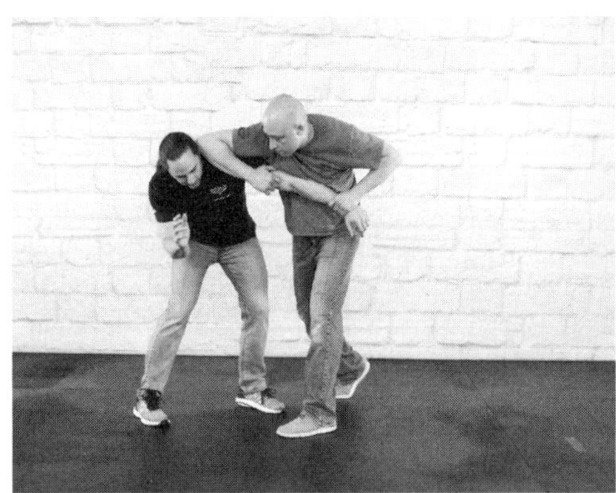

This series depicts a forward-arm trap combined with an over-the-top elbow strike.

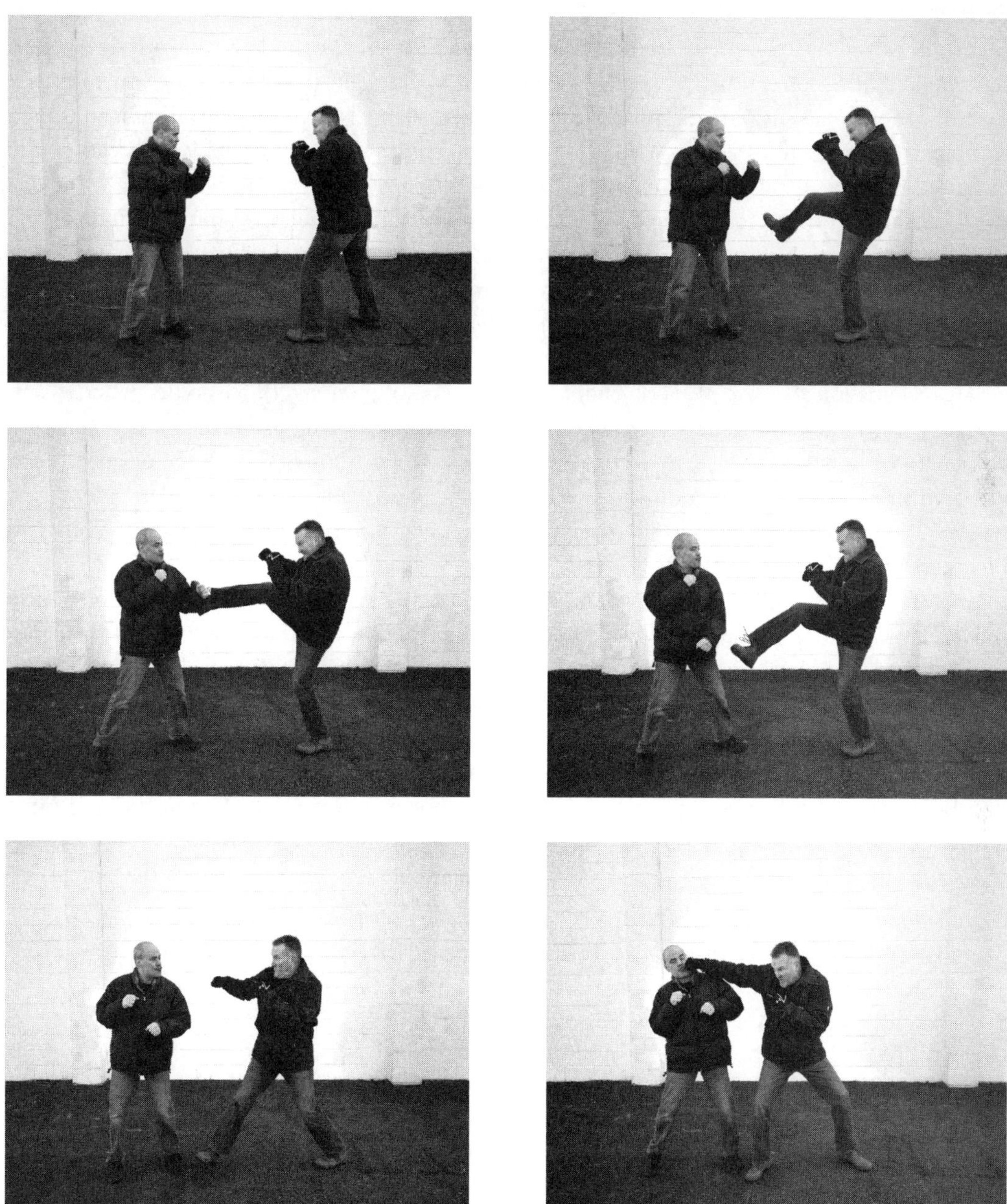

This series depicts a forward-arm trap by using an inside slap kick to knock the opponent's arm down to transition seamlessly into a straight punch combative.

Feinting

Feinting a combative—faking a movement to draw a reaction—baits an adversary into reacting against a phantom attack. This creates an opening in his defense for you to attack his vulnerable anatomy. An example of an upper-body feint is feigning a straight lead punch to draw the adversary's reaction while you then stop mid-movement to deliver instead a fully executed right cross punch. An example of a lower-body feint is feigning a straight kick to the adversary's groin to get him to drop his hand in defense but then mid-movement diverting your kick into a high roundhouse kick to his head. The IKMA curriculum emphasizes about a dozen core feints. Feints are one key tactic to defeating a skilled adversary—as I have personally witnessed in my many years of training in Israel against some of the best hand-to-hand-combat fighters (*lochamim*) in the world.

Your feint must be a real tactic though only partially completed; it should include limb and torso movements with accompanying facial theatrics. Feinting can also include changing your level of attack by attacking high, then low, and then high again, or the opposite. You can also attack one side of an opponent's body to force an opening on the other side. Alternatively, you can attack his body in such a way that it exposes a subsequent vulnerability to be taken advantage of in your next attack.

Master how to feint without overcommitting your limbs by utilizing shoulder bobs, hip movements, switching your feet, along with compact hand movements of only a few inches to deceive your adversary into thinking you are doing one combative when, in fact, you are orchestrating another. Feinting uses a correct half movement to disguise an attack from a different angle or limb. Feints require using footwork, the legs, arms, trunk, and the eyes, in one continuous flowing movement. A kravist recognizes the openings his feints will create and how to use those openings efficiently to create more openings. To force a parry using a feint:

- Don't wait for the parry to break your feint movement as you deliver the actual combative strike.
- Extend the feint far enough and with enough conviction to force the opponent to react. Attacks that rely on more than one feint can be perilous, as the opponent can catch you in between your half-movements.

The most common mistake with feints is poor timing and execution.

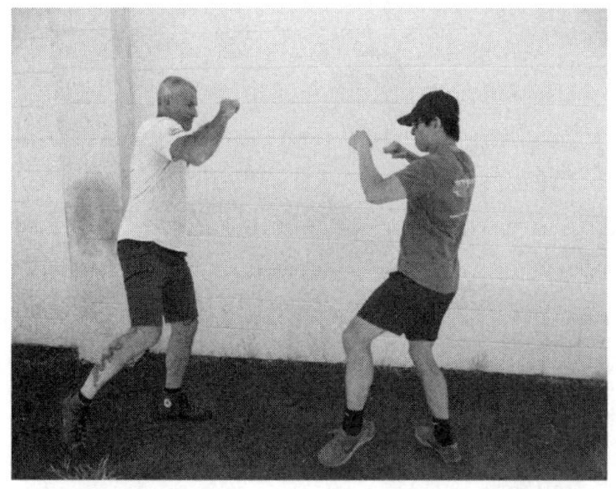
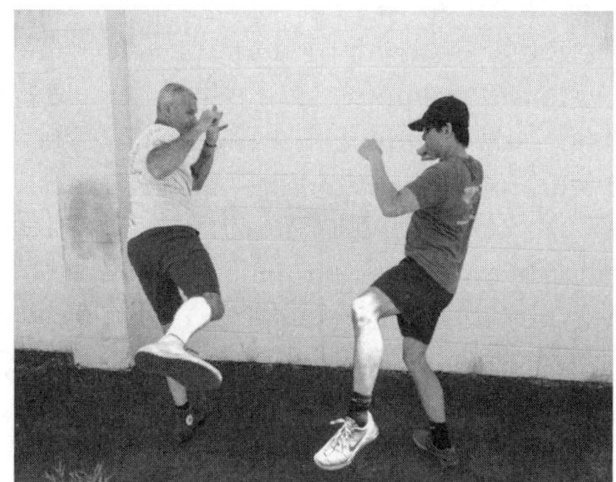
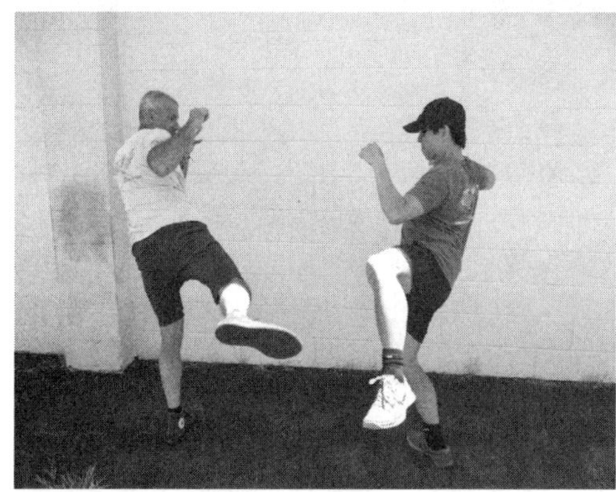
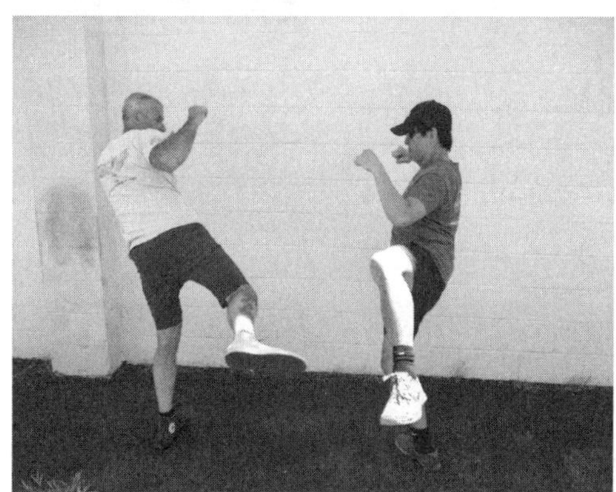
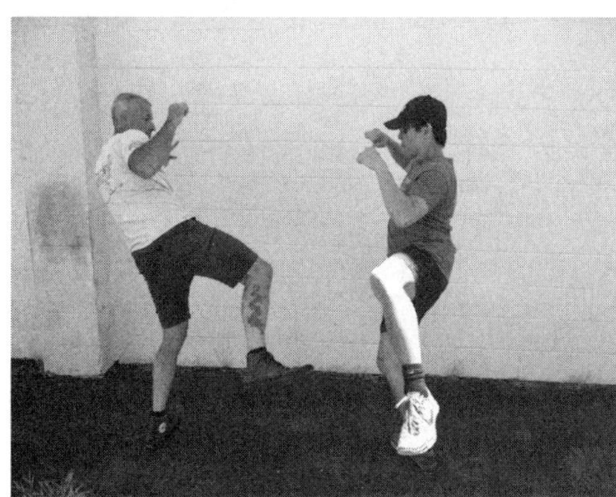
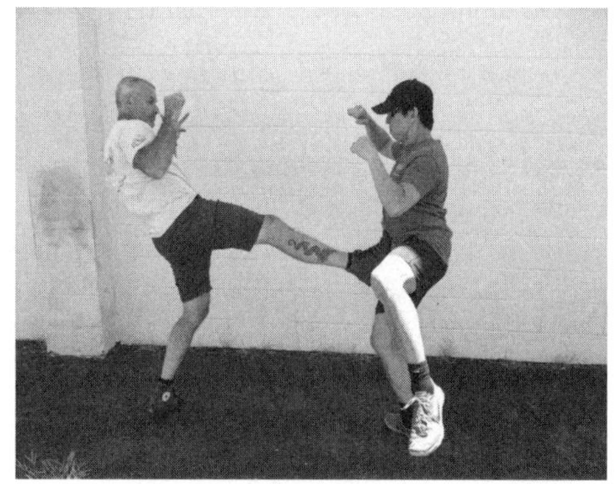

This is an example of a rear roundhouse feint kick into a straight kick. The key to this type of combative is performing a convincing half-movement to commit your opponent to a defense, thereby creating a vulnerability or opening elsewhere on his body. In this case, the defender commits a shin-to-foot interception, leaving his groin open to attack. The kicker seamlessly changes the form and trajectory of the feigned roundhouse kick to powerfully land a straight kick to the defender's groin.

Additional Strategies

Launching something into or covering an aggressor's eyes can wholly disorient him and he will reflexively disengage (albeit temporarily.). See the section "Using Reflections, 'Selfies,' and Other People's Reactions to Detect Rear Threats" in chapter 3. Baiting an opponent requires the highest skill to catch the opponent at his most vulnerable.

Attack-defend-attack combatives are designed to anticipate a fight one step ahead. The combatant launching an attack is prepared to also defend and immediately change his method of attack to target an opponent's exposed anatomical vulnerabilities.

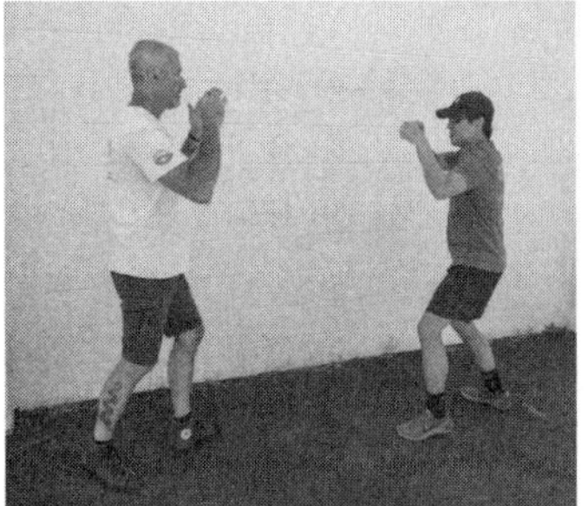

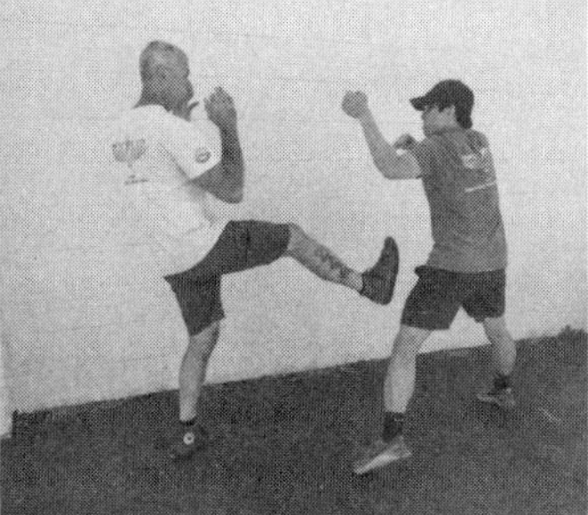

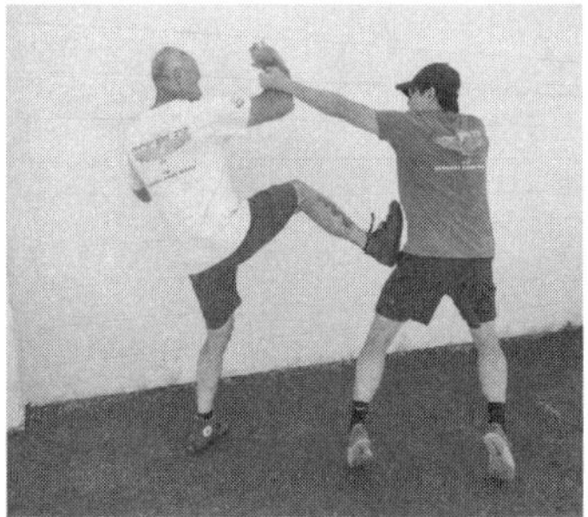

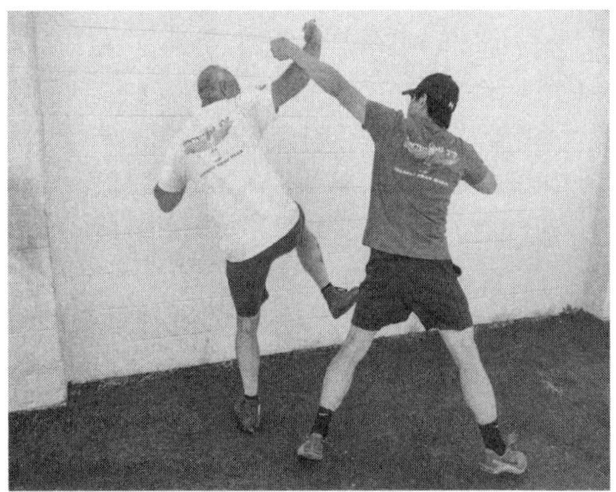

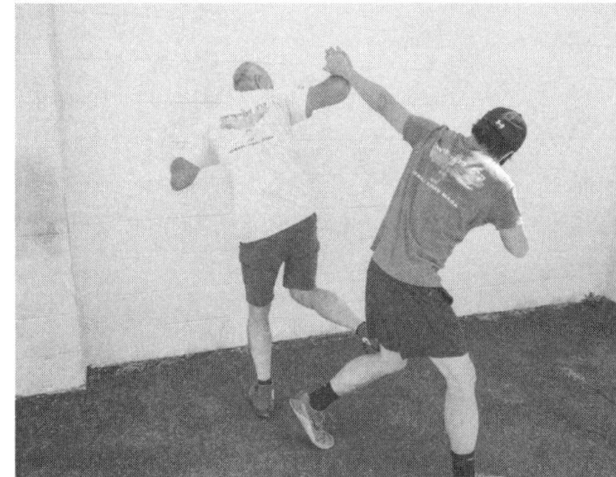

In this attack-defend-attack scenario, the man on the left launches a straight kick while the man on the right attempts to side step the kick and simultaneously punch his adversary in the head. The man who launched the offensive kick counters by intercepting the punch and seamlessly rerouting his straight kick to a side kick to take out his opponent's knee.

When Possible, Use the Same Tactics Both on the Ground and Standing

Krav maga ground survival is best defined as "what we do up, we do down" with additional specific ground-fighting capabilities. Krav maga generally tries to use the same effective tactics in similar situations. This often translates to what we do standing, we do on the ground with modification. These side headlock examples, both standing and on the ground represent krav maga's emphasis on using the same tactics whether standing or on the ground (as circumstances permit).

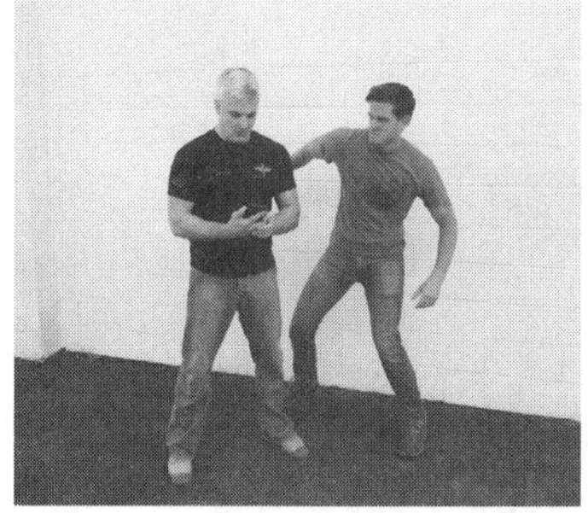
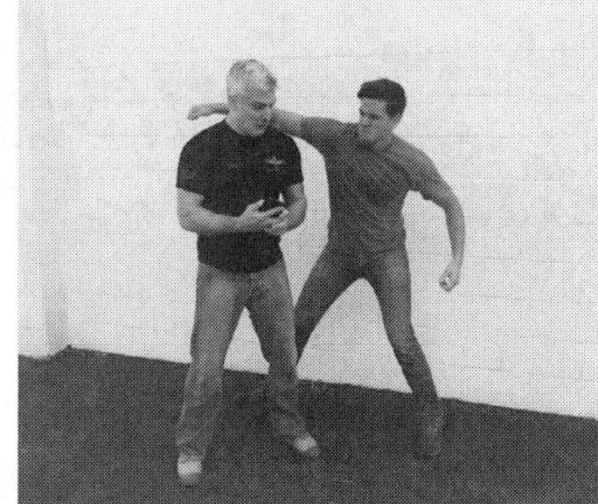
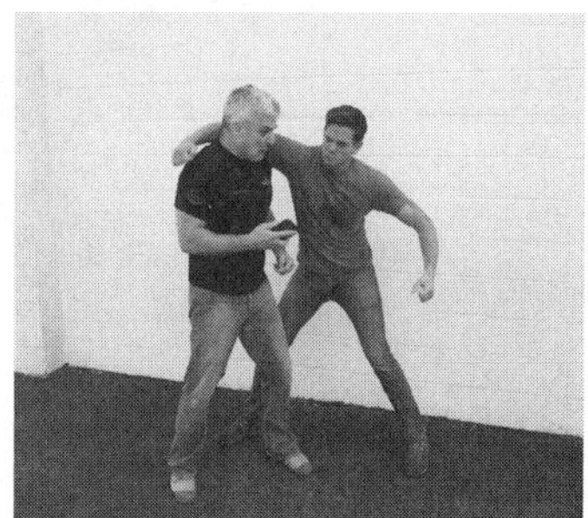
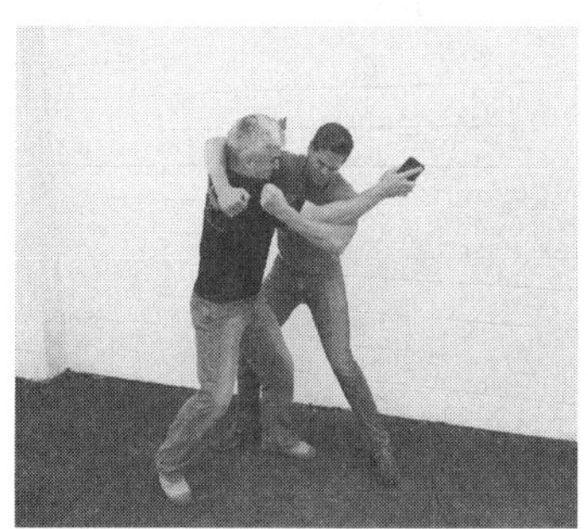
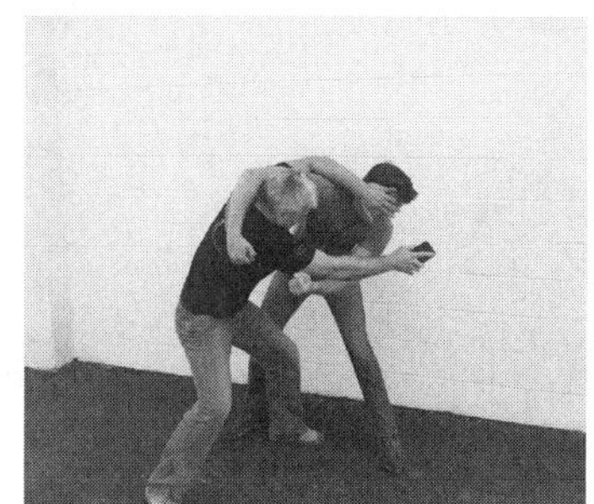
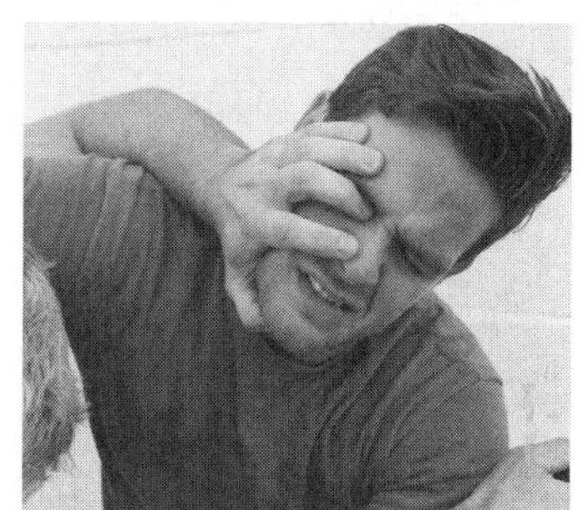
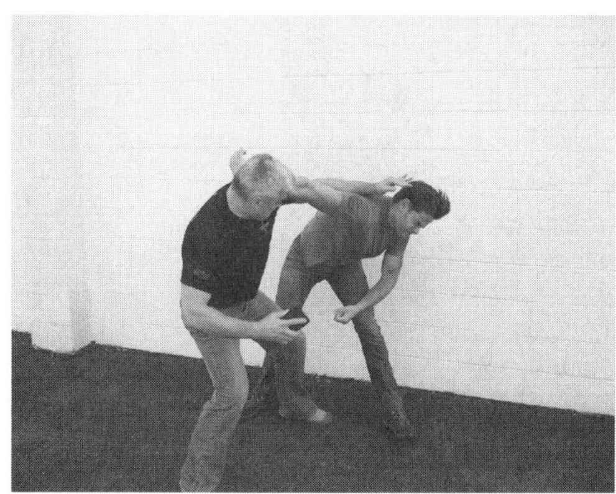
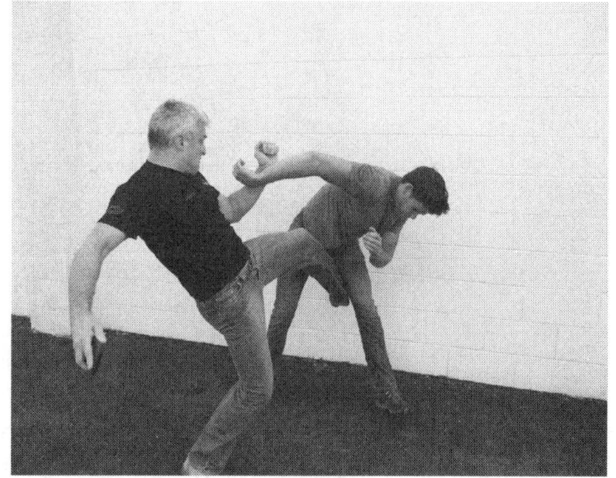

This is an example of defending against a standing combined side headlock and simultaneous punch to the head. For this defense, stab your front inside arm by shooting it past the attacker's biceps while your rear arm snakes around the back of the attacker's shoulder to apply an eye gouge. Follow up with other combatives as necessary.

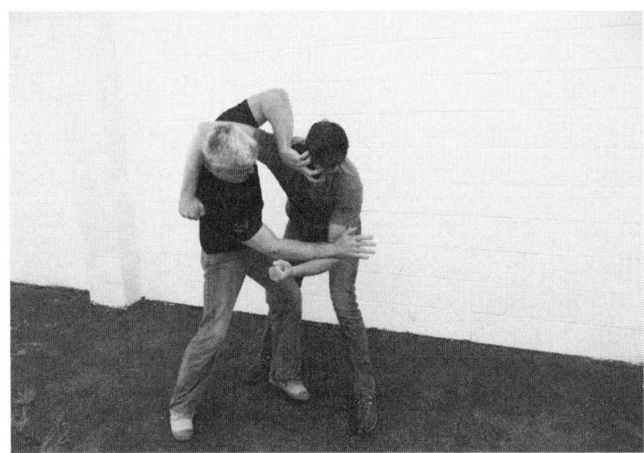

This is an alternative counterattack if you had your mobile device in your nearside left hand.

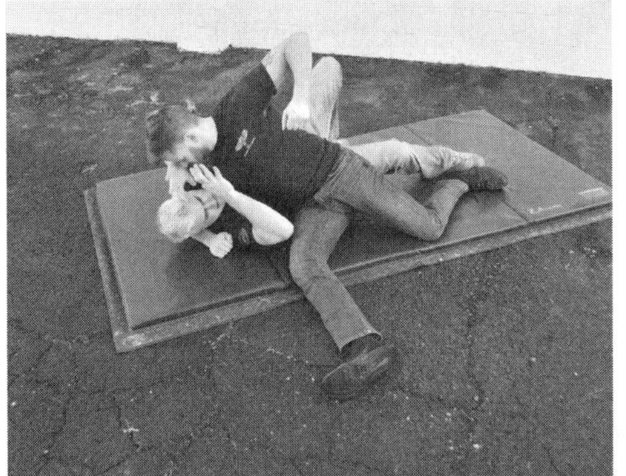

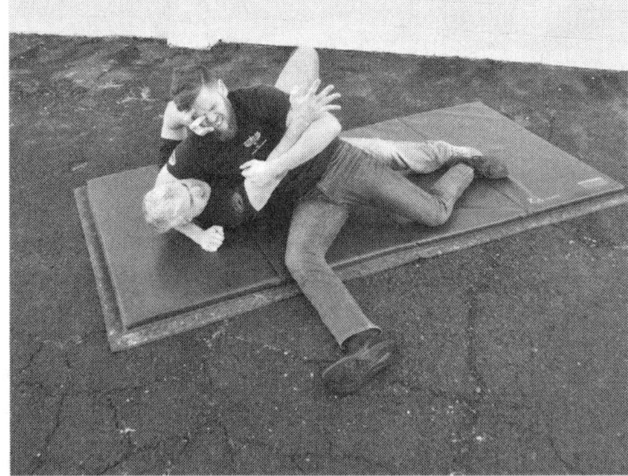

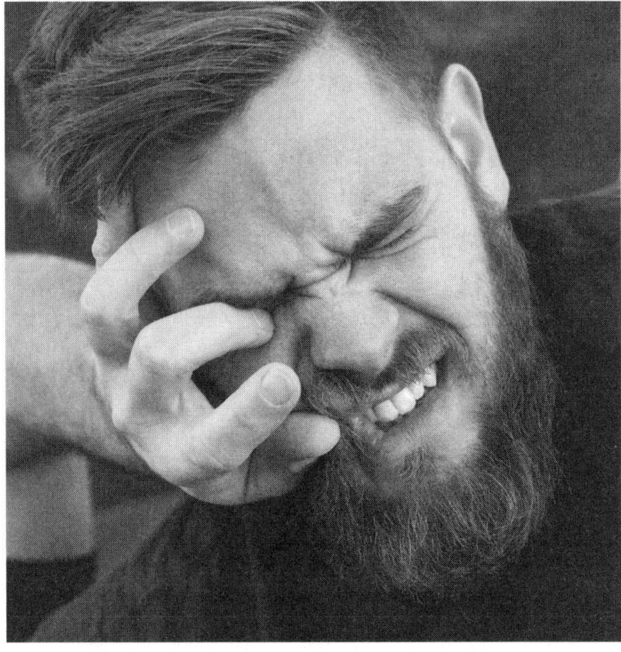

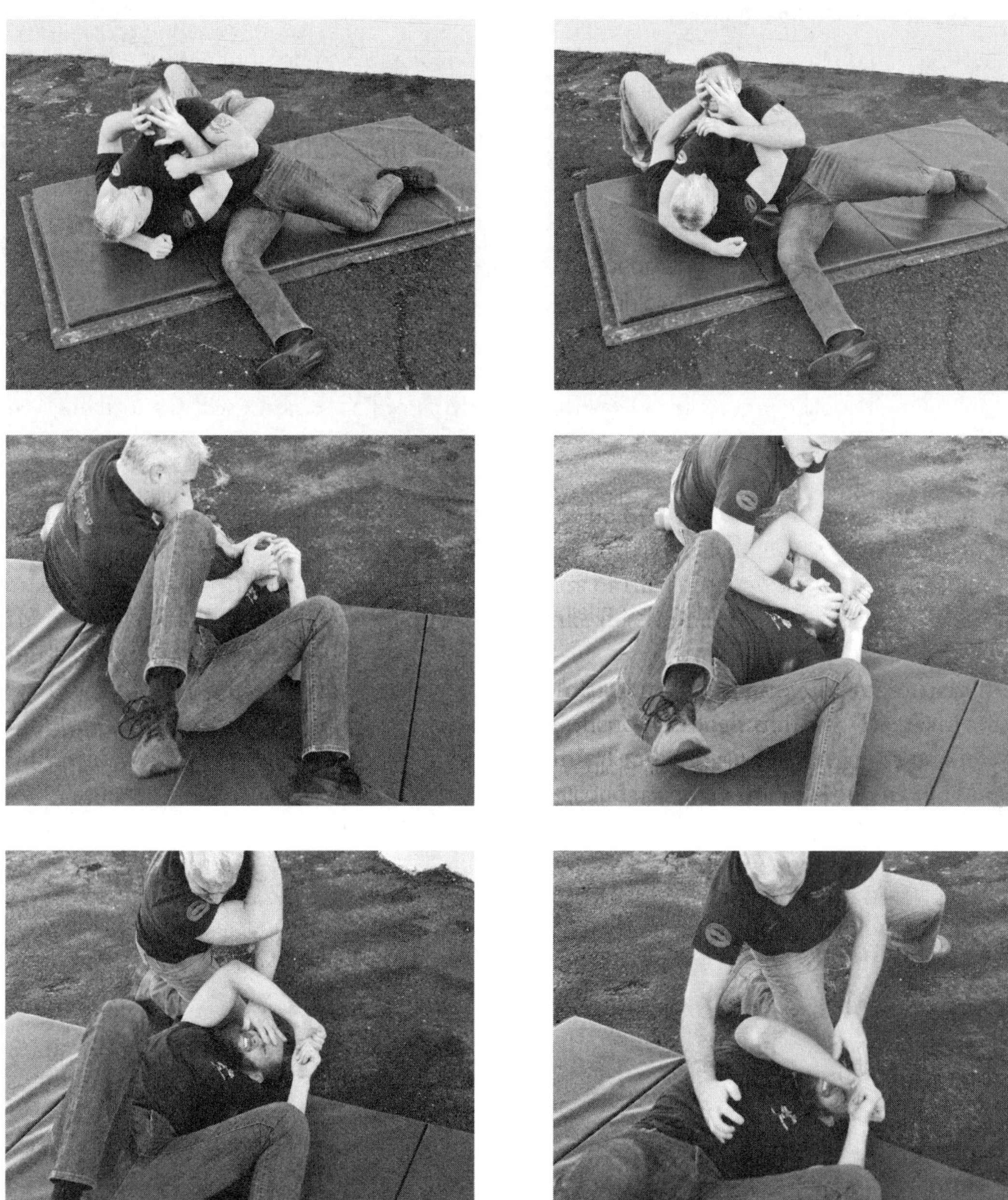

This series represents defending against a combined side headlock and simultaneous punch to the head when on the ground. Almost identically to the standing defense against such an attack, shoot your front nearside arm past the attacker's biceps while your rear arm snakes around the back of the attacker's shoulder to apply an eye gouge. Follow up with other combatives as necessary. To repeat, the strategy is: "when possible, what we do up we do down."

Strategy against Multiple Opponents

The truism that street violence is desperate and unpredictable could not hold more true than when facing multiple assailants. If anything defined krav maga, it was Imi and his students in Bratislava facing multiple attackers. In developing krav maga, Imi took into account his own experiences of often being outnumbered by multiple assailants in the city. Therefore, contending against multiple (un)armed attackers became a linchpin of his krav maga thinking. In his later years Imi approvingly observed Haim develop and expand krav maga's ground survival tactics. The one point Imi constantly emphasized, which Haim also reinforces, was the danger of multiple opponents converging on a defender who is grappling with one of the opponents while on the ground.

Defending against multiple opponents, to be sure, is a desperate situation and one in which many people cannot win. Determined, experienced adversaries will try to flank and get behind you to catch you unaware. A team of aggressors will move and lurk beyond your line of sight to ambush you. Such a scenario is often showcased by animal predators. For example, lions excel at hunting larger prey in a pack or pride to coordinate a team ambush.

The odds are stacked against you (especially when weapons are introduced). There are two types of groups you might have to confront: a preplanned attack group and a spontaneous attack group. The preplanned attack group intends to attack you regardless of what you might say to de-conflict. The spontaneous attack group may be on the fence and you may be able to talk your way out of it or at least gain enough advantage to be able to initiate a preemptive counterattack.

Facing multiple assailants, let alone multiple armed assailants, is an extremely perilous situation. Preemptive debilitating combatives are highly effective tools to begin narrowing the odds in your favor. Additional core principles involve deflection, redirection, evasive footwork, and upper-body movements combined with simultaneous or near-simultaneous counterattacks to overwhelm the assailant. These survival tactics are designed for multiple threats, allowing a defender to incapacitate the assailants, and, when necessary, commandeer weapons for the defender's use.

If you cannot immediately escape, there are two cardinal rules you must try to follow: (1) do not place yourself between two or more assailants and (2) do not end up on the ground. Tactically, to defend against multiple assailants, whenever possible, use flanking maneuvers. In other words, if an assailant initiates to your left or right, engage him while using footwork *to put him between* you and any other assailants. If facing three or more assailants, even if you were attacked by the assailant in the middle, still move to one of your flanks—do not go down the middle. Try never to engage an assailant if a defense would put you in between two or more assailants. On rare occasions, you might not have the choice but to go between them and split them. Techniques and tactics do not change, but you must modify your defenses to keep an opponent between you and any other assailants as long and as often as you can.

Imi Lichtenfeld and Haim Gidon emphasize using optimum combatives to debilitate an opponent, especially when you are defending against multiple assailants. Whether your preferred combative is a long-range kick, eye rake, or punch, every combative must count. You must maximize your power and reach to debilitate an opponent both viciously and effectively in preparation for the next opponent's violent onslaught. Of course, if you debilitate, maim, or—if necessary and *in extremis*—kill an opponent quickly and decisively, his colleagues may think better of tangling with you; however, you may also increase their resolve to harm you. The bottom line is that, if you consider a multiple-assailant assault imminent and a threat to your life, act violently and with extreme prejudice. In any objectively reasonable force legal analysis, multiple assailants represent an extreme and very possibly deadly threat.

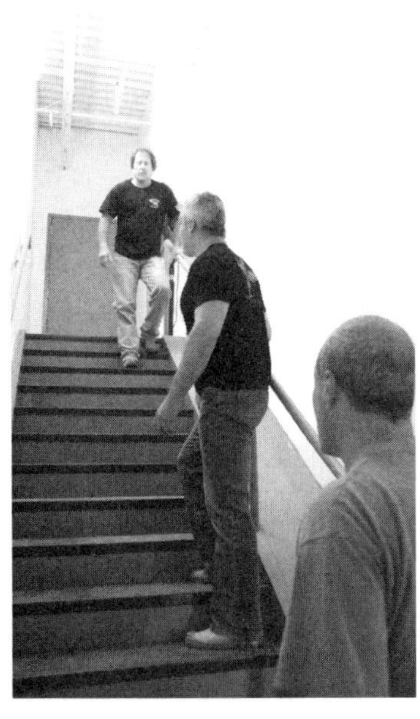
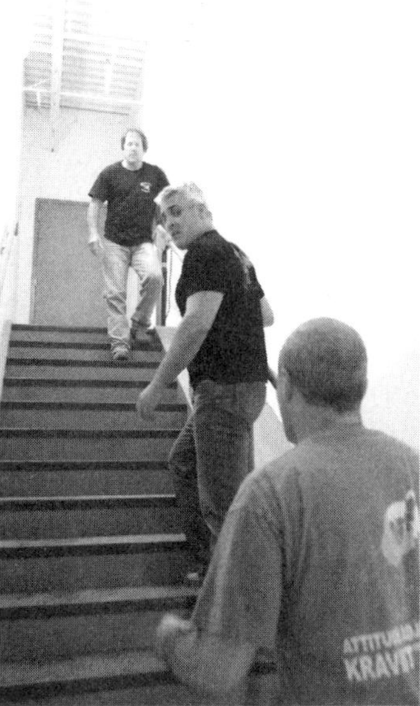
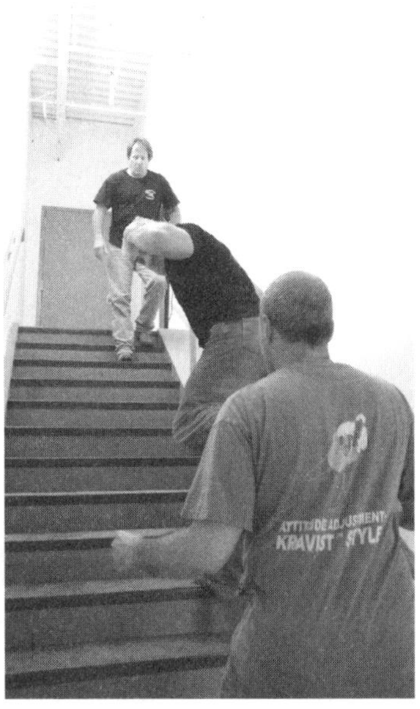
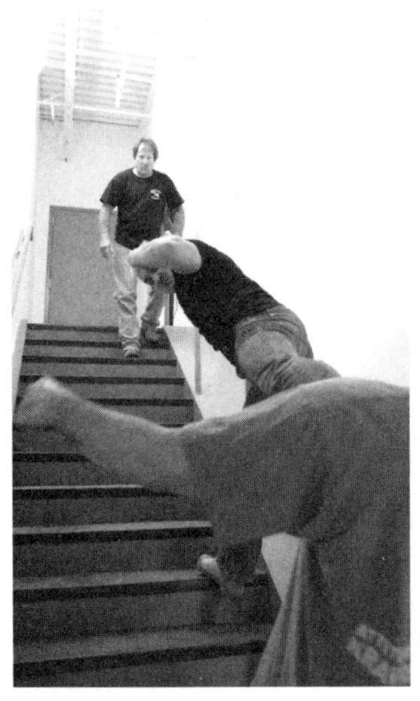
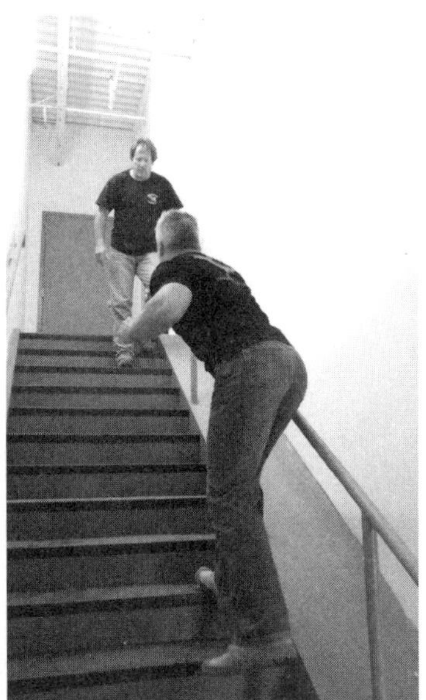
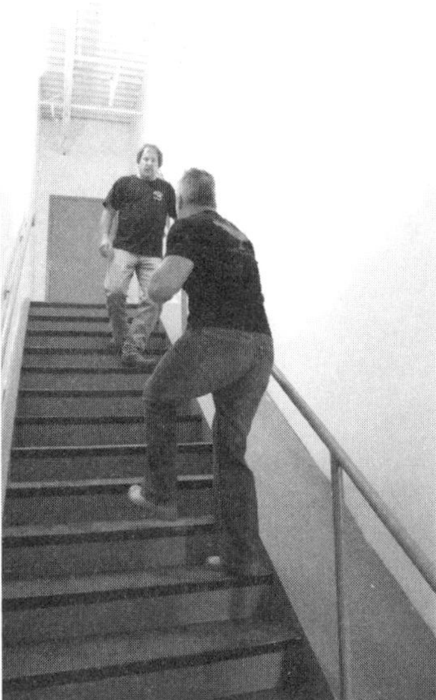

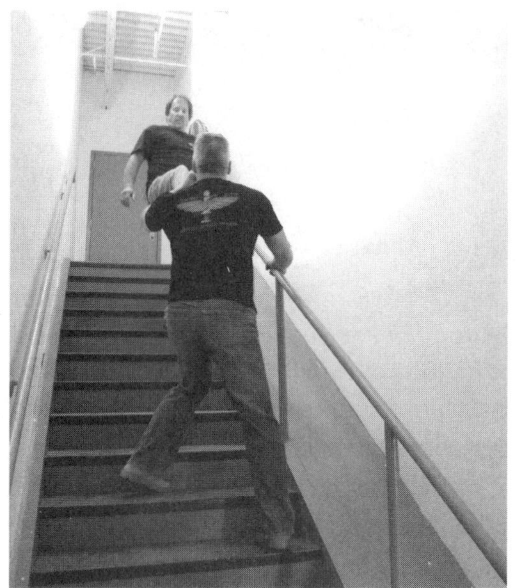
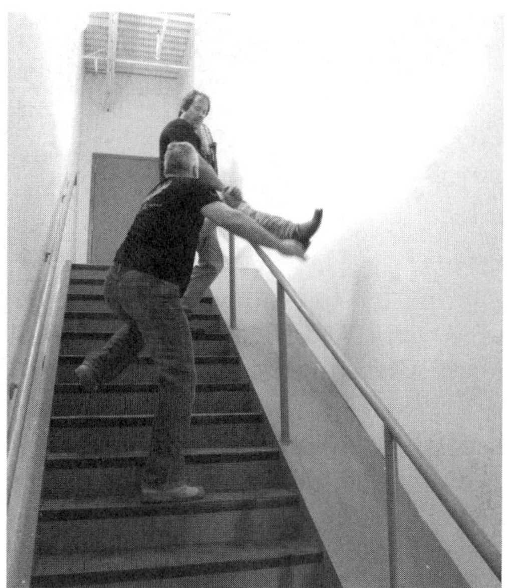
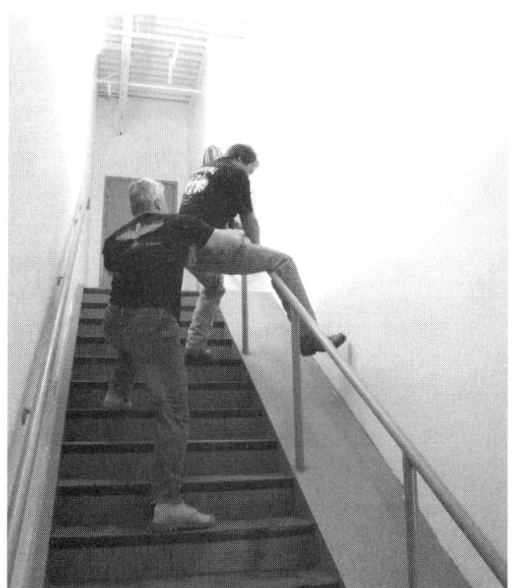
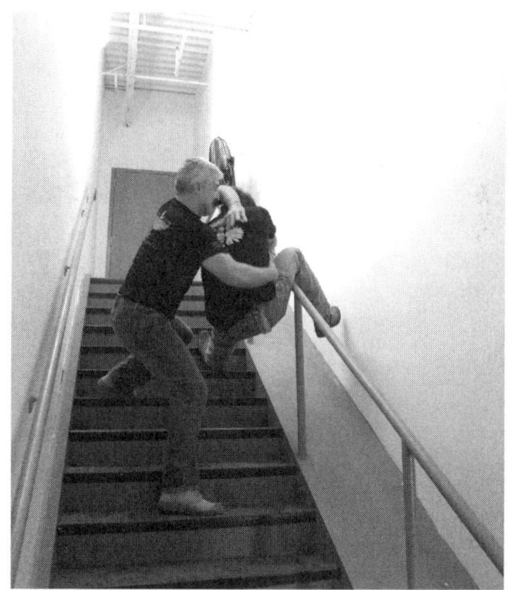

This series depicts defending against two assailants in a staircase, one above you and one below you. Strategy dictates that you engage the closest opponent (similar to most multiple-assailant scenarios). In this example, the opponent at the bottom of the staircase is more proximate, allowing you to engage him with a sidekick to send him sprawling down the stairs. Then contend with the other opponent.

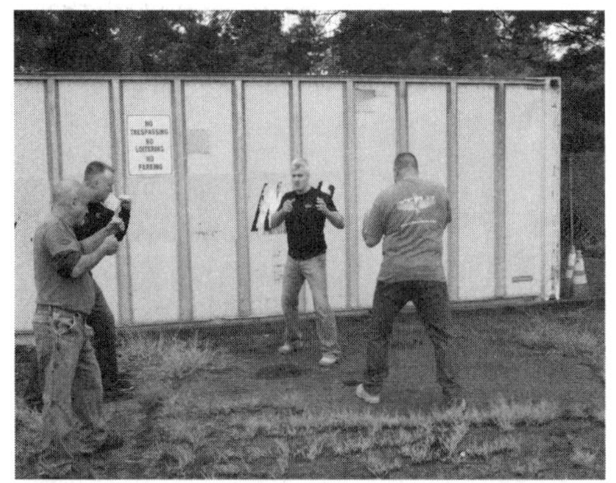

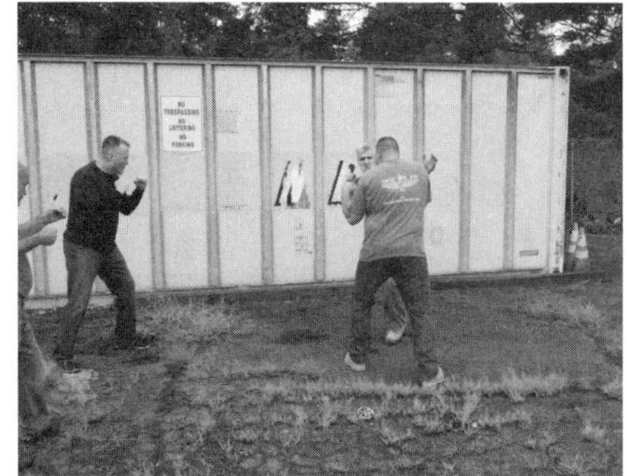

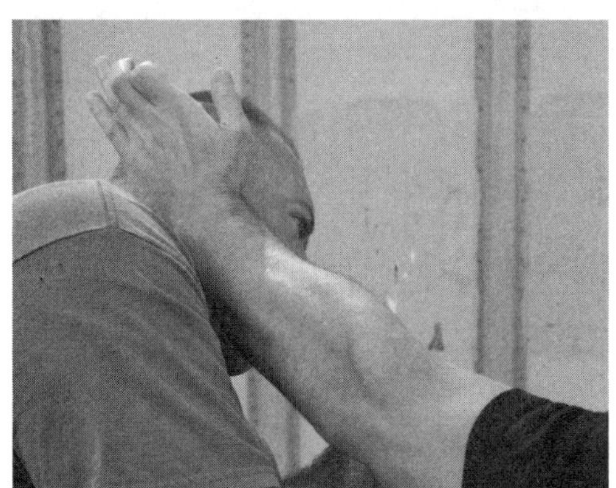

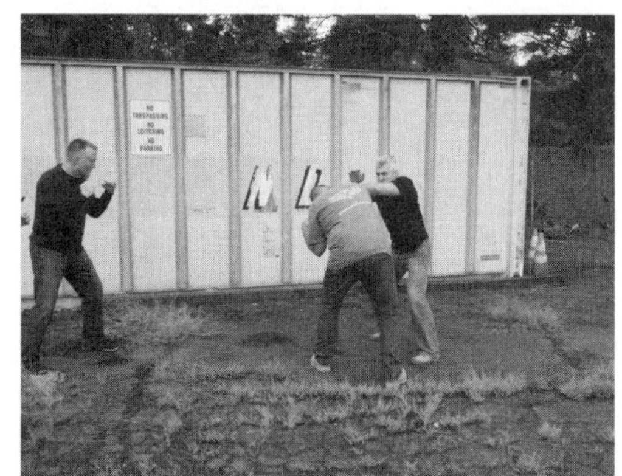

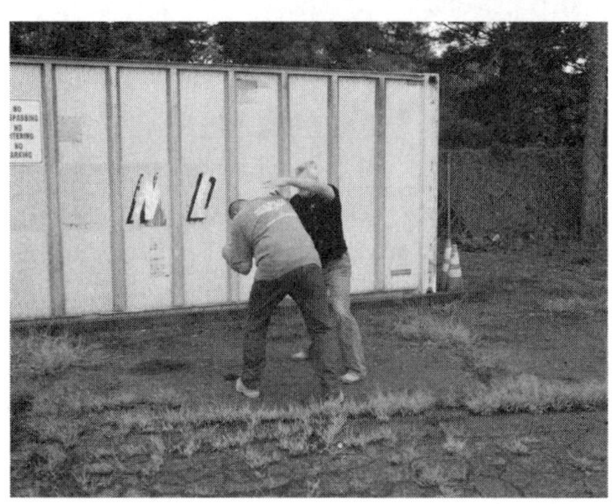

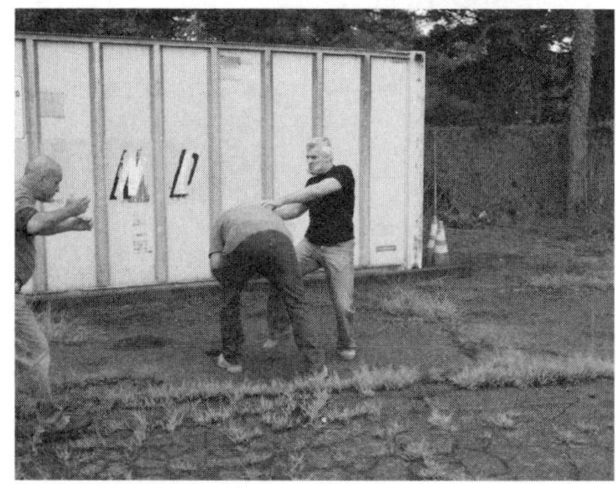

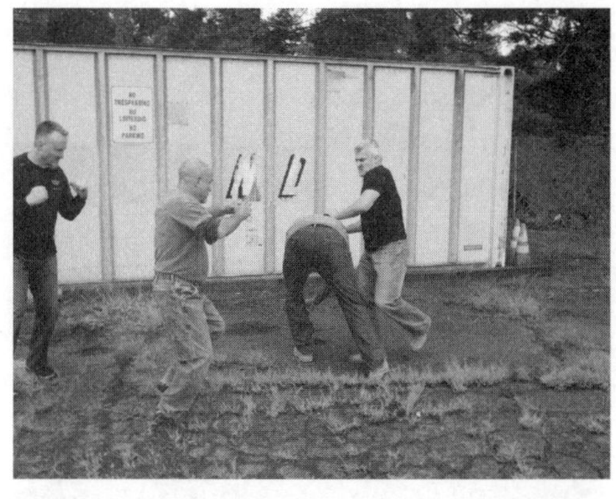

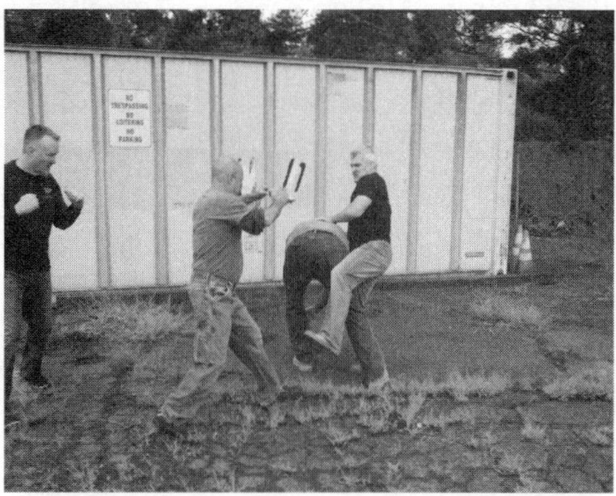

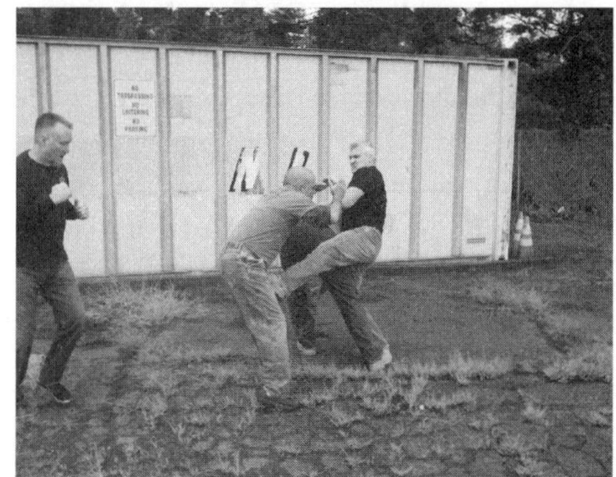

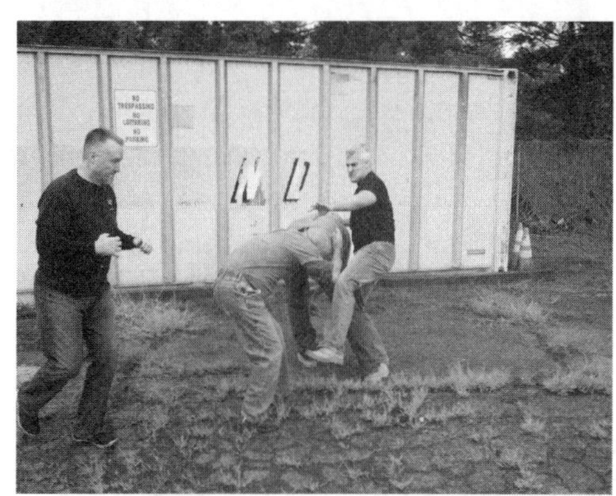

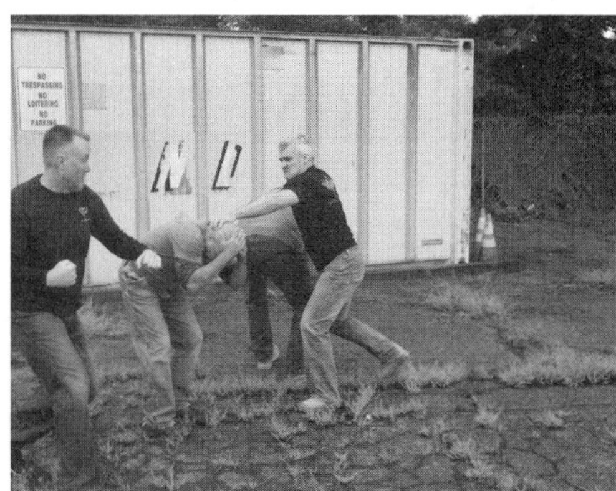

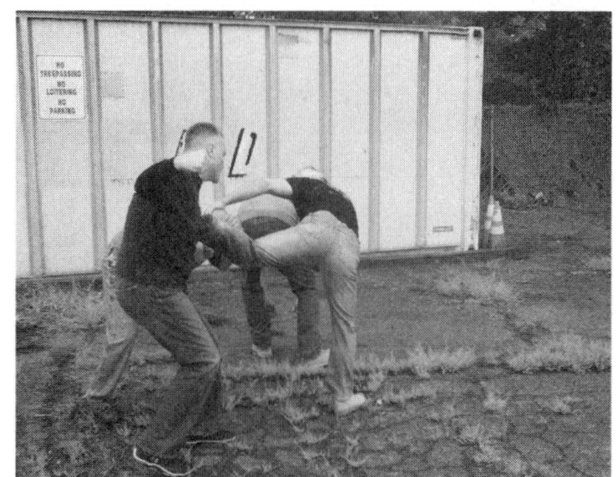

This series represents defending against three assailants. Strategy dictates you do everything you can to neither end up in the middle of active multiple assailants nor simultaneously engage more than two assailants. Preemptive long-range debilitating kicks and flanking movements (when possible) are usually the key.

Having a skilled group of attackers lined up is fleeting, so you've got to make every combative count (the essence of all krav maga strategy). You must also be aware of tunnel vision and those seeking to flank you for an ambush or blindside attack.

As with any fight, it is paramount that you keep moving. Do not give the assailants a stationary target or any opportunity to coordinate their attack. The key to fighting multiple armed and unarmed adversaries is to neutralize one threat at a time, moving brutally and efficiently, when possible, to the deadside of one of the opponents. Remain mobile and moving on the balls of your feet to prevent becoming a stationary target so that you are able to administer debilitating combatives whenever and however you can while not spending any longer than necessary hobbling and disabling a single opponent.

The deadside often provides you with a decisive tactical advantage. In select circumstances, you may have to go through them (see anti-group elbow strike #10 in *Krav Maga Combatives*). This strategy should revolve around your capabilities and preferred tactics involving long, medium, and short combatives combined with evasive maneuvers. Positioning becomes even more important when facing multiple assailants. Inexperienced assailants will often and fortunately group together. If you use correct tactical positioning (seldom if ever between two assailants), you limit the assailants' abilities to harm you.

There is a limitation on how many assailants can occupy the same space to get at you. It bears repeating that when facing multiple attackers, engage only one threat at a time, using combined optimum combatives and movement, forcing the closest attacker between you and any others. Once superior position is achieved, the opponent will have minimal ability to defend or to counter your retzev attack. Remember, retzev, because it uses all parts of your body and incorporates multiple facets of fighting, provides an overwhelming counterattack. The simple fact is you must take out each adversary ruthlessly with whatever vulnerable anatomical targets you can target.

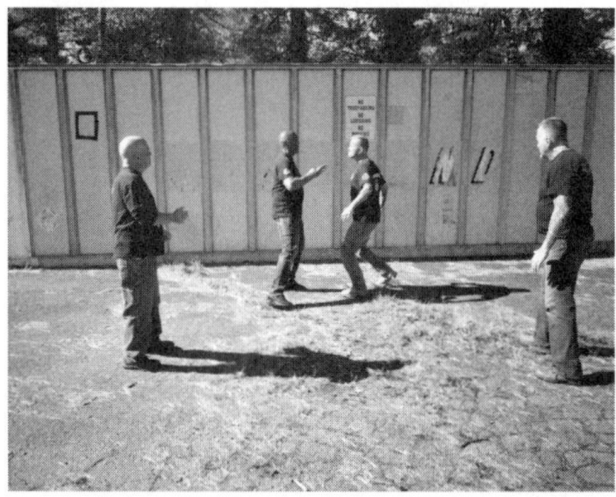

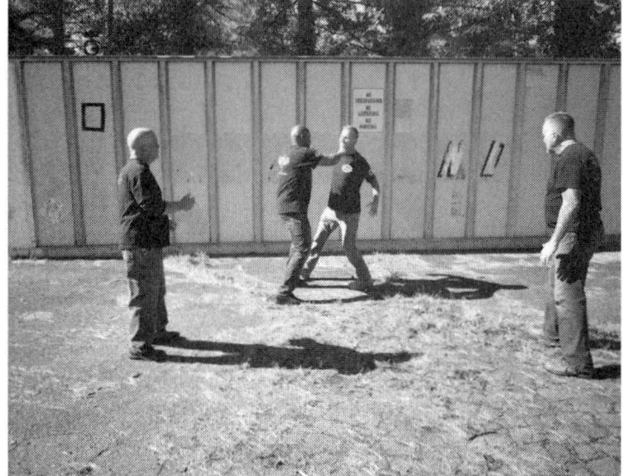

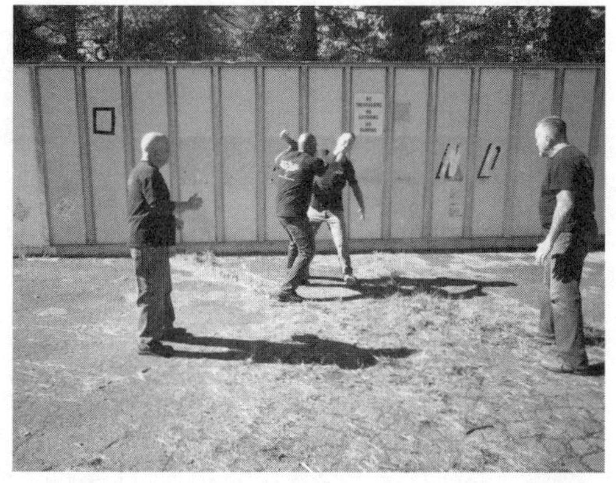

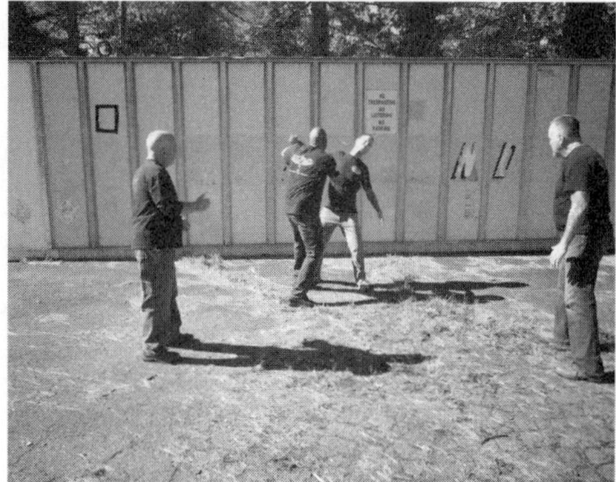

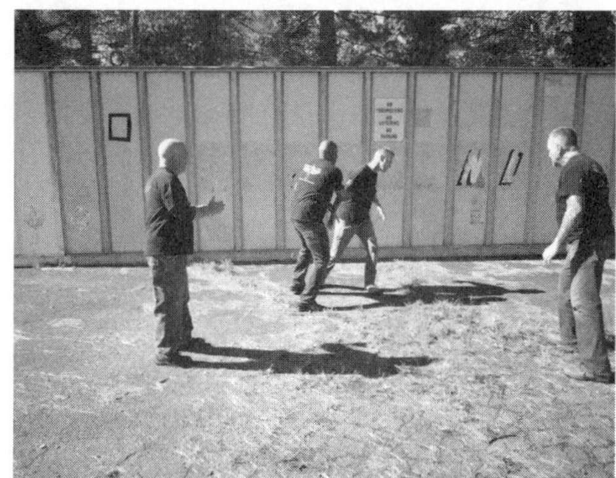

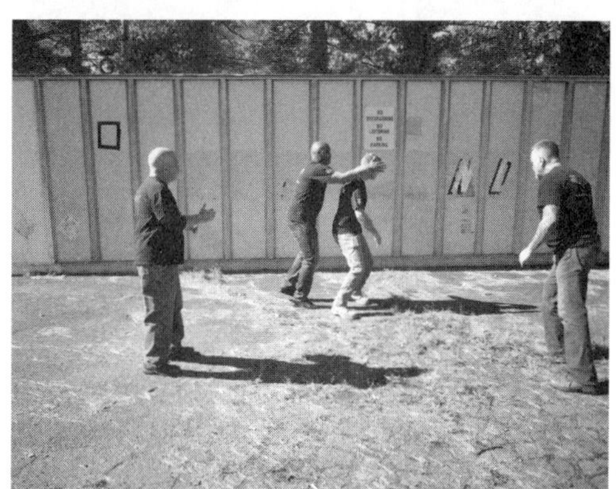

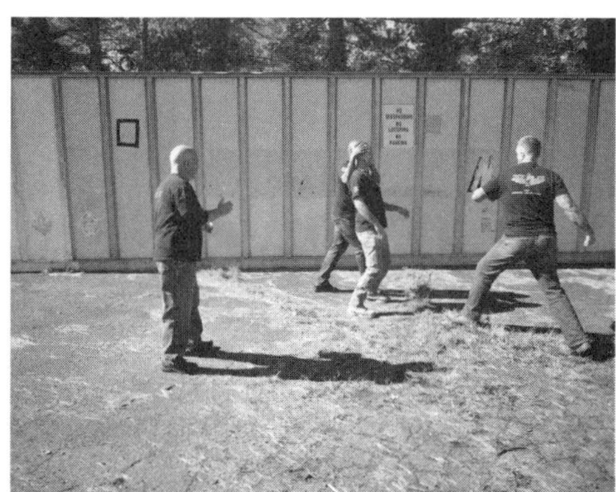

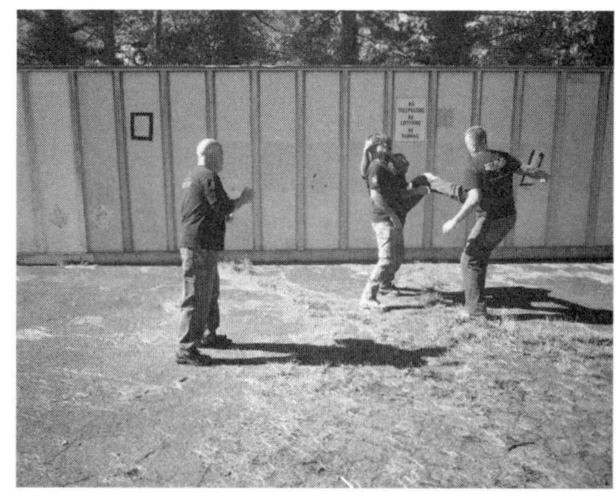

series continued on next page ...

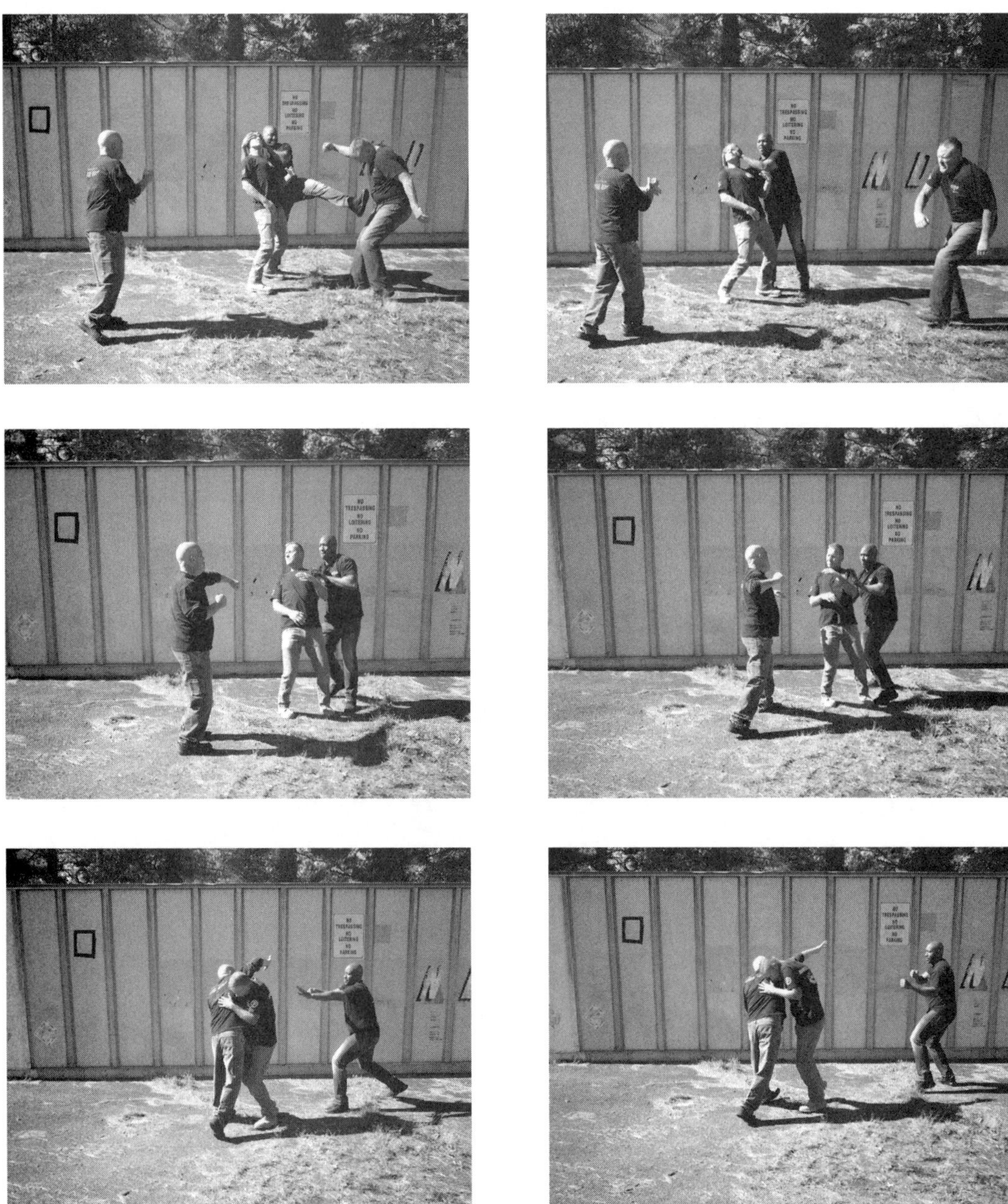

This series again represents defending against three assailants. Strategy dictates you do everything you can to neither end up in the middle of multiple assailants nor engage more than one assailant at a time. Stunning and spinning one attacker to face the next attacker is a highly effective maneuver allowing for long-range debilitating kicks while providing a shield between the defender and other attackers.

On-the-Ground Strategy against Multiple Assailants

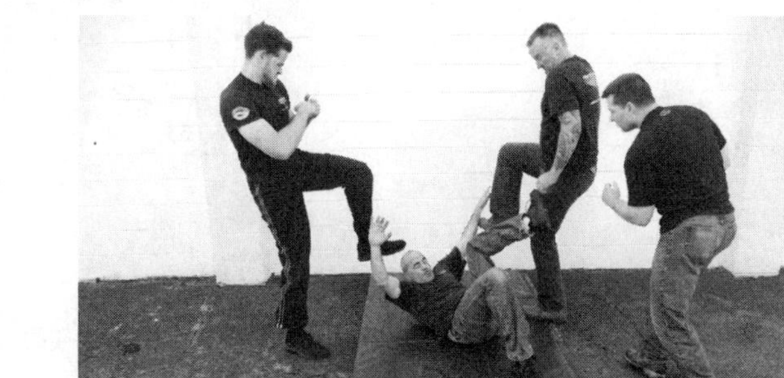

This photo represents the danger of being stomped by multiple assailants. Strategy: do everything possible to avoid going to the ground. Remember, a fight does not have to end up on the ground if you know how to prevent being grabbed or entangled.

As noted, you do not want to be on the ground *at any time* if you can help it, particularly against multiple assailants who are likely to stomp you. The dangers cannot be overstated, which is why your standup tactics must be optimized. If you cannot fight one person well, you will almost certainly not contend against three people well. Herein lies the danger in ground survival systems that assume going to the ground is a *sine qua non*.

Additional information on defending against multiple attackers is also available in *Krav Maga Professional Tactics* (YMAA 2016), chapter 7.

Counterattack Strategy: Lower-body and Upper-body Ranges

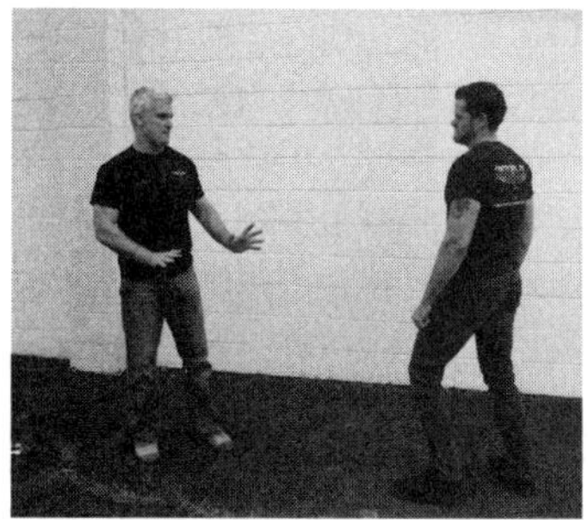

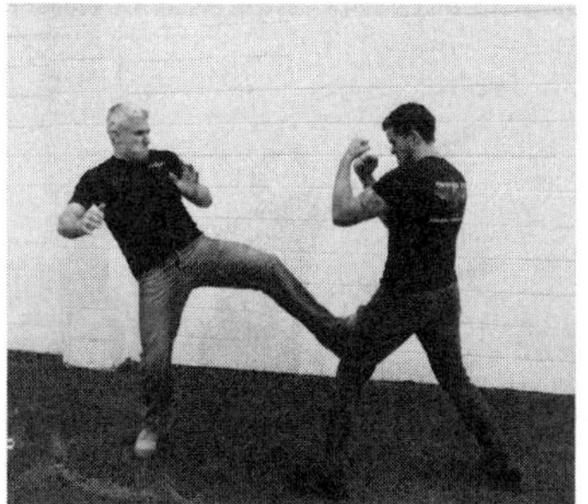

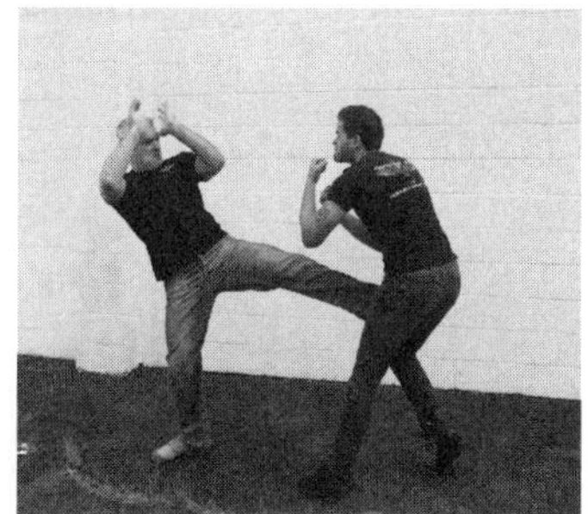

This is an example of a long-range preemptive straight kick against any type of upper-body threat or attack. Note the strategy here: the defender has already made up his mind to deliver a debilitating straight kick no matter what the attacker does. In other words, this combative will work against any type of menacing encroachment or attack.

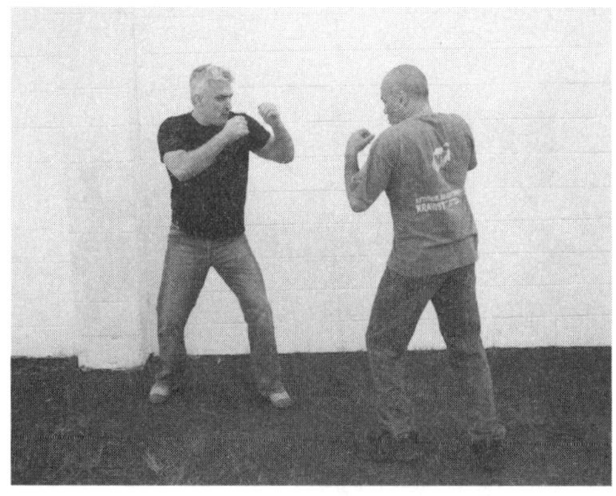
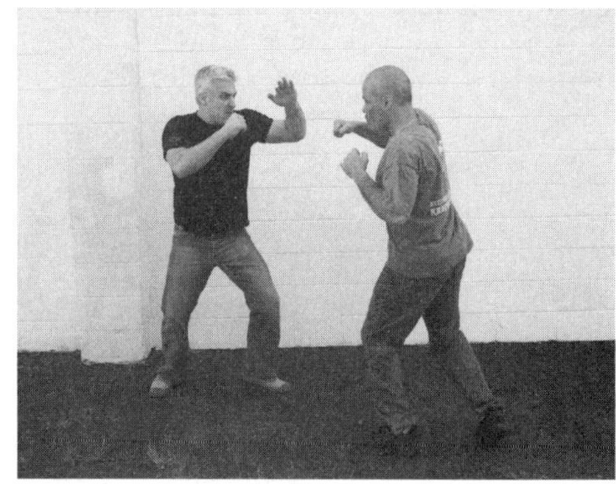
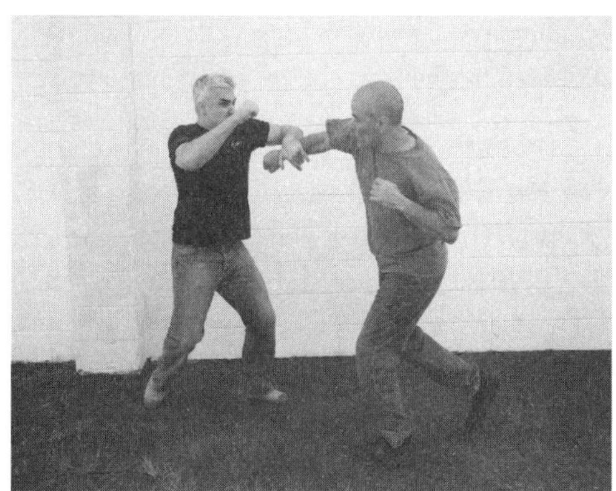
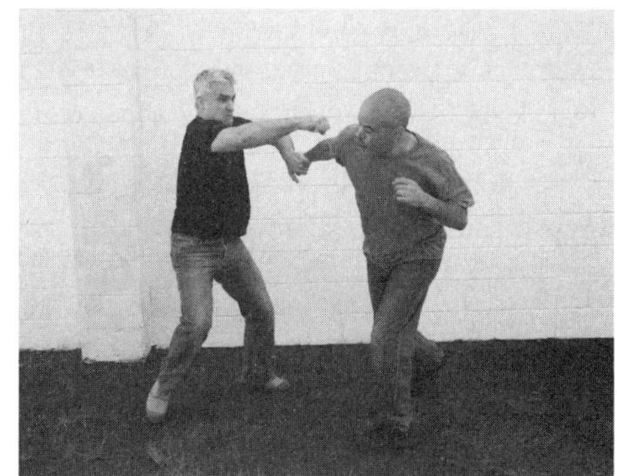
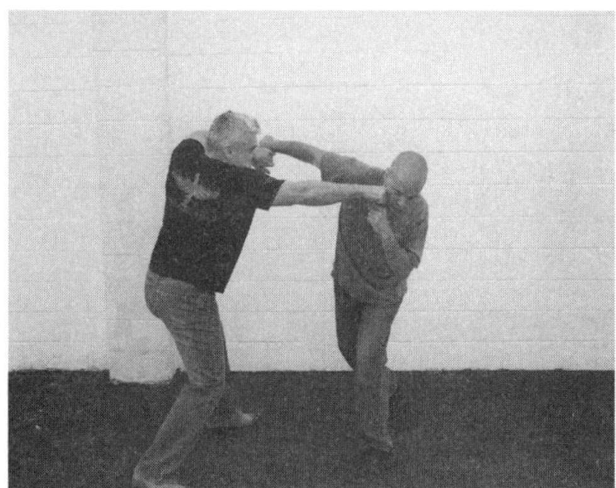

This series represents using a medium-range straight punch hand-scoop defense while stepping away from the attack. As you step off the line, deliver a near-simultaneous straight counterpunch.

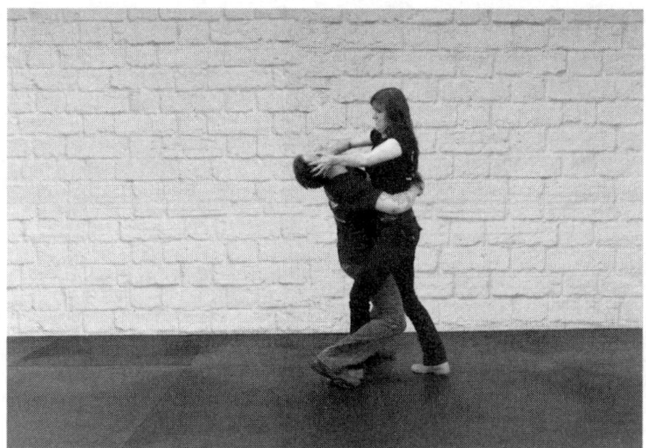

This is an example of a grappling-range double-eye-gouge defense against a frontal bearhug when your arms are free.

One of the most important aspects of winning a violent confrontation is range: the proximity of the attacker and defender. Range and evasive body defenses are integral parts of any fight strategy. Related to this is the time-distance connection between the attacker and defender that affects the action-reaction cycle. Some essential concepts regarding attack distance:

- Understanding defensive reaction time against long-distance attacks and against short-distance attacks is crucial to understanding the reactionary response deficit (action trumps reaction). Keep in mind that an attack can be launched and reach a target in under one second. The following attack speed/time-lapse observations were made by the Federal Law Enforcement Training Center in conjuction with Bruce K. Siddle's research:
    - — An attacker can launch straight punch to the head from passive stance in as little as 1/10 of a second.
    - — An attacker can launch a straight punch to the torso from a passive stance in as little as 6/100 of a second.
- The distance principle: any attack from a close enough range might reach a target regardless of how fast one can parry, block, or possibly evade. Again, action beats reaction.
- If defenders can control distance and position while improving their body position for counterattack, they stand a good chance of prevailing in an unavoidable violent encounter.
- Dominate the violent encounter by controlling the attacker's distance and position along with tactical targeting.

Tactical Footwork and Body Positioning Strategies

During the course of our training, we had the great opportunity to work with the United States Secret Service Academy instructors, all consummate professionals. In discussing best defensive-tactics theory and practices, I had the chance to ask M., the lead USSS instructor (one of the most insightful, capable, and experienced instructors I've ever had the honor of meeting) what he thought was the most important factor for a successful outcome in physical confrontation. In a word, M. deftly answered: positioning. I could not agree more. Your strategic positioning in a violent conflict is overwhelmingly the deciding factor. Positioning while standing is obviously dictated by footwork, while positioning on the ground is often dictated by your hips. In any position, you must do your best to protect your vital anatomy. Once again, whenever possible, krav maga emphasizes moving to an attacker's deadside.

A few notes on footwork:

- Correct footwork allows you to push off both balls of your feet and land on the opposite ball of your stepping foot (not your heel). Do not telegraph your movement by needlessly shifting your weight onto your supporting leg in preparation for your stepping leg, thereby moving your body away from the direction you intend to go. Remain light on the balls of your feet (your metatarsals) at all times.
- Sound footwork allows you to flank or circle an opponent and avoid being a static target. You can move forward and laterally more quickly than your opponent can move to the rear (or laterally to the rear), and moving in this way keeps you off his line of attack.
- Forward and backward shuffling footwork is a highly effective tactic that enables you to maintain your fighting stance when moving in and out and around your adversary.
- A tai sabaki (semi-circular) step is generally one of the quickest footwork techniques to change an angle toward an adversary, get off the line of a linear attack, or take an adversary down with a joint lock.
- Using good footwork to stay in combat motion disguises your strikes.

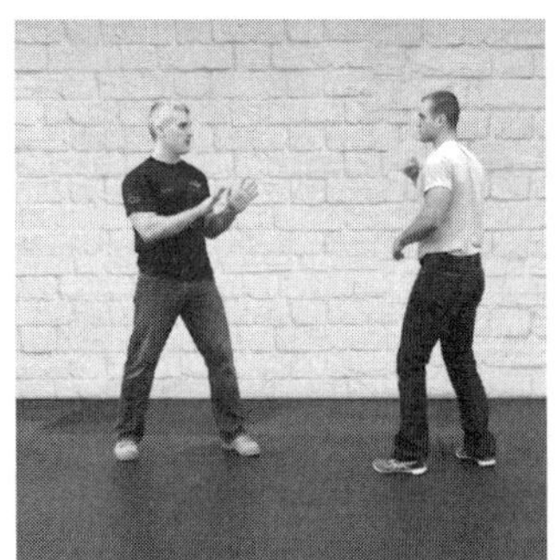
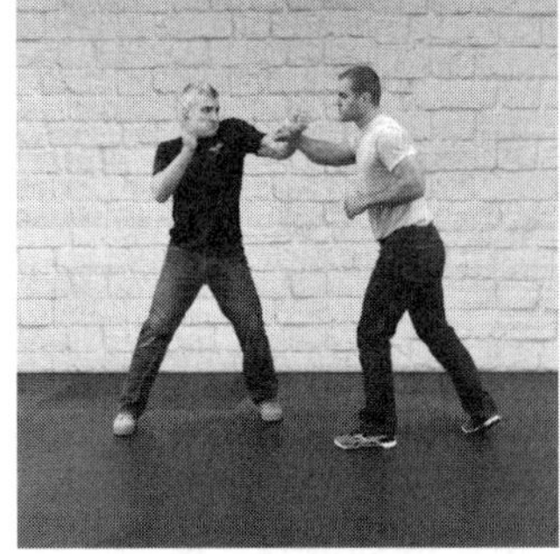
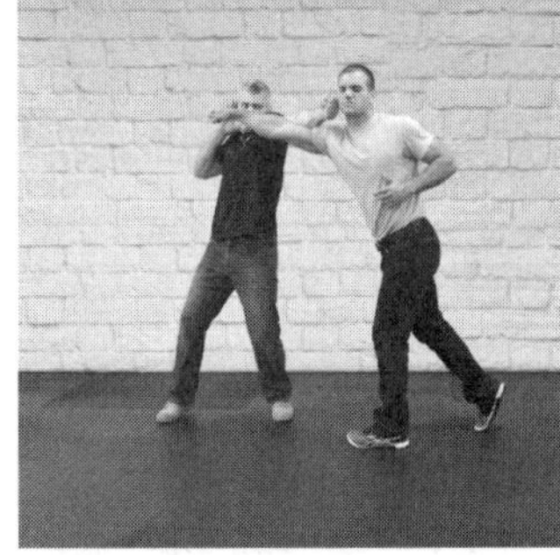

This series represents defending a straight punch by stepping off the line attack combined with an over-the-top counterpunch.

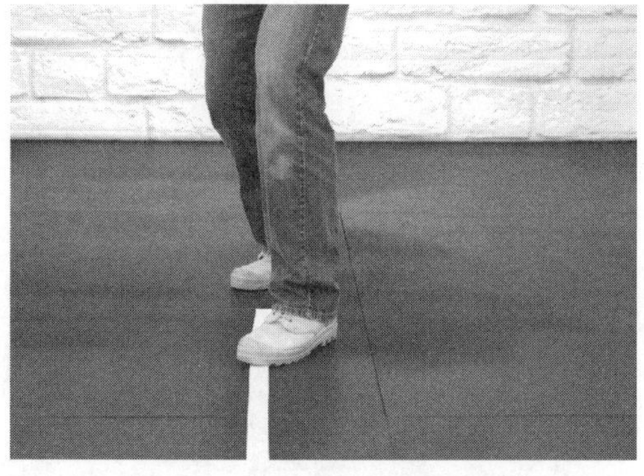

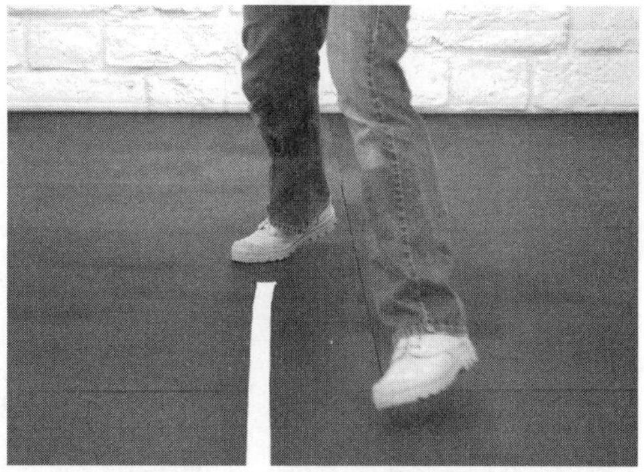

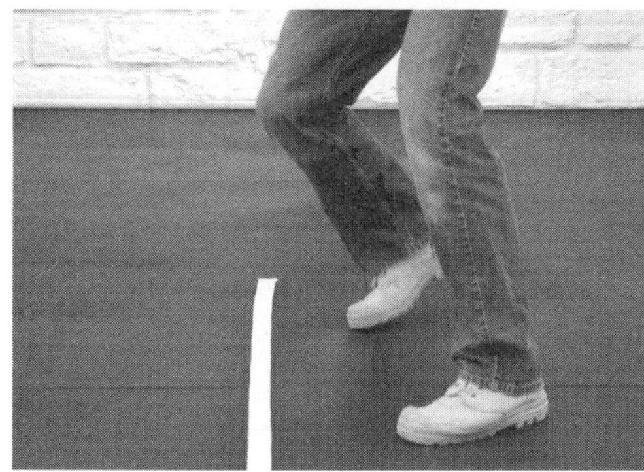

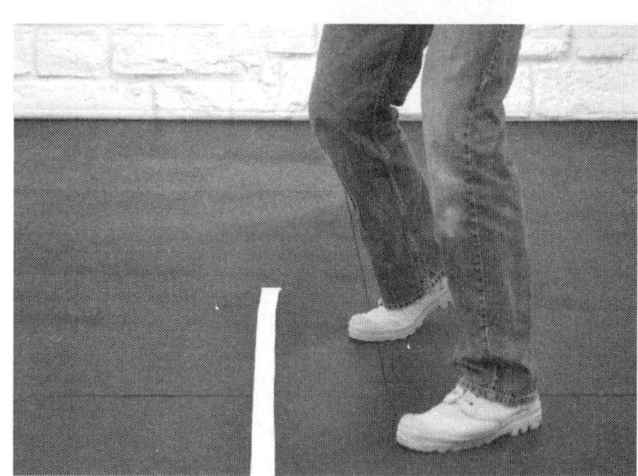

Representative footwork in stepping off the line of attack.

Note the footwork, stepping off the line of attack, for this over-the-top counterpunch defense against a straight punch.

Krav maga recognizes that training time is usually at a premium. This was Imi's underlying premise and his mandate in creating the Israel Defense Force's military krav maga program. A few core expandable tactics applicable to the most common scenarios had to be developed, tactics that could be instinctively harnessed and used on the battlefield. In a civilian setting when we have little time to train students who may not have the benefit of future krav maga training, we take the same approach (though, importantly, with non-lethal emphasis). As an example, the following defense was developed for the law enforcement community and civilians who have limited training time.

This representative tactic is for those who must master just a few tactical movements that can defeat a myriad of upper-body attacks, including straight and hook punches along with pushes—three of the most common physical assaults. Notably, this tactic will work against any linear attack, including straight kicks from either leg, provided you move off the straight line of attack. The defense takes into account that 85 percent or more of the world's population is right-side dominant. Therefore, the majority of attackers will use the right arm to initiate an assault. You will step off the line of attack one way and one way only at approximately a 45 degree angle while delivering a simultaneous counterattack. Here are a few examples of the defense in action with counterattack options.

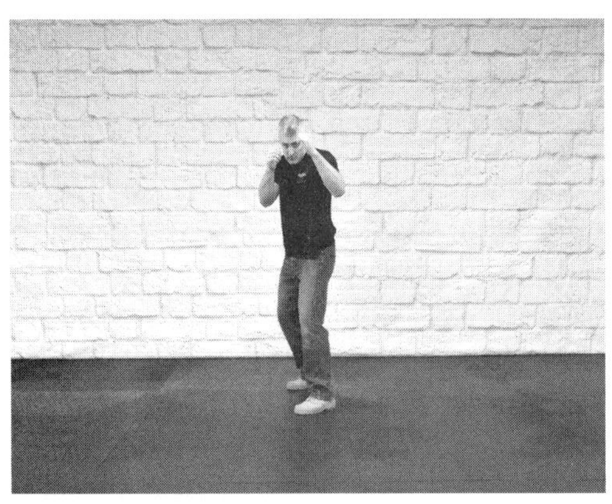
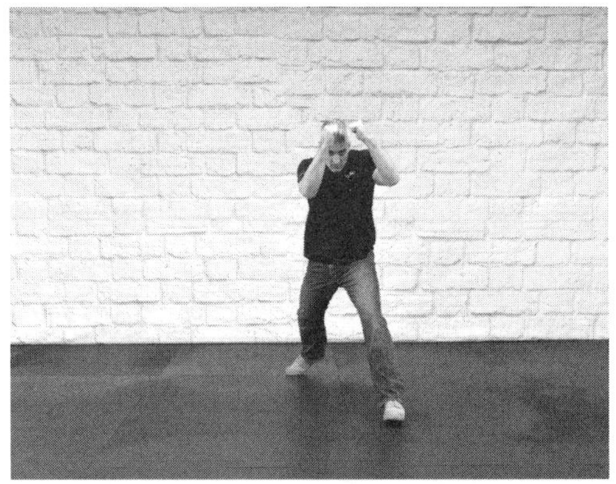
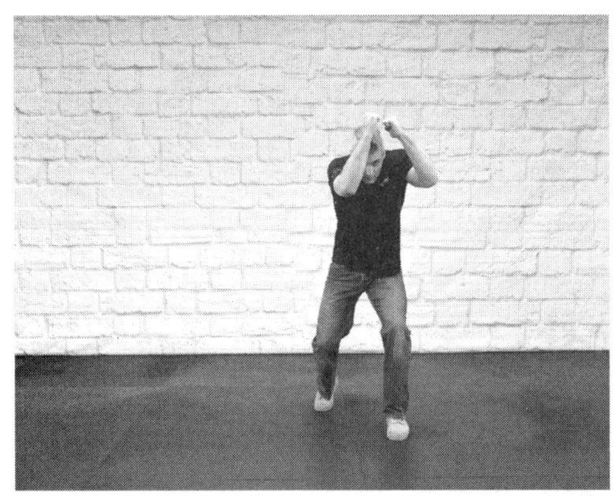
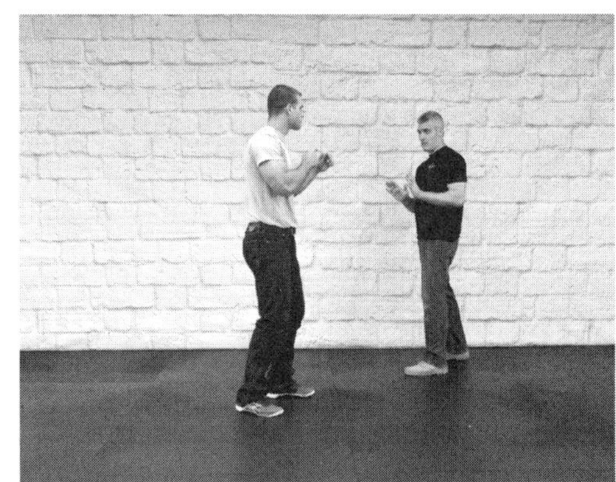
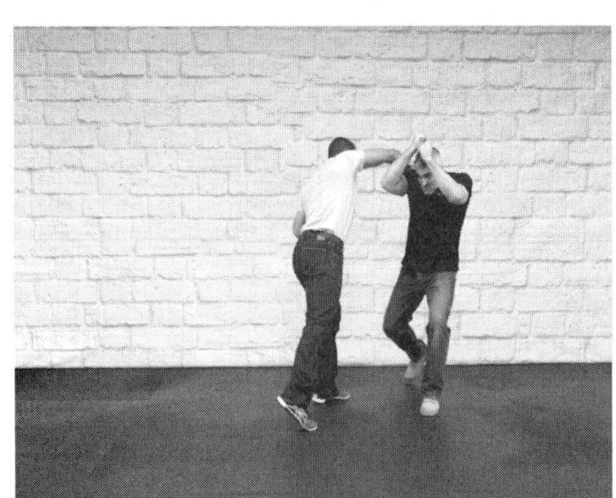
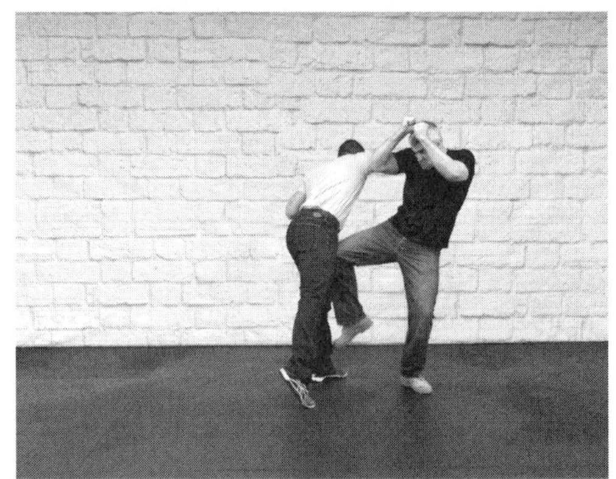

To thwart a straight right punch, take a 45-degree forward step to your left. As you step you will deliver a simultaneous knee counterattack with your rear leg. Move off the line attack with both feet. As you burst forward, raise your arms in a strong position with your forearms facing outward to serve as a defensive shield. The punch should glide off your nearside forearm. Note: by forcefully raising your arms, you will protect your head while also helping to generate forward momentum. Deliver a straight or modified straight knee to the attacker's groin or nearside thigh to debilitate him. Follow up with retzev combatives as necessary.

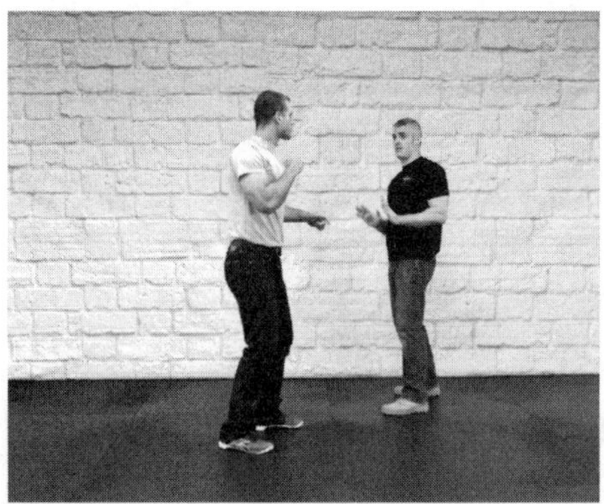

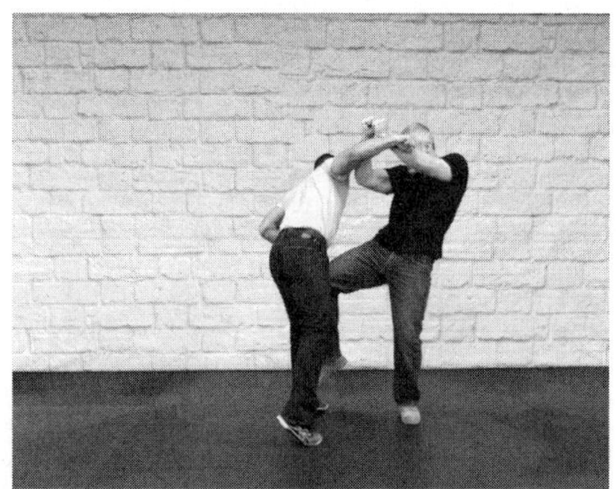

Against a right hook punch, once again step off the line of attack using a 45-degree angle forward step to your left. As you step, deliver a simultaneous knee counterattack to the attacker's groin. Be sure to move both of your feet off the line of attack. As you burst forward, raise your arms as a strong defensive shield to intercept the incoming punch. By raising your arms, you will protect your head while also helping to generate forward momentum.

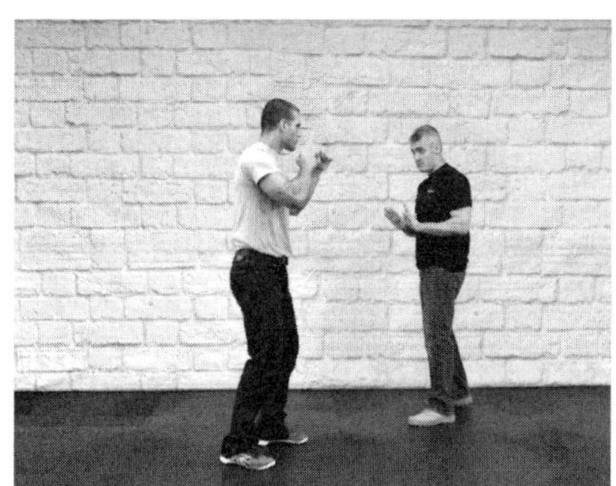

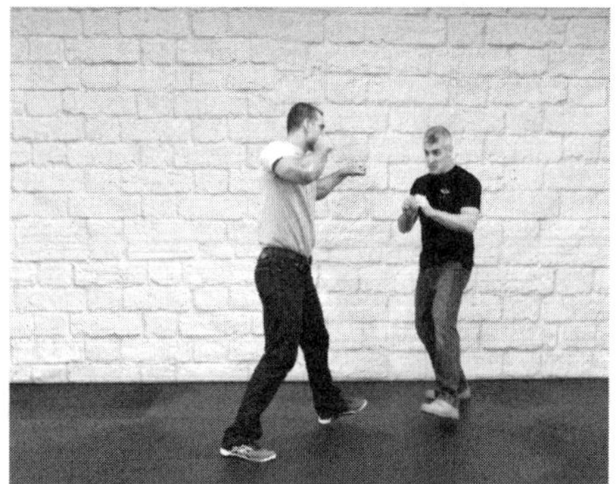

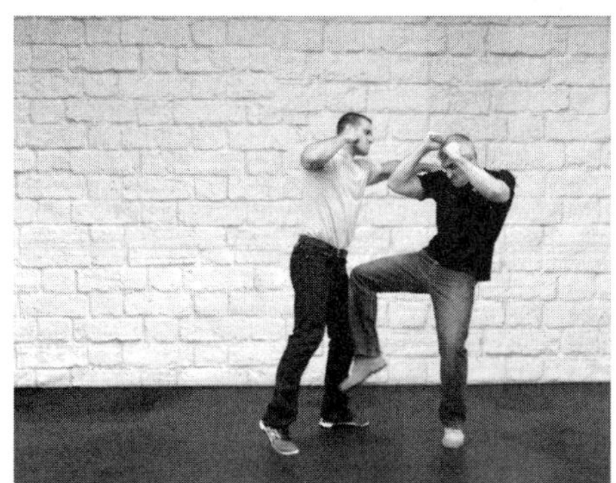

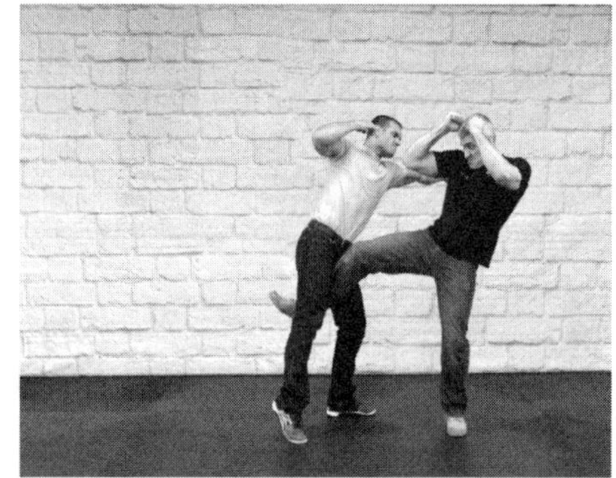

Against a left straight punch, step off the line of attack on a 45-degree angle to your left using a forward step while delivering a simultaneous straight-kick counterattack. Move with both feet to get off the line of attack. As you burst forward, raise your arms as a strong defensive shield. The punch should glide off your nearside arm. By raising your arms, you protect your head while also helping to generate forward momentum to step off the line of attack. Deliver a straight shin kick to the attacker's groin to debilitate him. Follow up with retzev combatives as necessary.

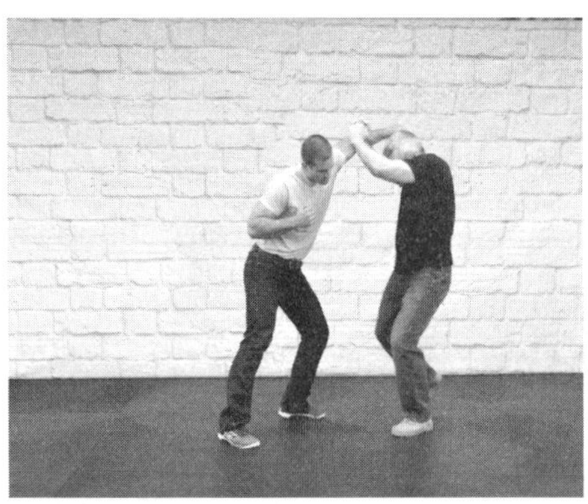

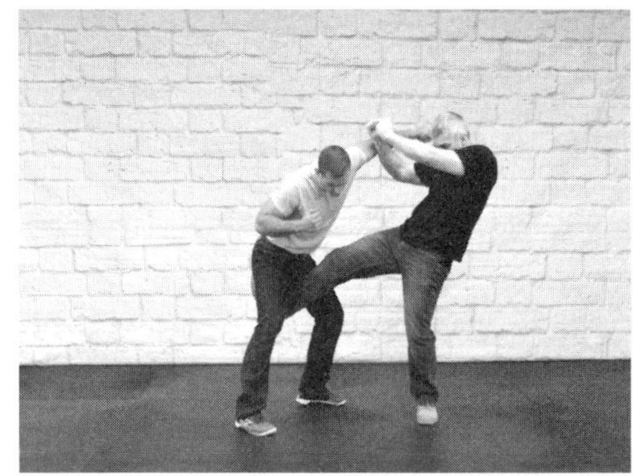

Against a left hook punch, again step forward off the line of attack on a 45-degree angle to your left. Deliver a straight shin kick to the attacker's groin to debilitate him. Follow up with retzev combatives as necessary.

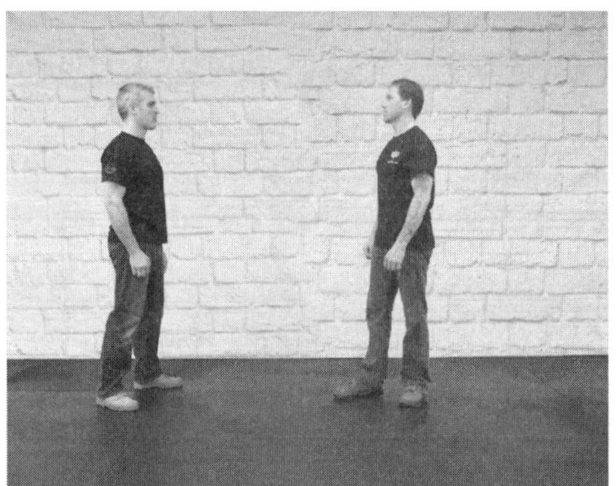

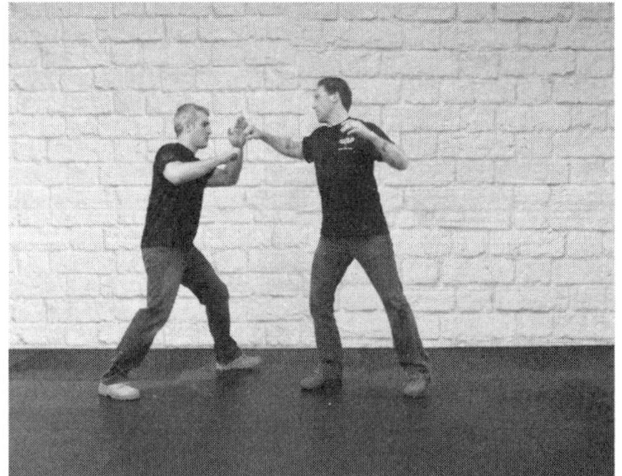

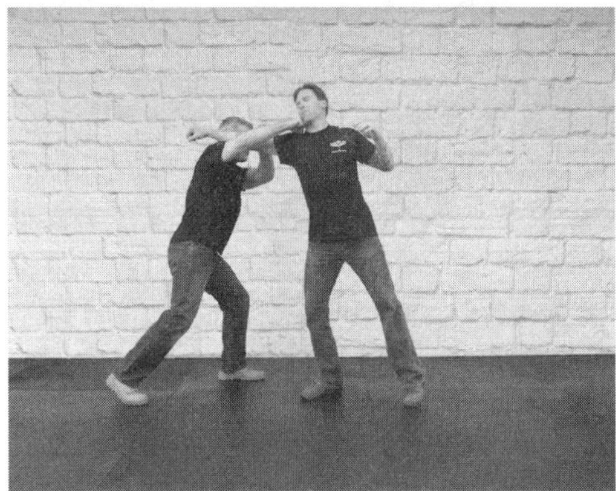

This series represents a combined sliding parry involving stepping off the line of attack against a straight punch.

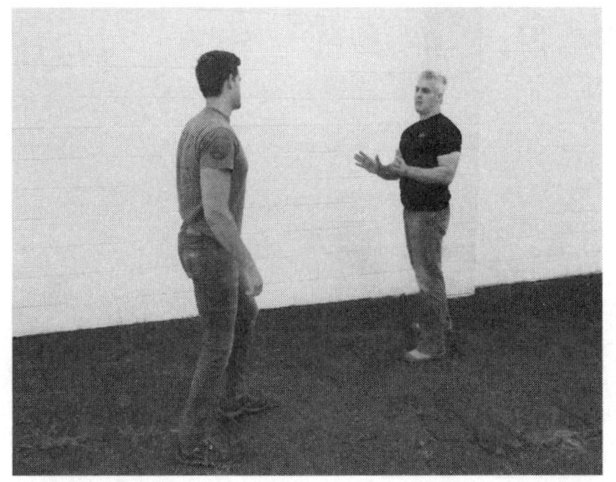

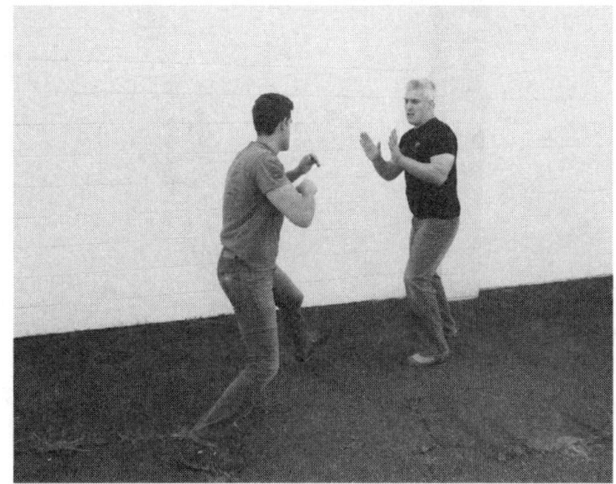

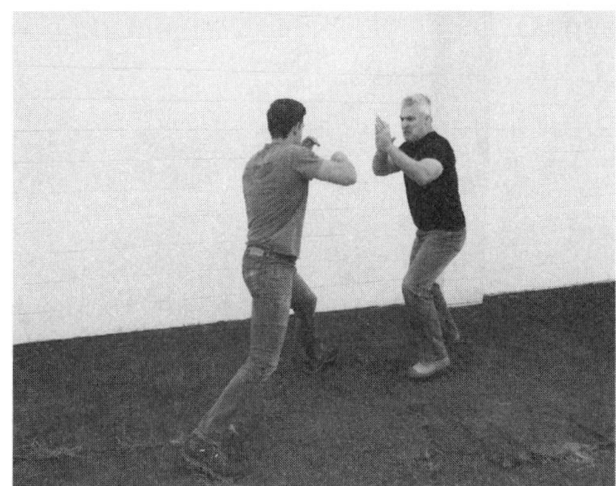

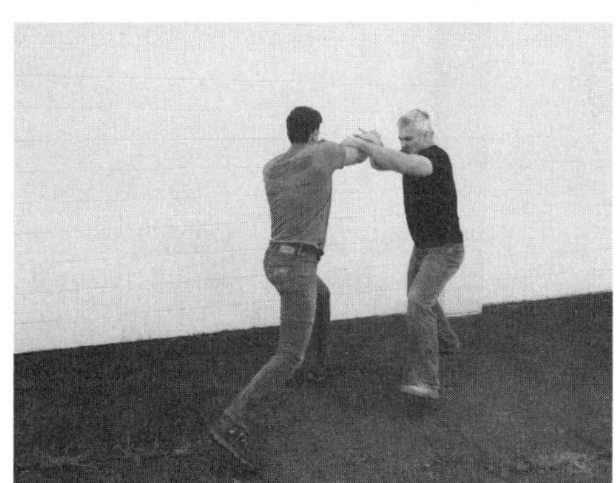

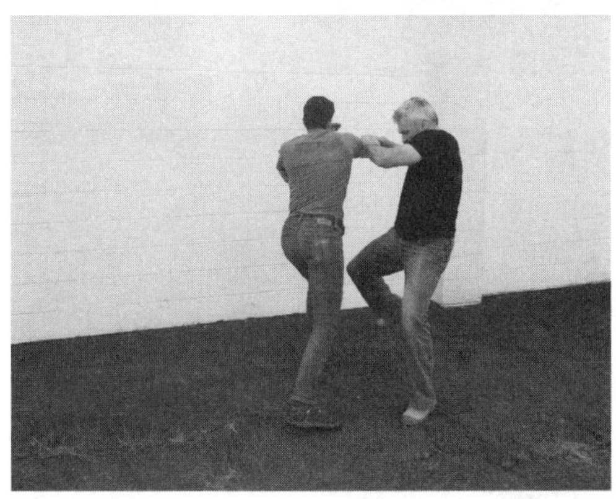

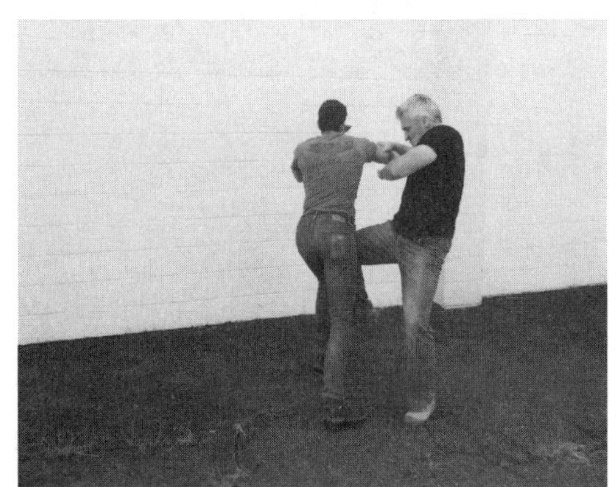

series continued on next page ...

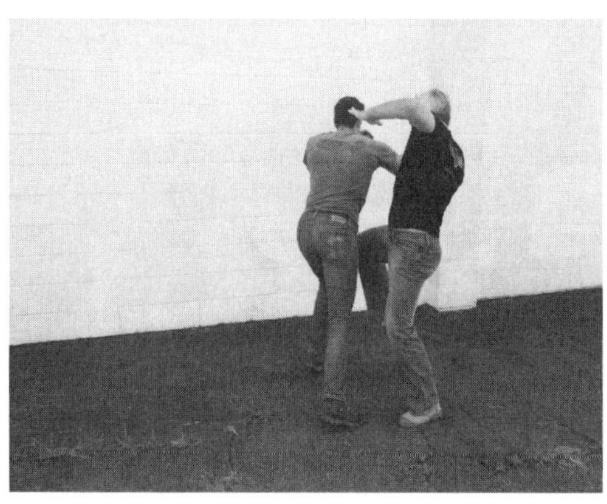

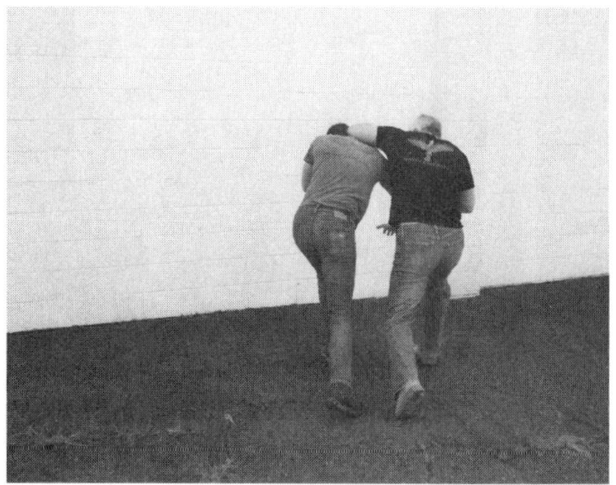

This series represents a combined, double-arm sliding parry against a straight punch accomplished by stepping off the line of attack combined with a knee strike.

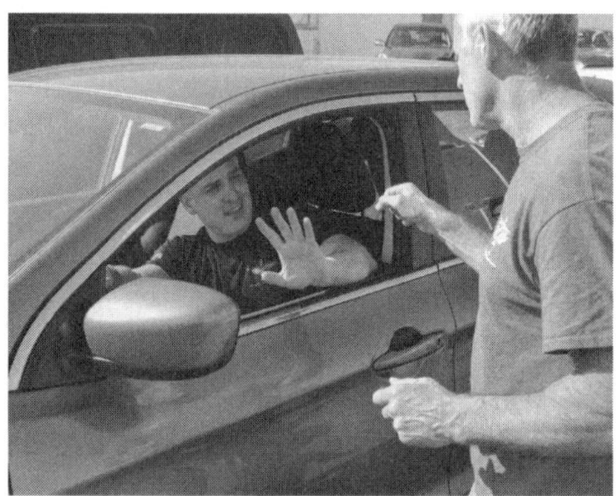

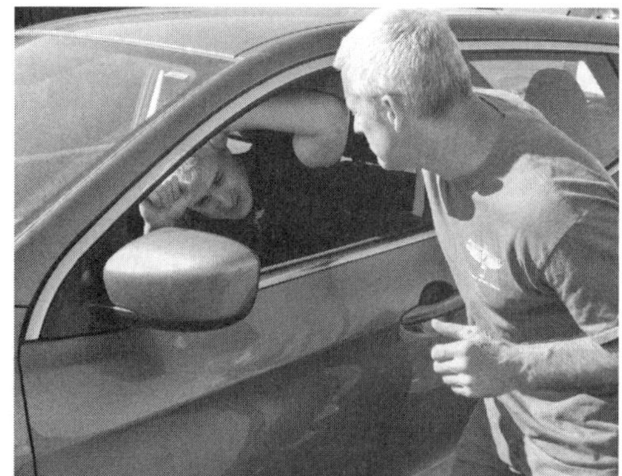

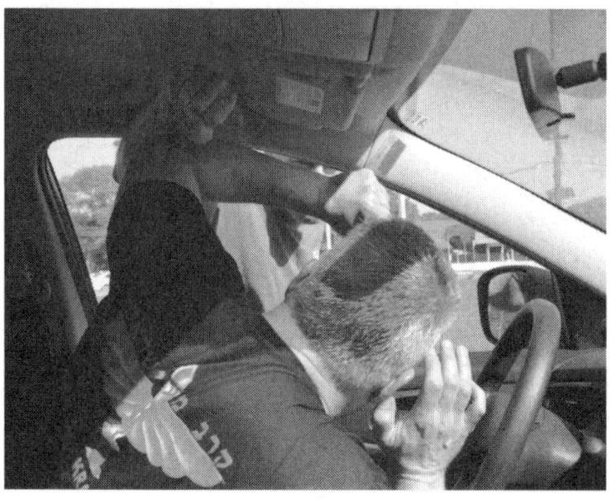

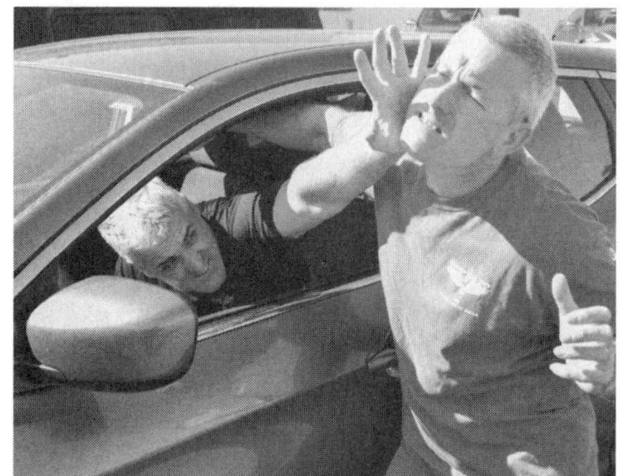

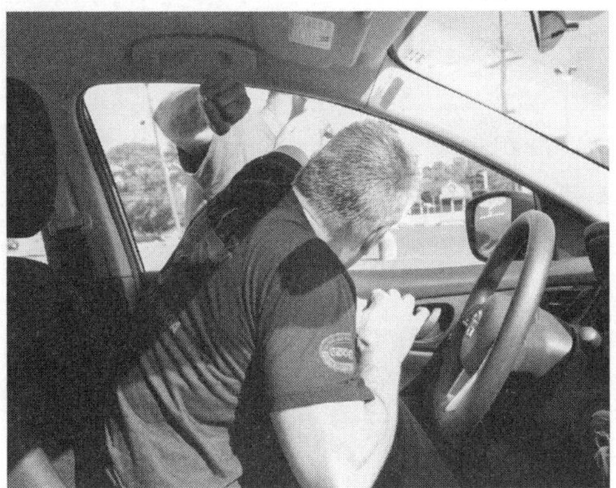

This series represents a combined body defense and arm deflection against a road-rage straight right punch followed by a same deflecting arm counterattack. Either exit the vehicle or drive away immediately to report the incident. Be aware that your seatbelt may restrict your movements, especially if it locks as a result of your abrupt defensive movements.

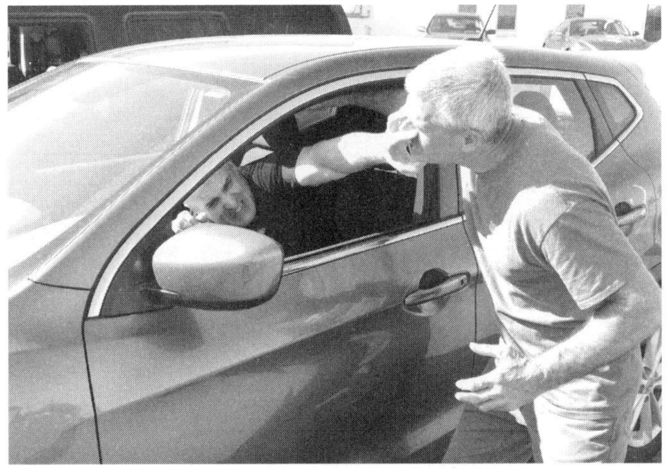

Here is an optional finger rake to the eyes (instead of a straight palm-heel strike as previously depicted).

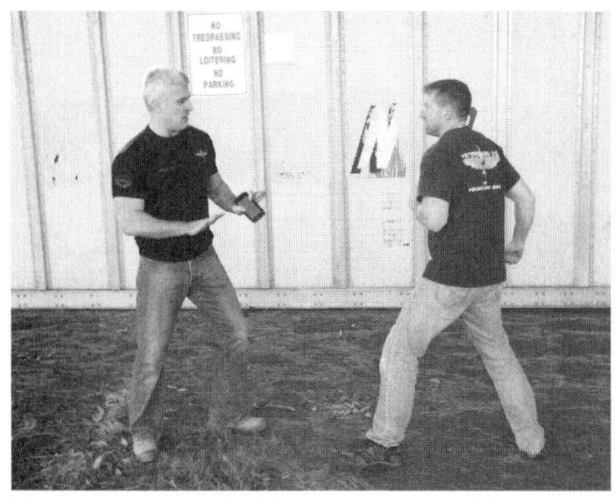

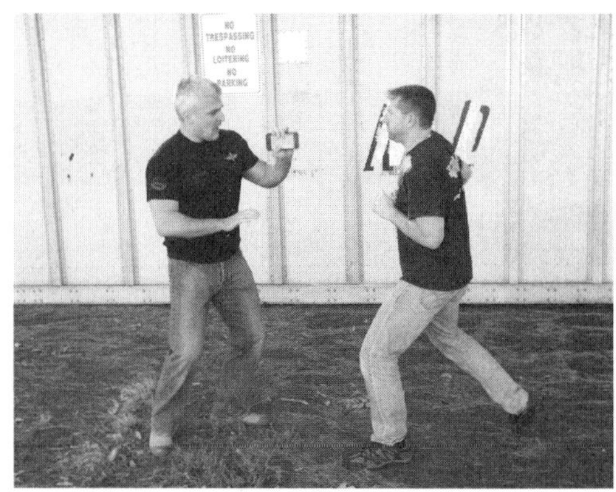

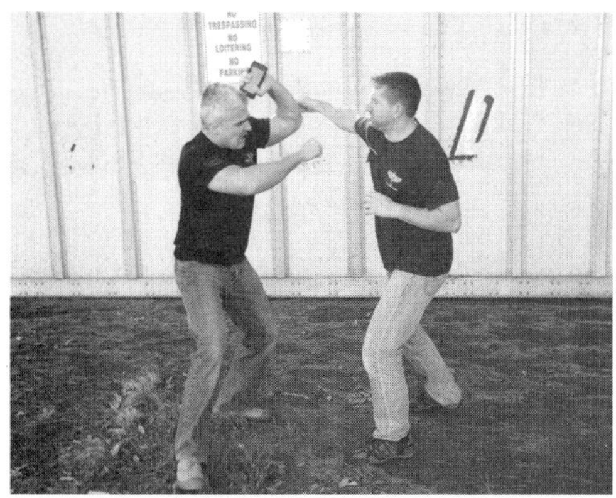

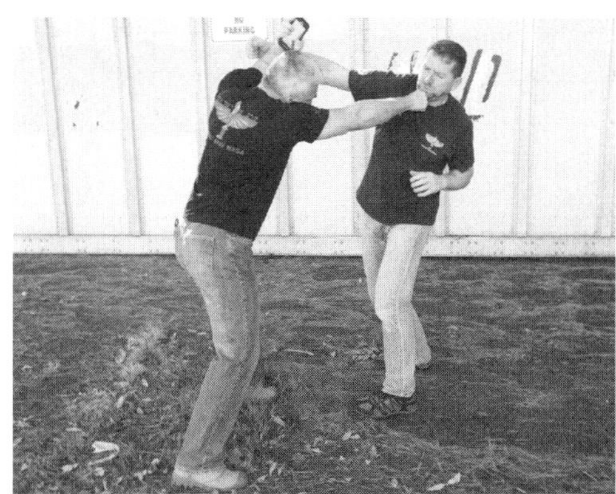

This series represents a hook punch gunting defense with a mobile device in hand accomplished by stepping off the line combined with a gunt defense and simultaneous counterpunch. Importantly, while you can step or burst directly into the punch, such a defense may fail against a stronger attacker with long arms.

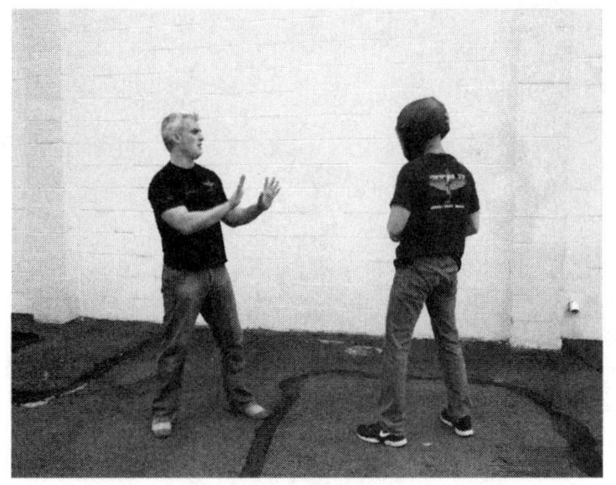

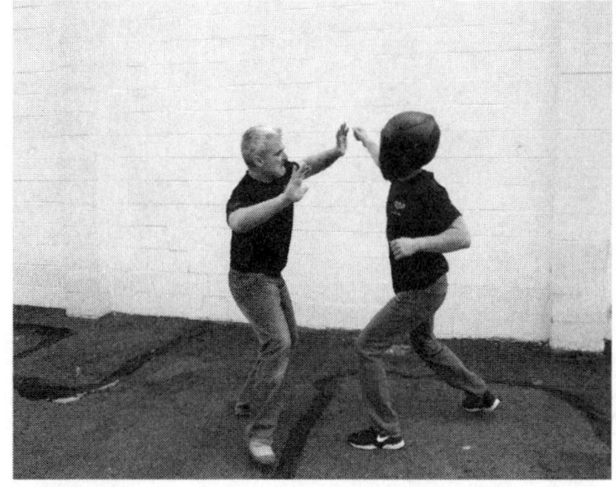

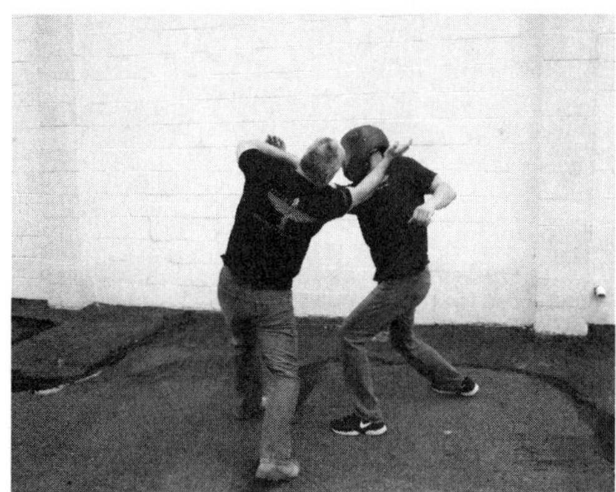

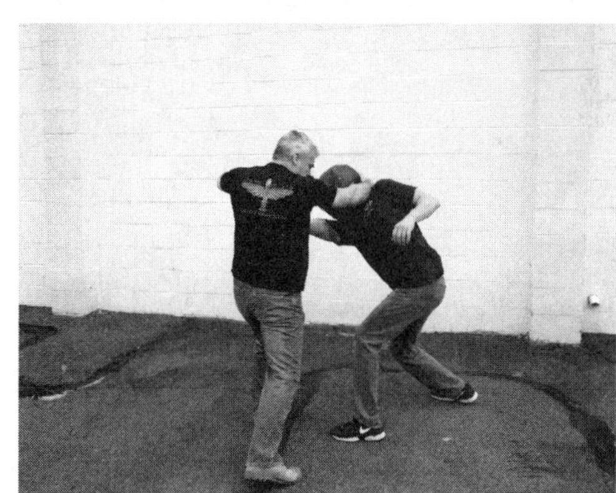

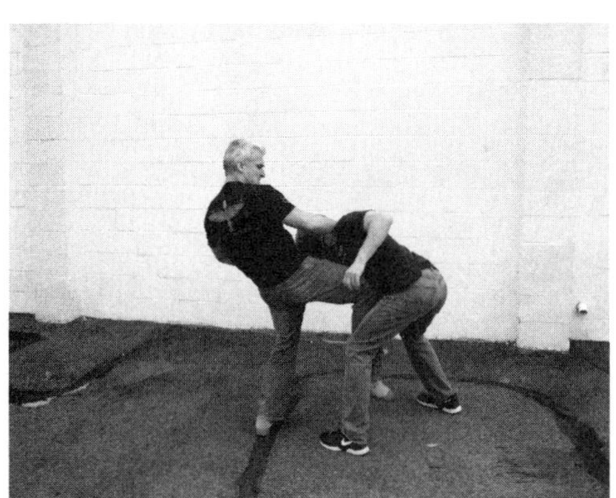

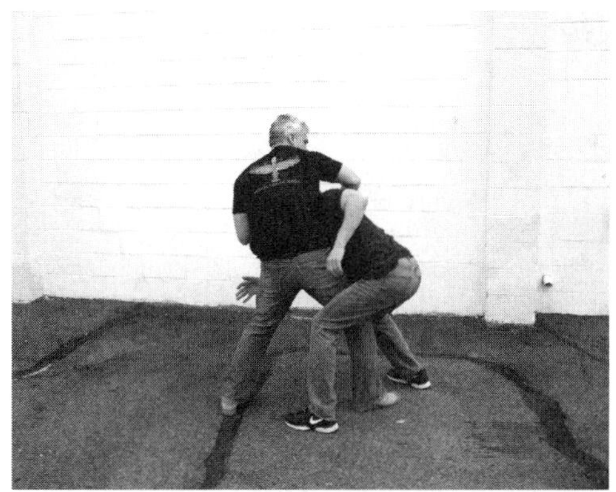

series continued on next page …

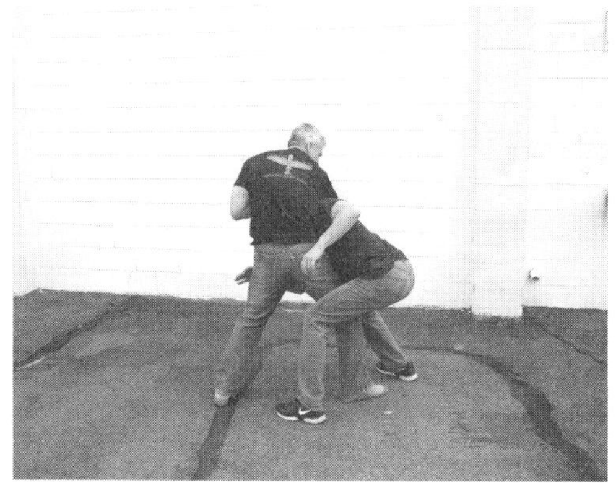

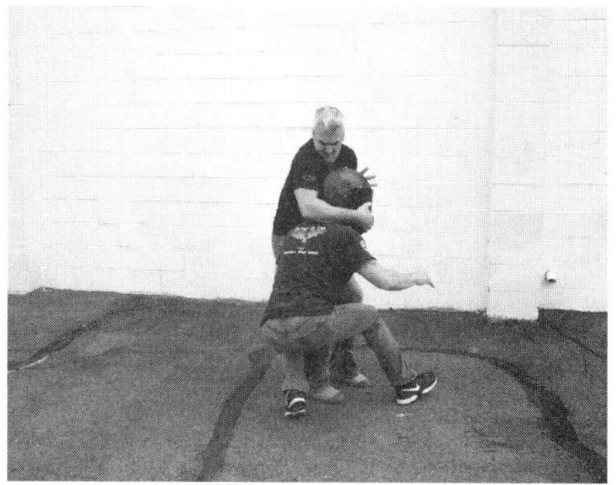

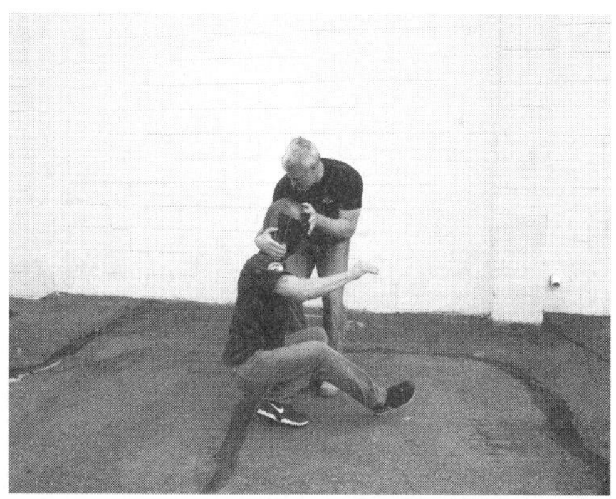

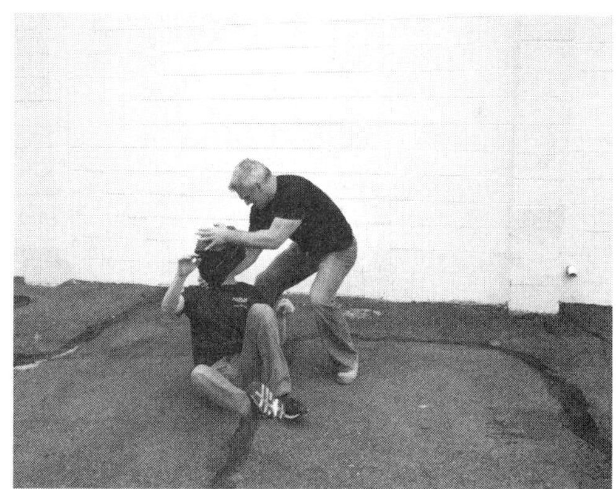

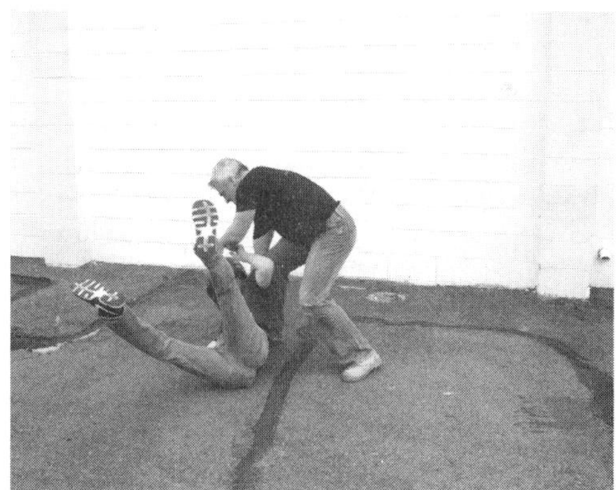

This series represents a hook punch defense accomplished by stepping off the line against a helmeted attacker combined with a chop, straight knee, and head-spin takedown counterattack. Note the footwork involved in stepping off the line of attack for this 360-degree outside defense against a hook punch. Importantly, while one can step or burst directly into the punch, such a defense may fail against a stronger attacker with long arms, and an inside chop counterattack is more difficult.

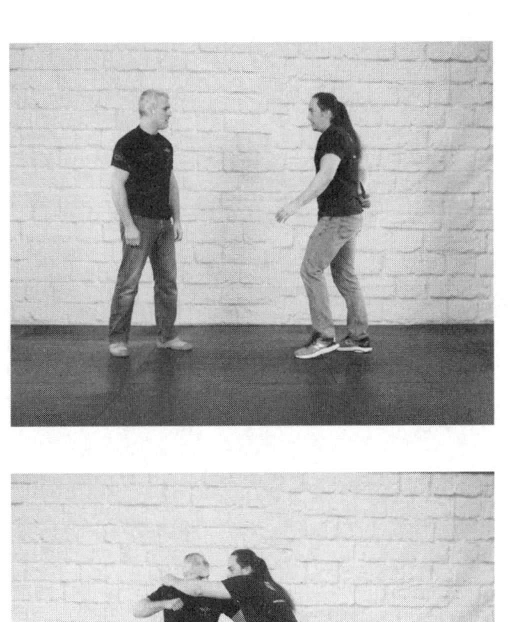

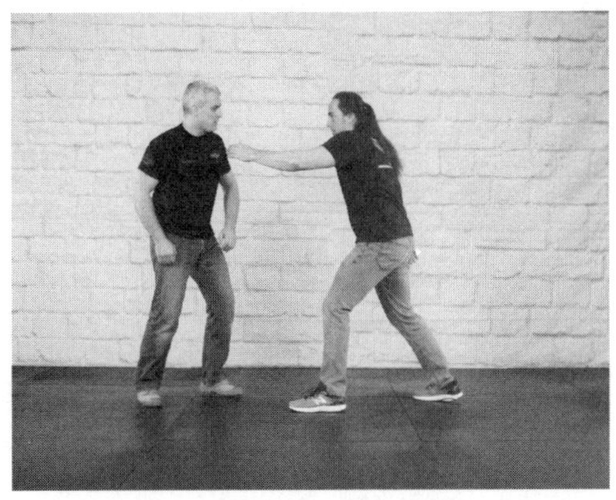

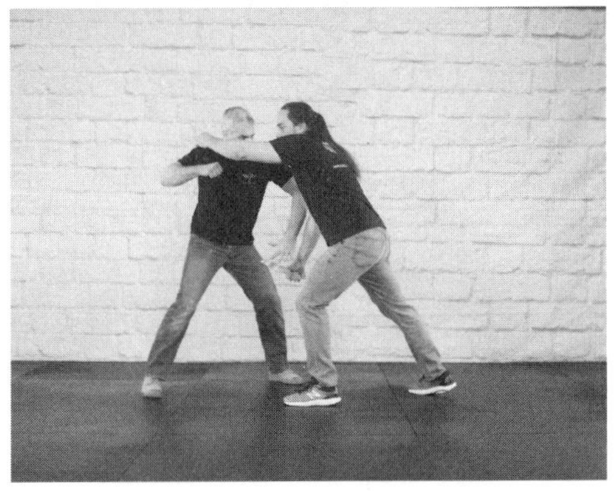

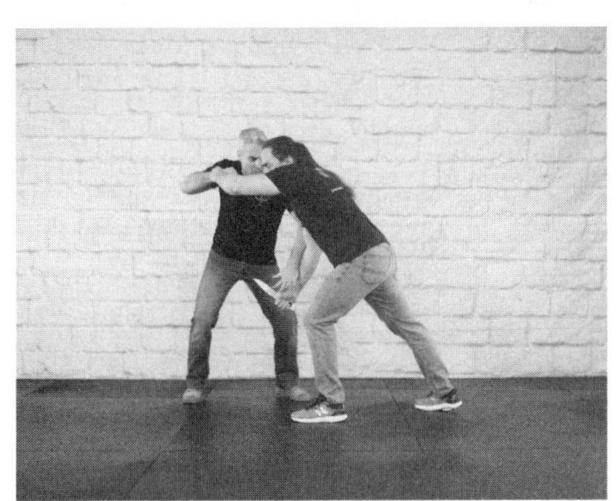

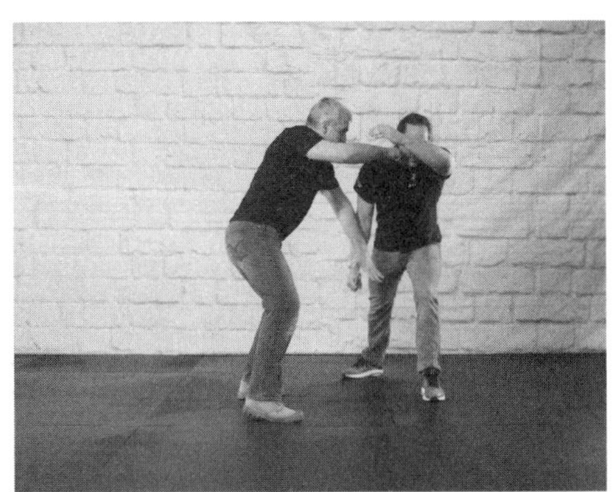

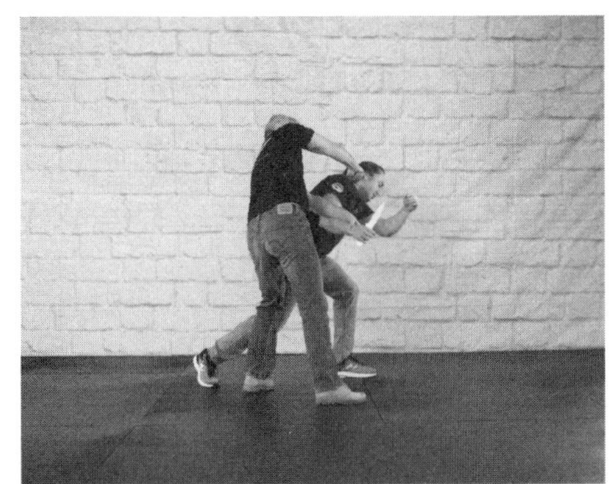

series continued on next page ...

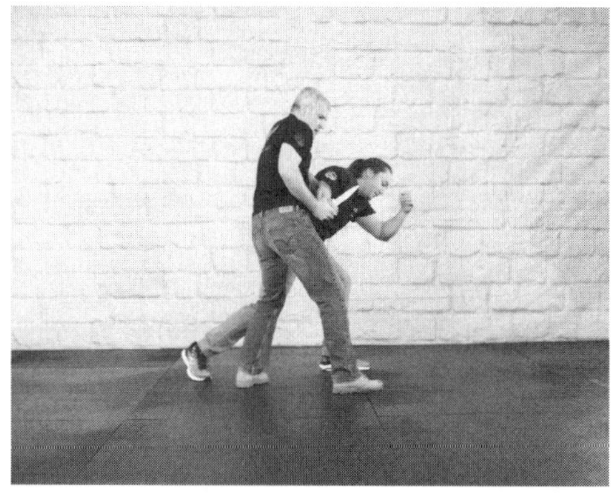

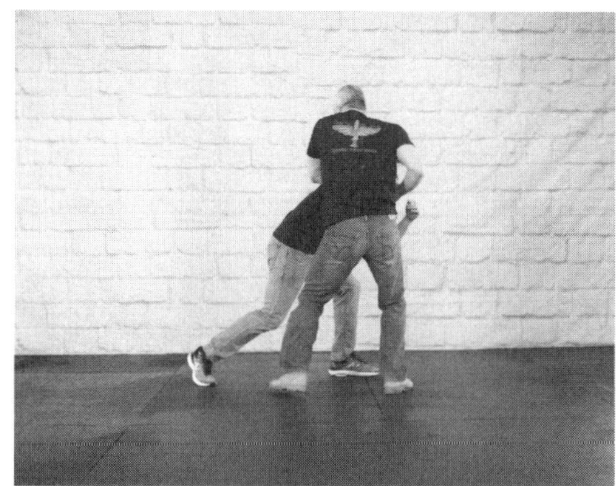

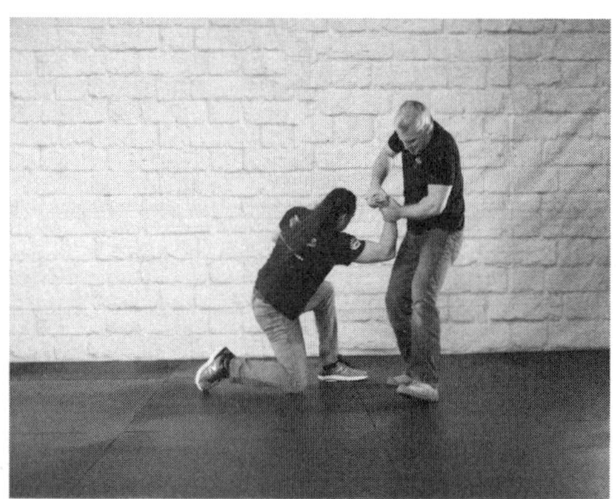

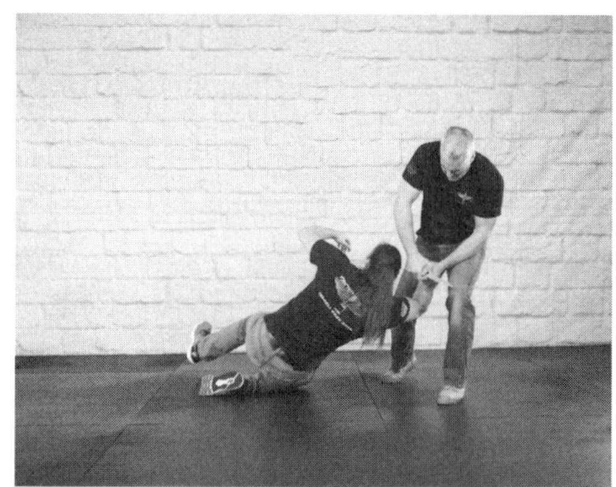

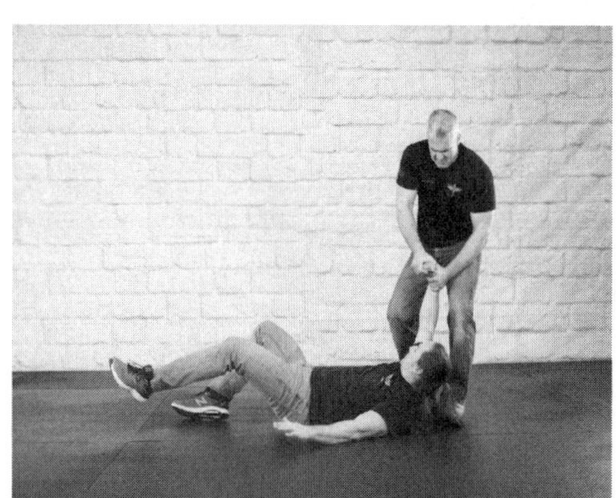

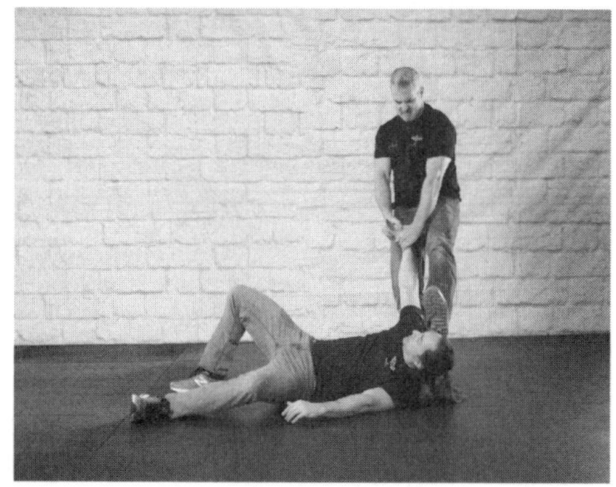

This series represents an attempted clinch grab and stab attack. An attacker will often grab a victim to limit the victim's mobility to escape or defend. On recognizing the attack, if you do not have time to strategically kick the attacker, you must step off the line to intercept the knife arm's up-thrust. As you step off the line of attack, simultaneously strike the attacker in the head. Use tai-sabaki cavalier #1 footwork to take him down and remove the weapon from his grip.

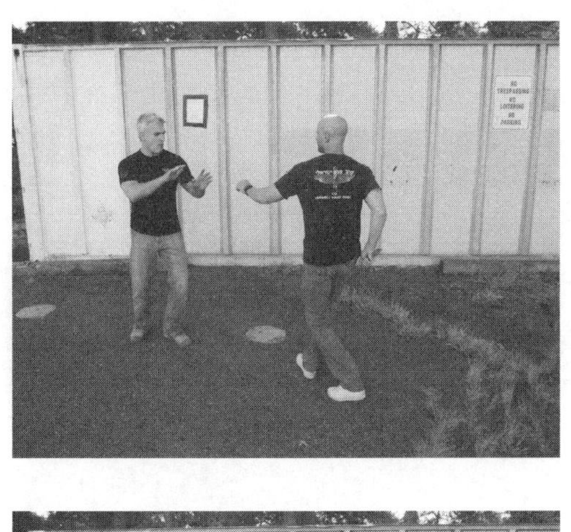

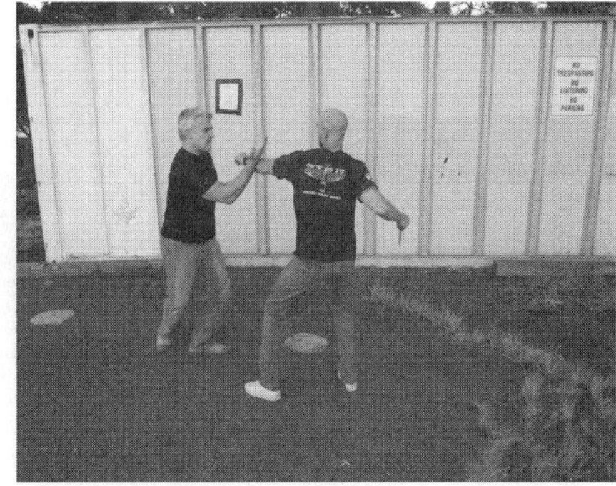

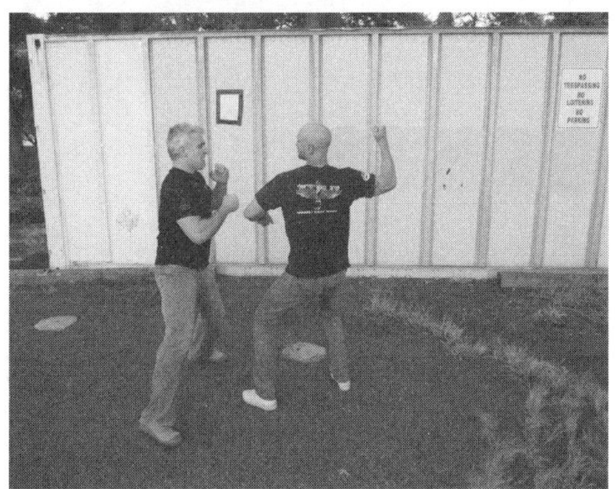

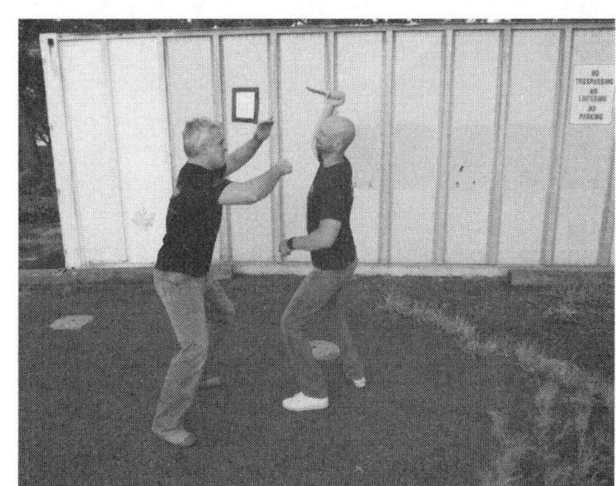

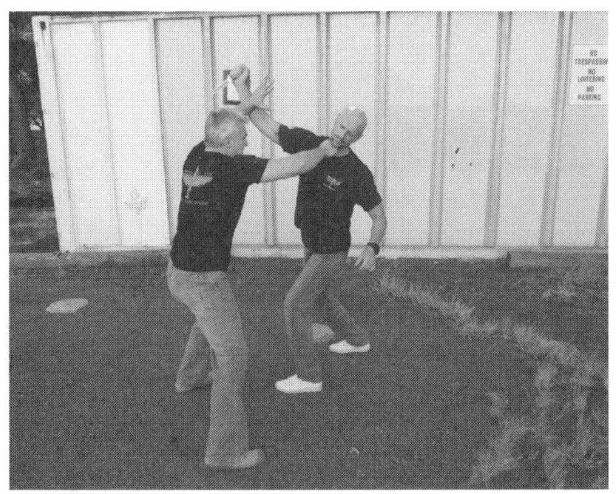

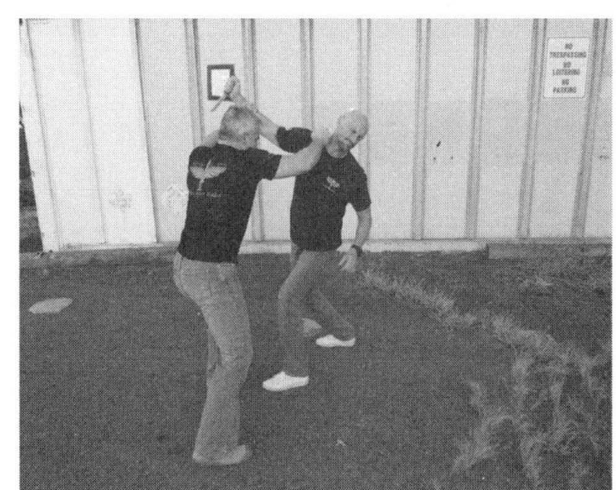

series continued on next page …

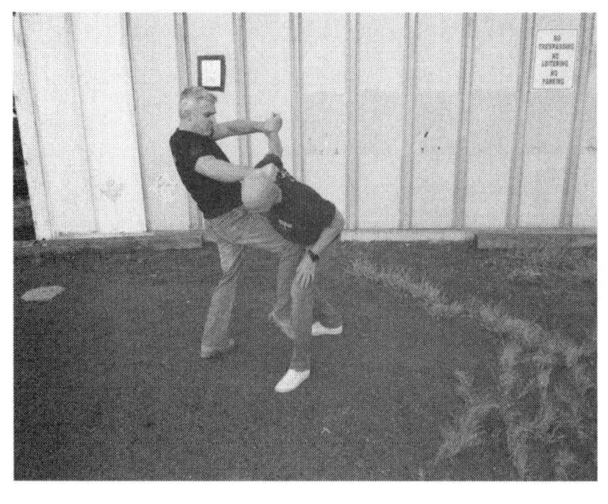

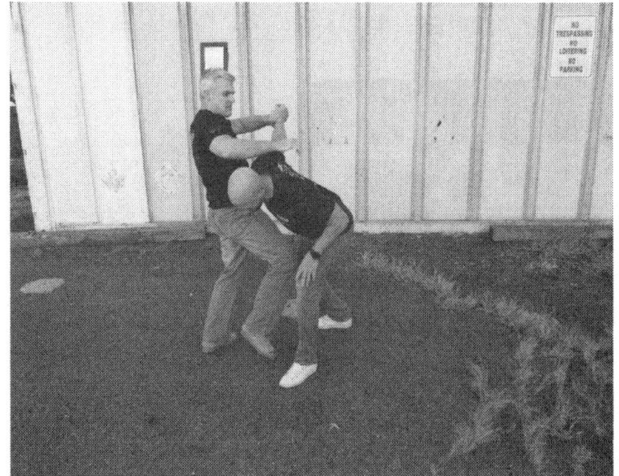

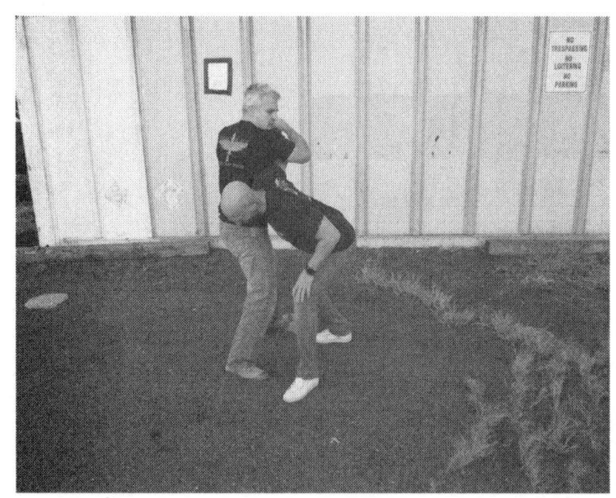

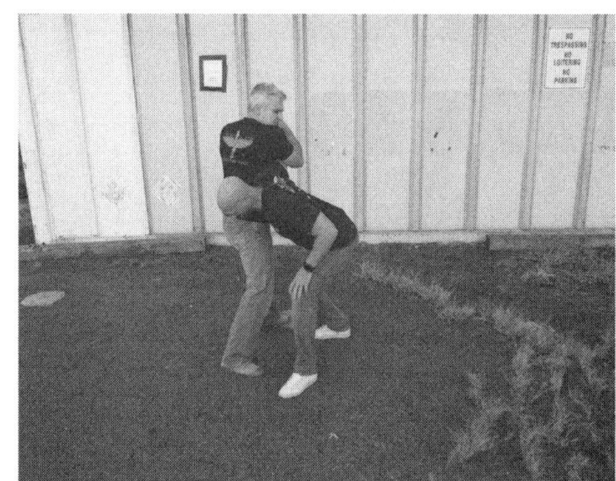

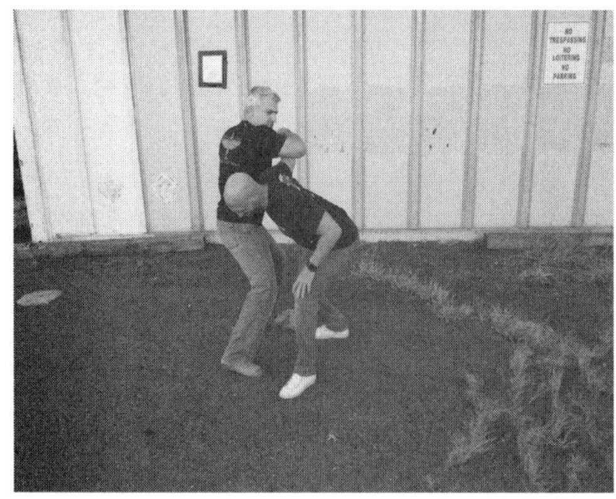

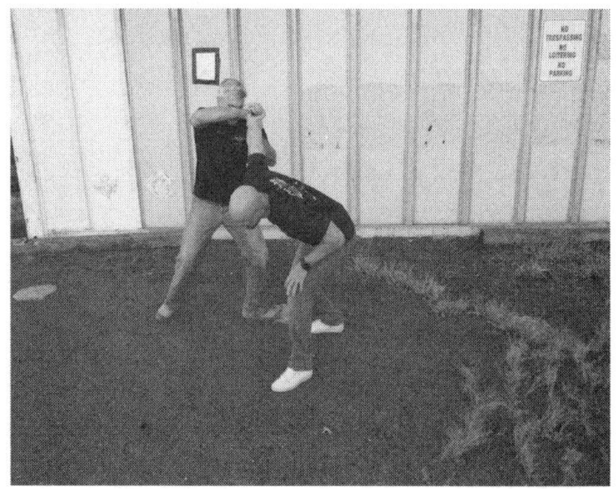

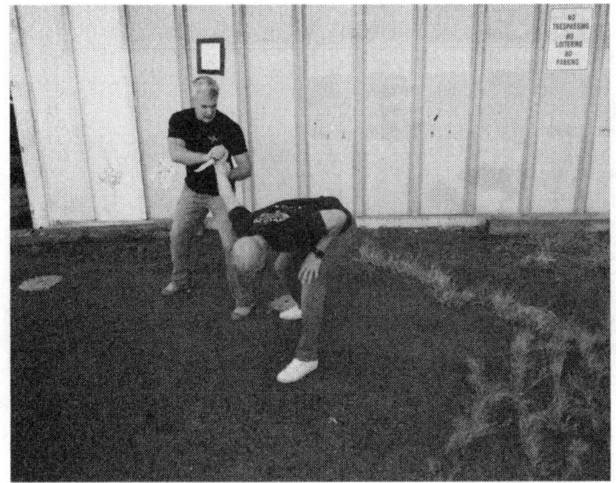

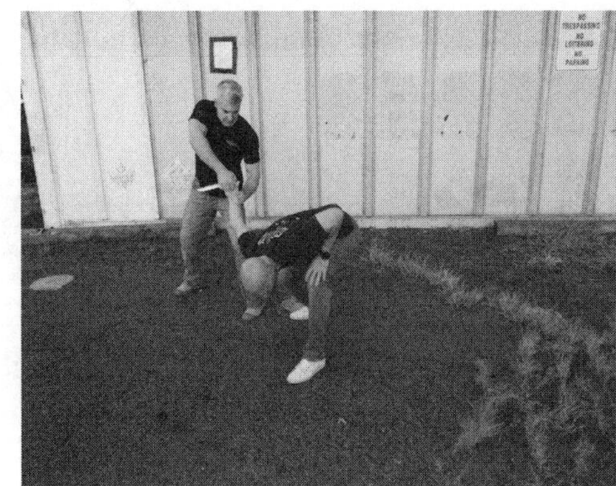

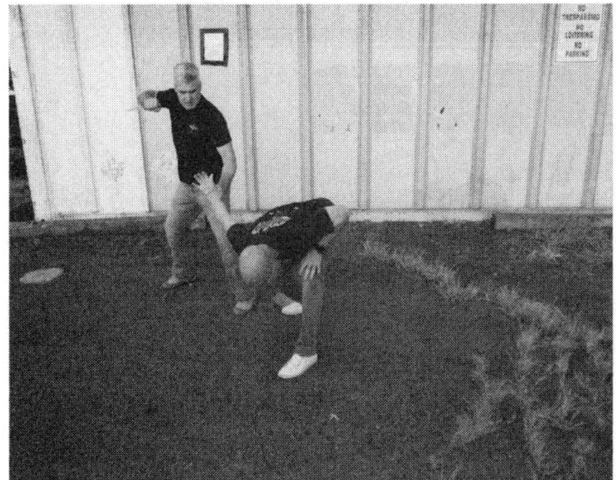

This series depicts a combined grab and overhand knife attack. Once again, an attacker will often grab a victim to limit the victim's ability to escape or defend. On recognizing the attack, if you do not have time to strategically kick the attacker, L-parry the initial grab attempt while stepping off the line to counter the overhead knife attack. Defend with a 360-degree outside defense combined with a simultaneous punch to the throat. Instantaneously secure his weapon arm by the wrist followed by an immediate knee strike to the groin. Remove the weapon using cavalier #2. Note: as in the previous examples above, while you can step or burst directly into the punch, such a defense may catastrophically fail against a stronger attacker with long arms and an edged weapon. Further note the tai-sabaki footwork to place the attacker into a cavalier #2 for knife removal.

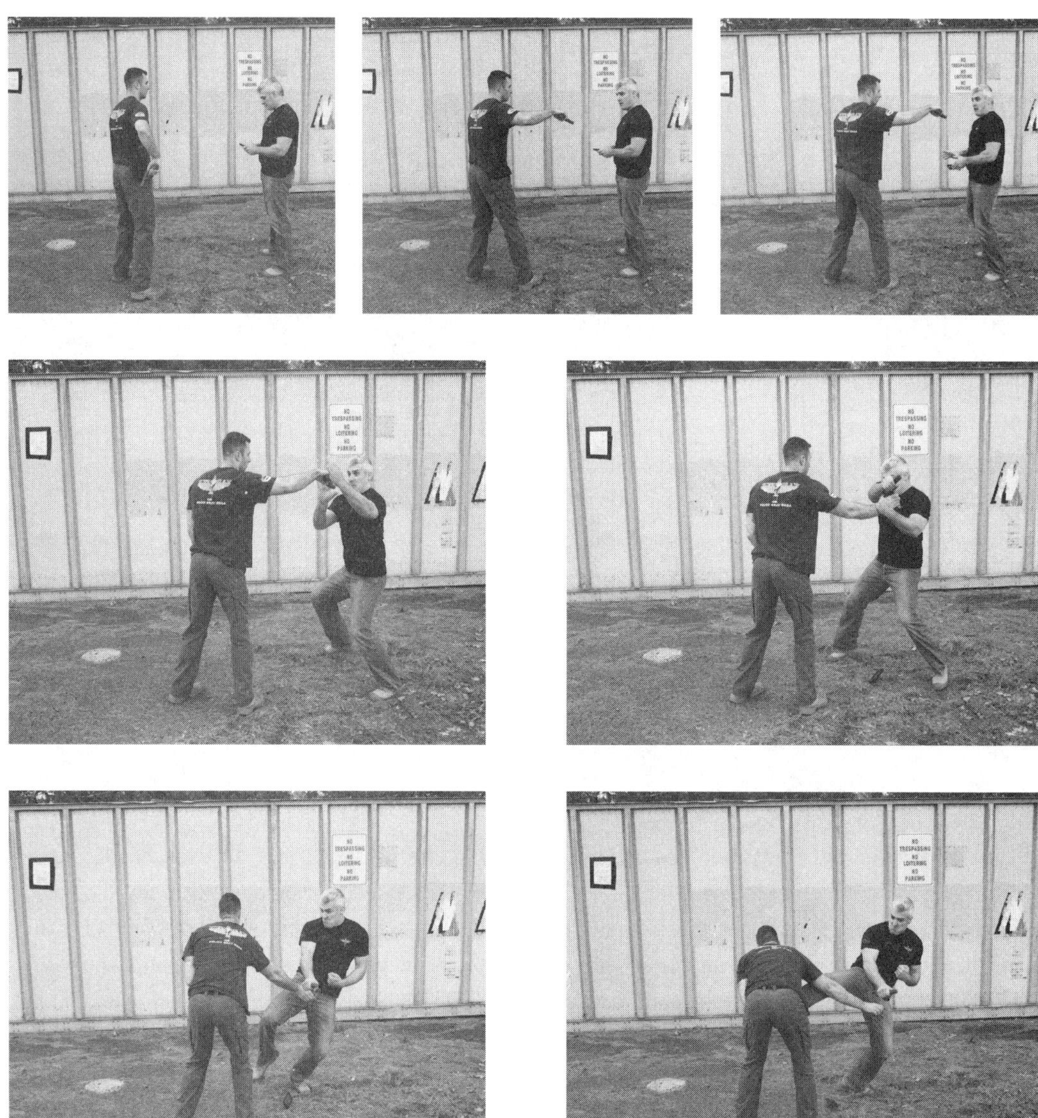

This series represents handgun defense #2 accomplished by stepping off the line, while simultaneously dropping your mobile device to execute the disarm. Note once again the crucial defensive footwork to get off the line of attack as you disarm the assailant combined with a straight kick to his groin with your outside leg (as the inside leg will be weight bearing).

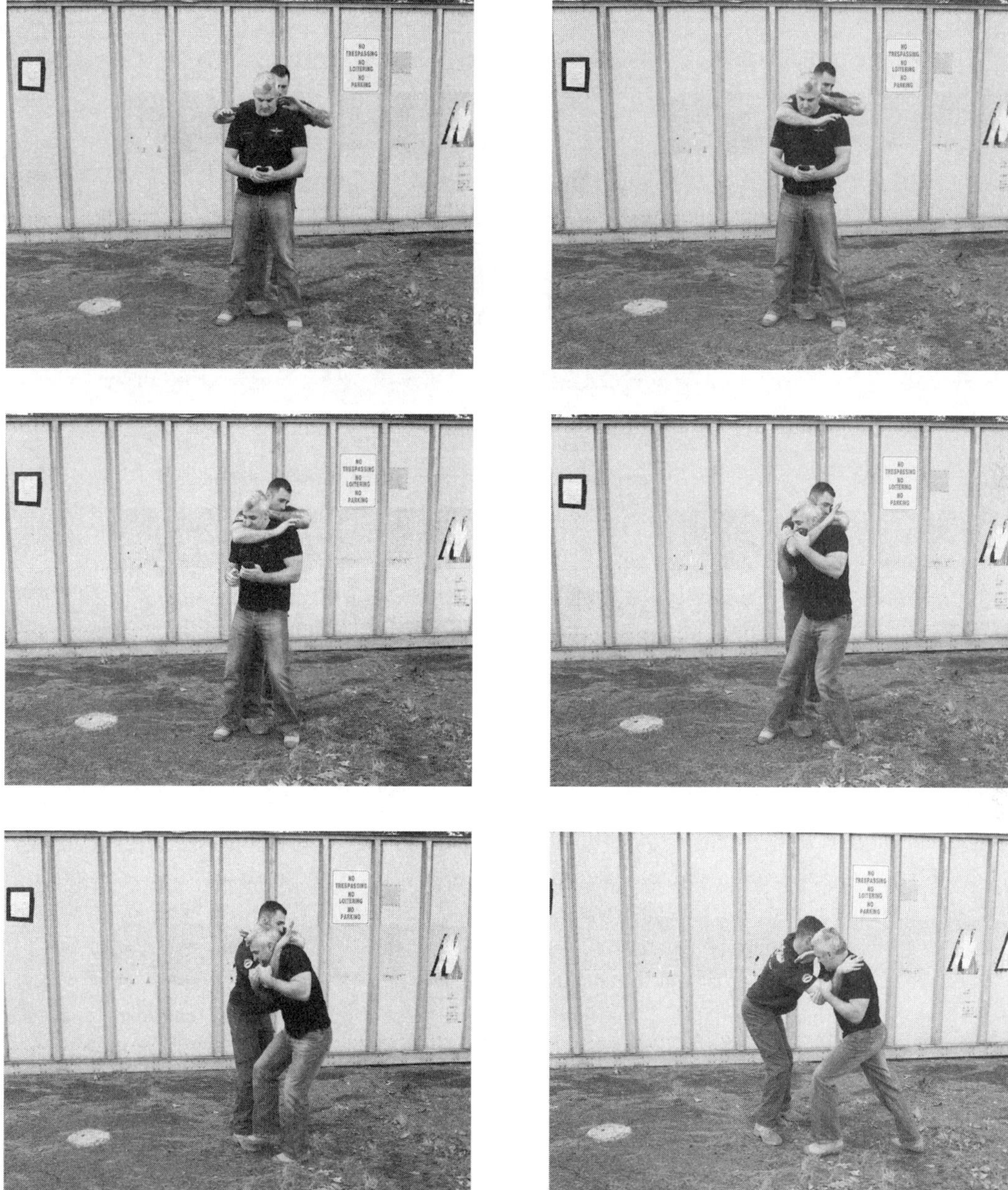

series continued on next page ...

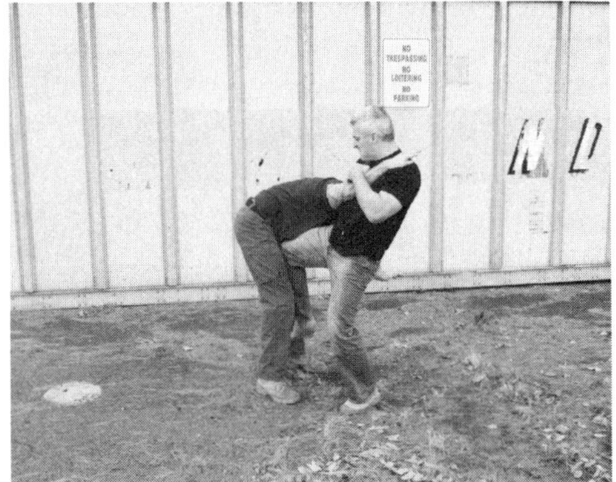

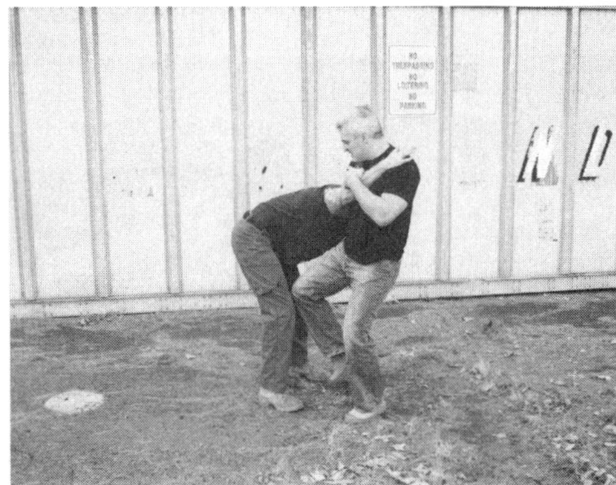

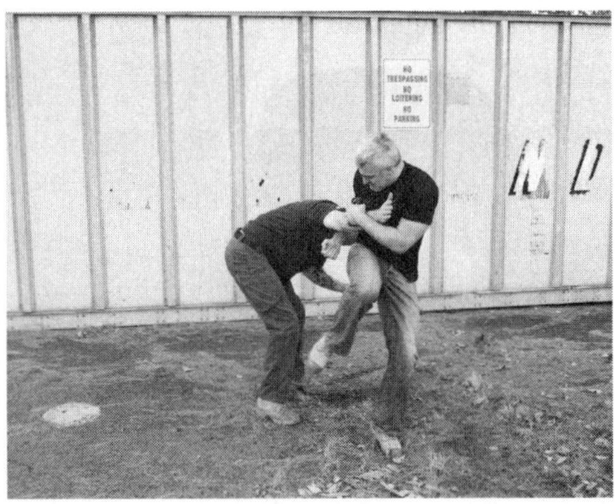

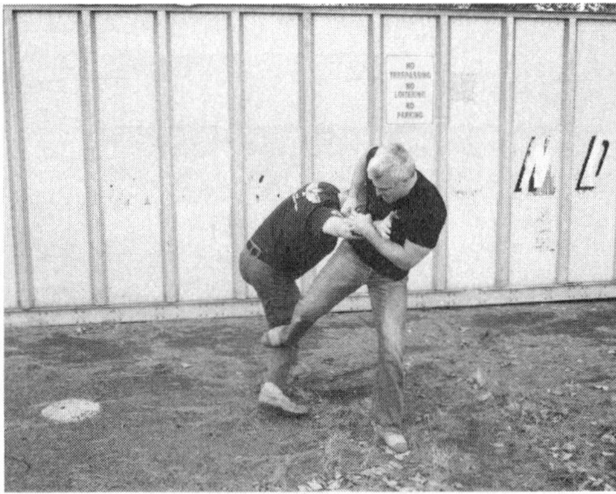

This series depicts defending a rear naked choke defense. Note the vital instantaneous, instinctive grab to exert counter-force against the attacker's arm before he can lock the choke on, coupled with the simultaneous footwork consisting of sharply crossing the right leg behind the left leg at roughly an 180-degree angle to break the angle of attack, while harnessing the body's core strength to break the choke hold or at least compromise the attacker's stranglehold grip, enabling you to effectively fight back. It cannot be emphasized enough the instinctive, instantaneous, and honed timing required to defeat such an attack the instant you feel an arm wrap around your neck. Krav maga emphasizes this particular right leg cross-behind step because 85 percent of all rear naked chokes are done with the right arm around the neck. This underscores the strategy of training to the threat. (Importantly, this right leg behind left leg crossover step will work against a left arm choke as depicted in a subsequent sequence.) This about-face footwork that defeats the attack also places the defender in a superior position to deliver a devastating knee to the attacker's groin or lower quadrant. If the attacker is able to lock the choke on and the defender does not initially succeed in breaking the attacker's hold, the defender can deliver a crippling sidekick to the attacker's nearside knee (the left knee not the outside right knee as the final photo depicts); or release one arm to pummel the attacker's groin; or step around to hook the attacker's outside leg for a kosoto-gake trip takedown; or step through using a modified ouchi gari counterattack targeting the attacker's inside leg to trip him. Each of these counterattacks requires at least one of the defender's arms to maintain strong counter-pressure against the choke.

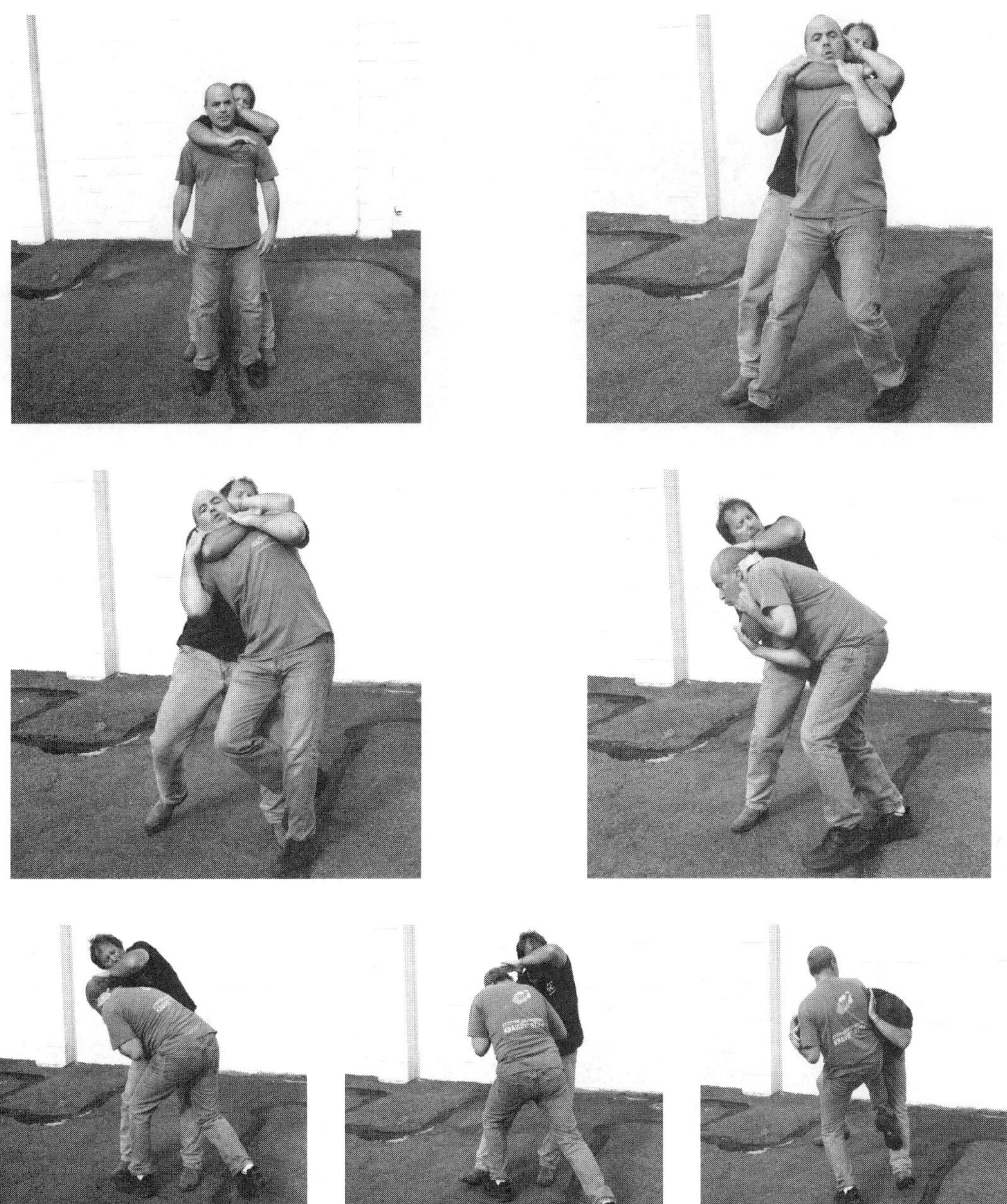

This series depicts defending a rear choke when being yanked backward. The crucial footwork of stepping naturally backward combines with a 45-degree cross-step of the right leg behind the left leg to break the angle of attack (same as the previous defense) while harnessing the body's core strength to break the choke hold. This counter-tactic places the defender in a superior position to deliver a debilitating knee to the attacker's groin or lower quadrant followed by additional combatives as necessary.

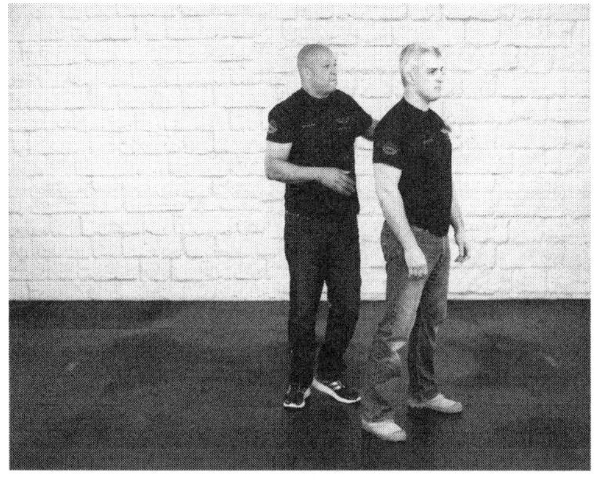

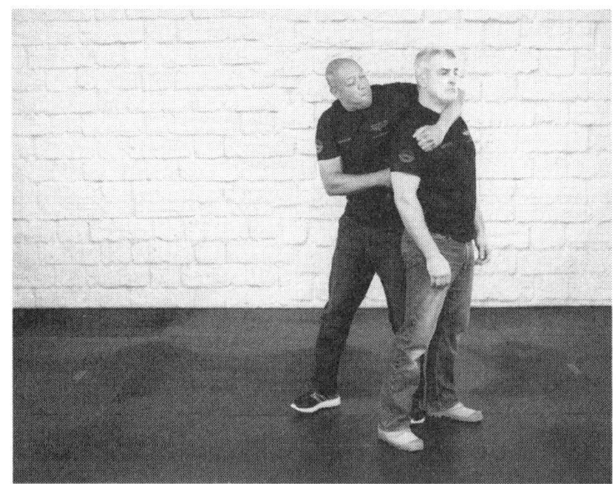

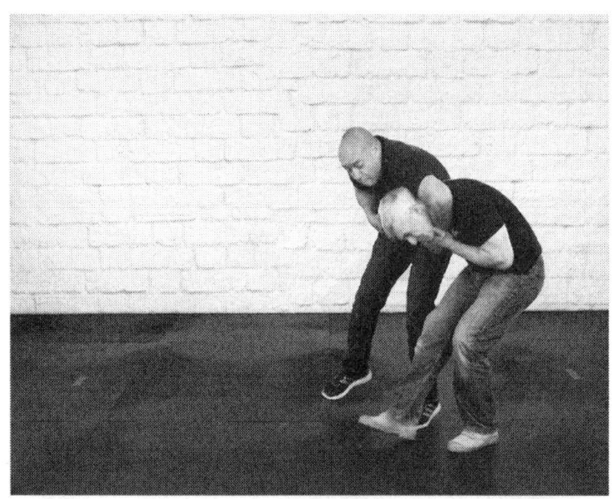

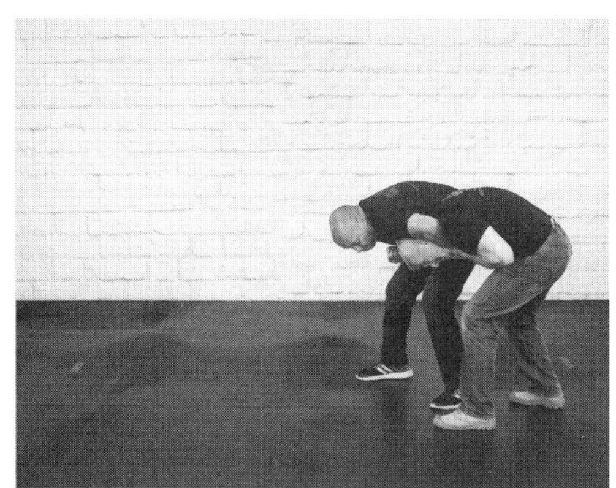

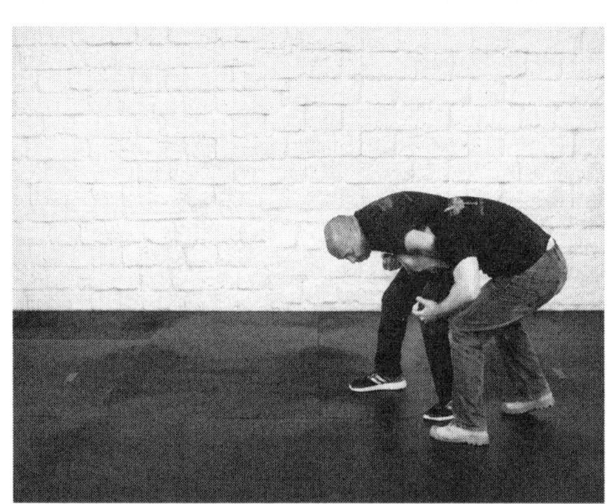

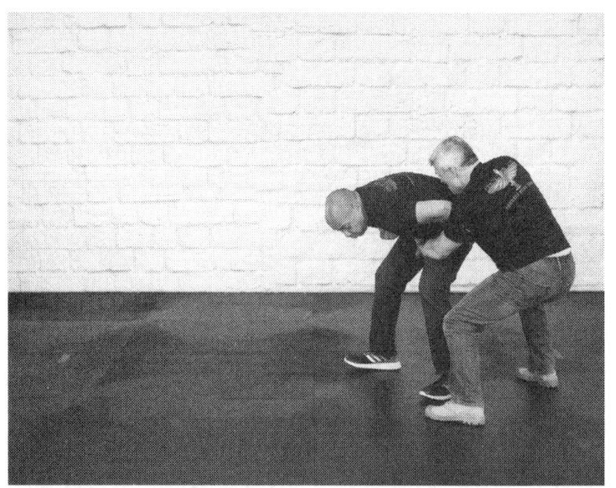

This series depicts defending a left arm choke using the same right-leg-behind-left-leg crossover step as the previously depicted choke defense tactics. Therefore, while the defender could cross the left leg behind the right leg to execute the defense, *training to move one way and one way only can provide a strategic advantage in a struggle*. In other words, by perfecting only one technique, you don't have to think.

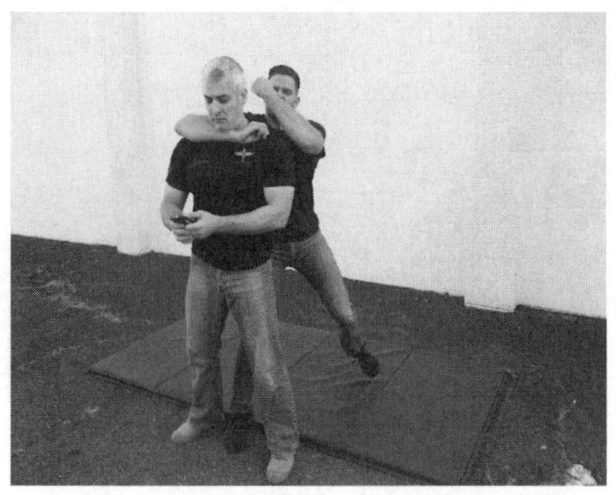

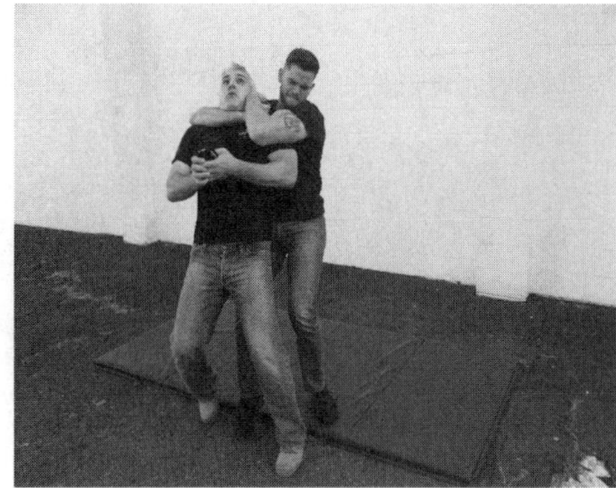

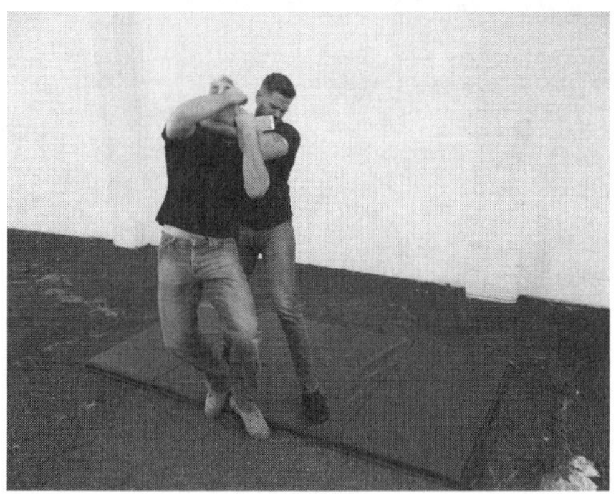

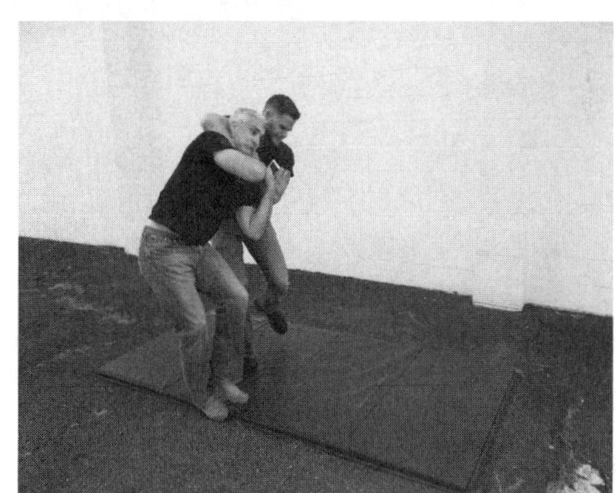

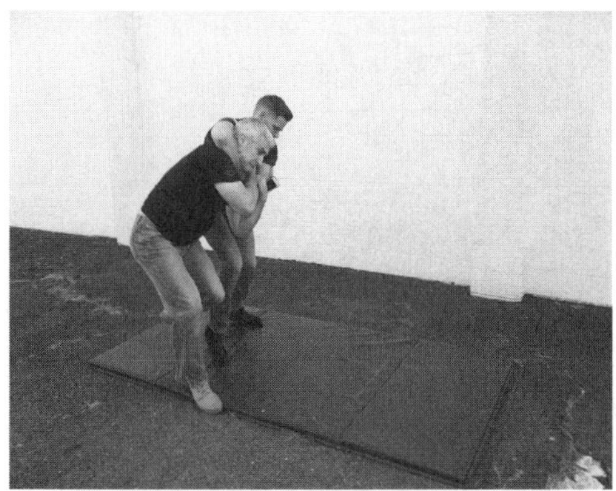

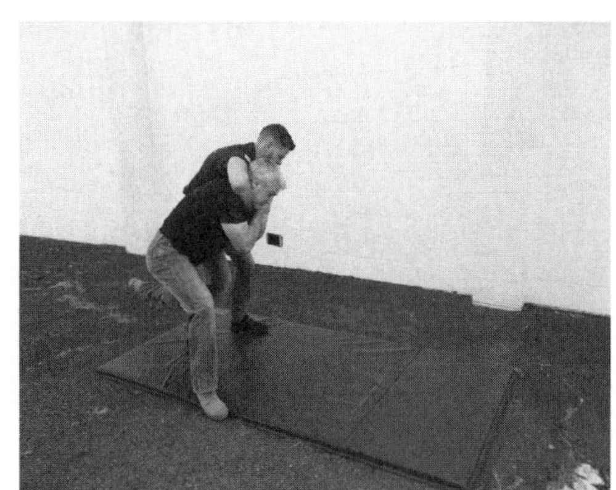

series continued on next page ...

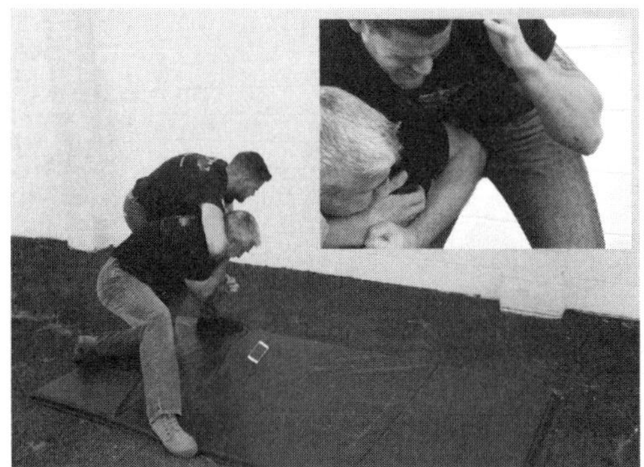

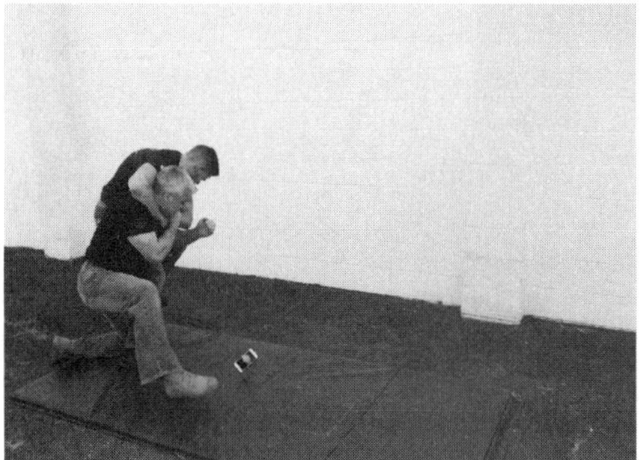

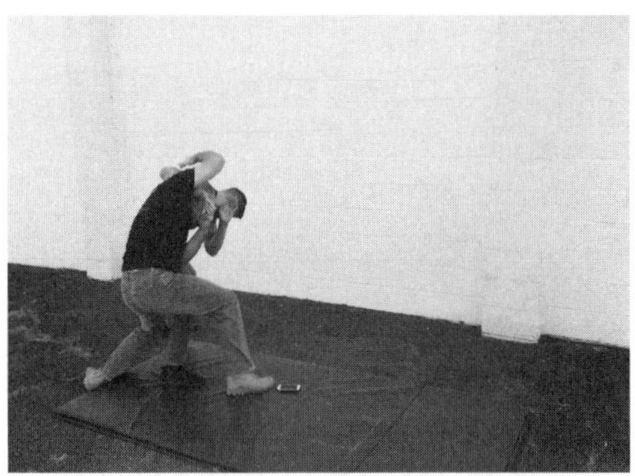

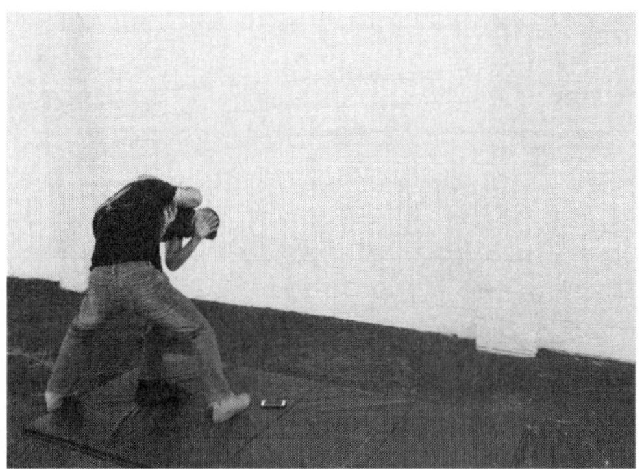

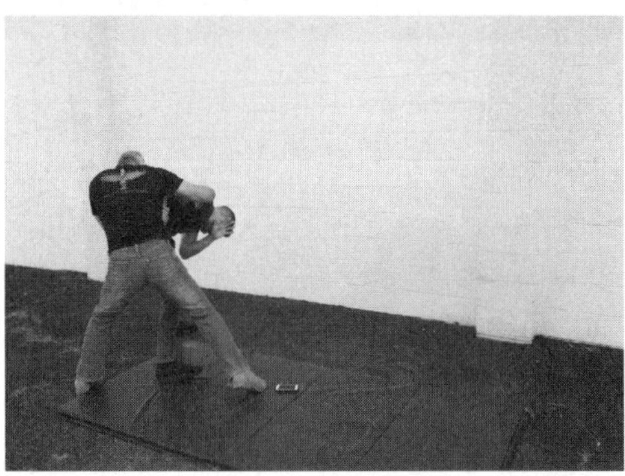

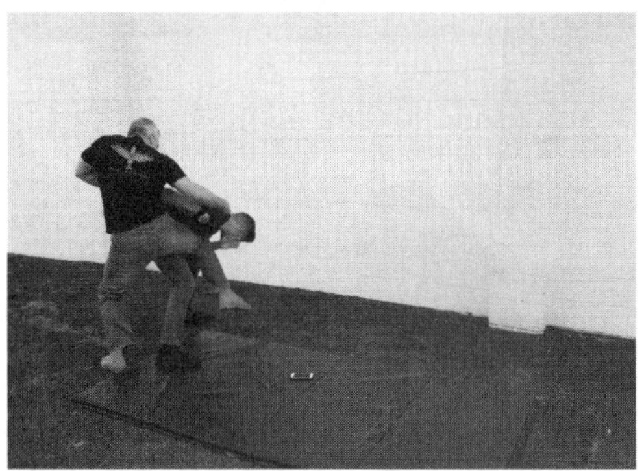

This series depicts defending a rear naked choke when the attacker has locked in the choke and is pulling you backward. In this case, the momentum pulling you backward forces you to cross your left leg. In other words, if you are choked from the rear and yanked backward, you may not be able to successfully cross your right leg behind your left (as depicted in the previous techniques.) Strategically, krav maga must always provide alternatives. The momentum of being pulled backward might make you stumble and thus require you to kneel down with your crossover leg. Once you have broken the choke angle with both of your arms supplying counterpressure, use a left rear elbow strike to the attacker's groin followed by additional combatives as necessary to break the hold while continuing to exert counterpressure with your right hand.

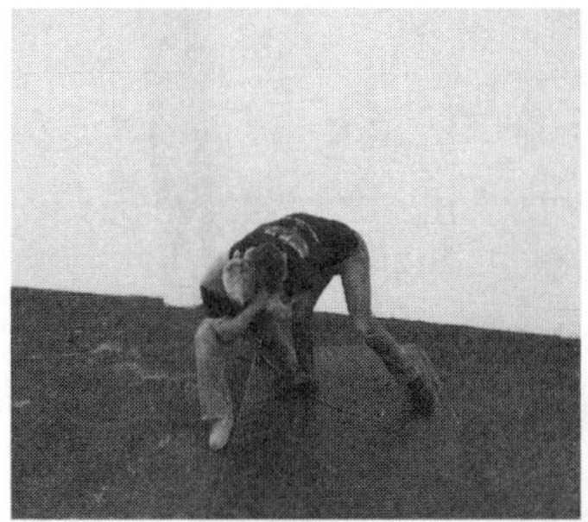

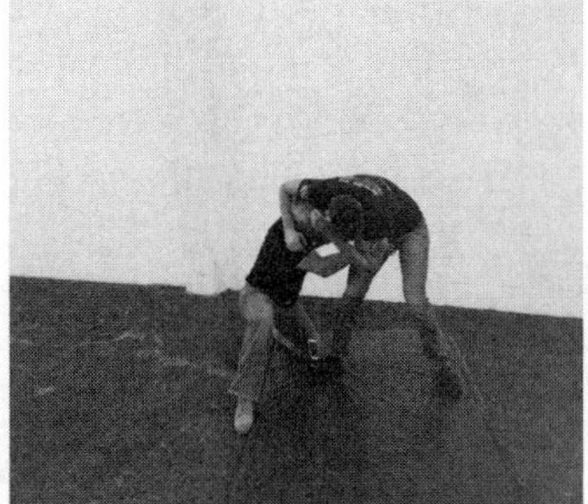

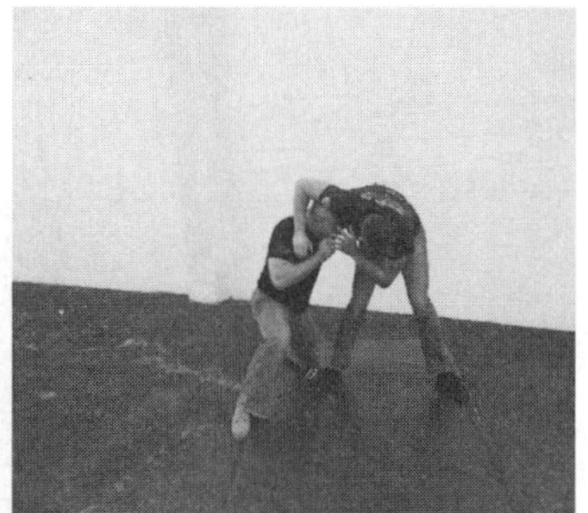

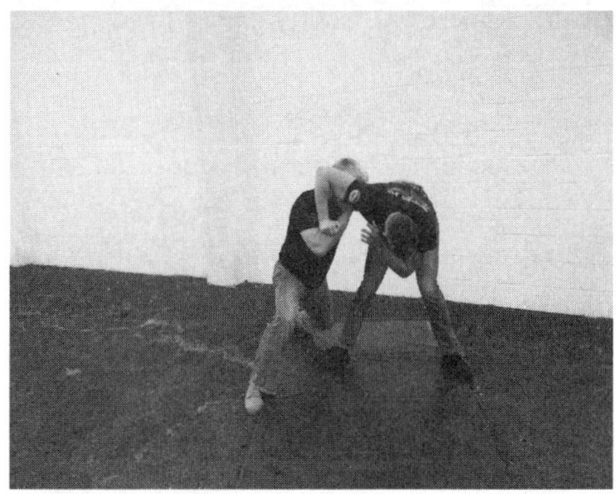

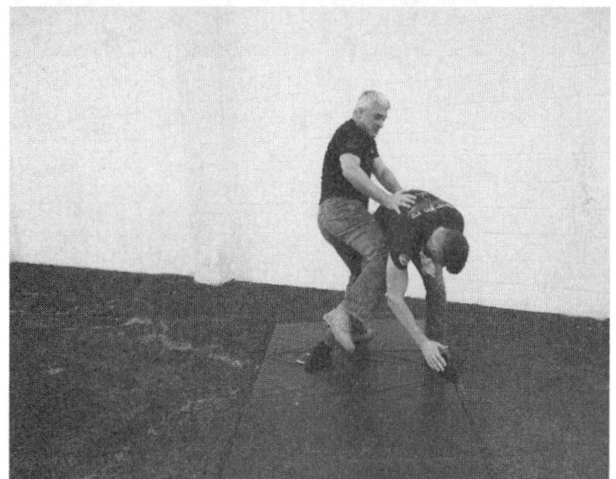

This abbreviated photo series depicts a forced knee dip defense against a rear naked choke when pulled backward and forced to the ground; however, you use a different counterstrike. Here again, you are forced backward and must dip your inside left knee as you stumble backward to move with and counter the attacker's pull. While securing and putting counter-pressure against the choking arm with your *left hand*, release your outside *right hand* to strike the attacker in his groin, followed by additional combatives.

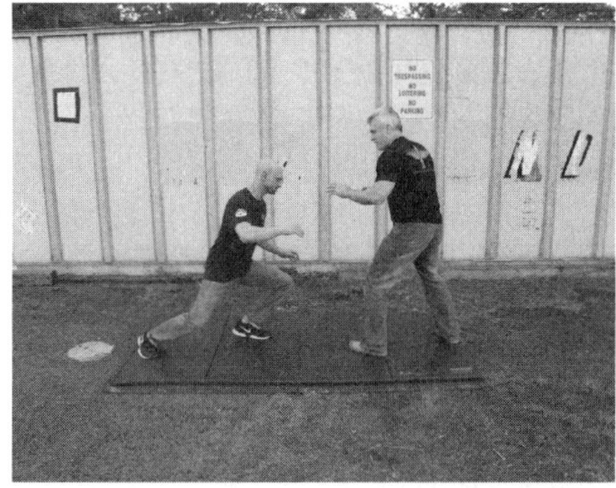

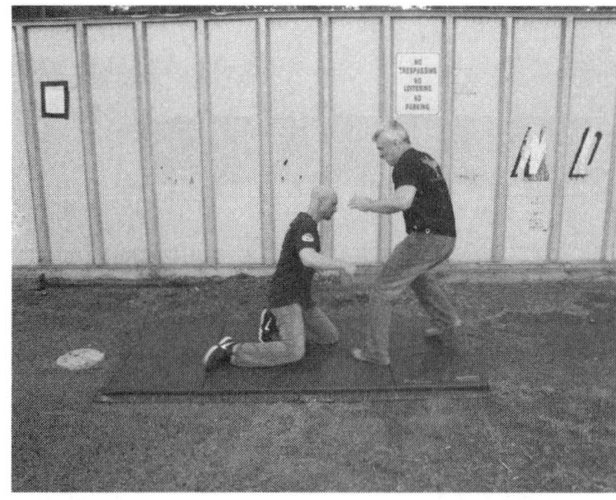

series continued on next page ...

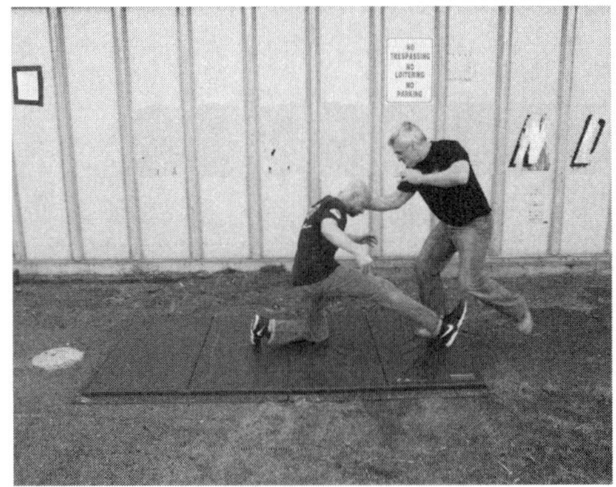

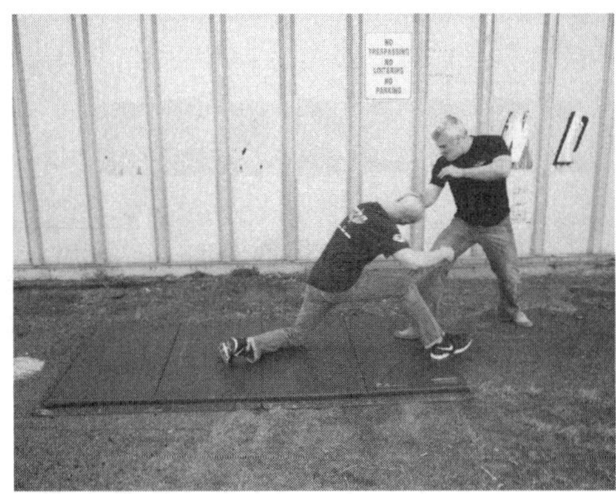

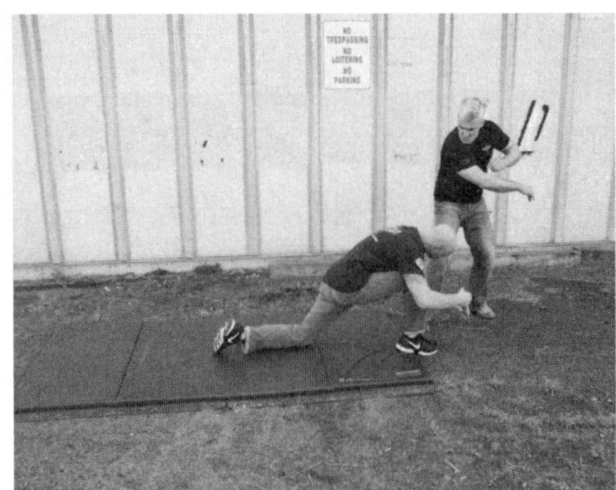

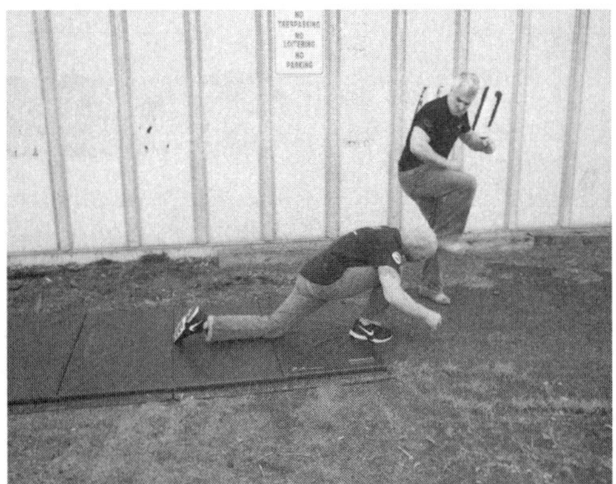

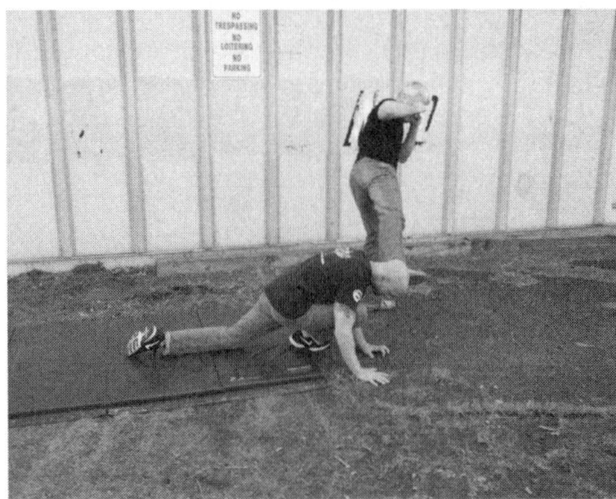

A popular takedown technique is a one leg or ankle pick where a grappler glides down to his knee to then step forward with his same knee to trip you. Defensive tactical footwork by retracting your front leg to an opposite outlet stance removes your targeted leg and generates momentum for a counter-attack such as a palm-heel strike to the ear followed by additional opportune combatives such as a kick or knee to the attacker's head.

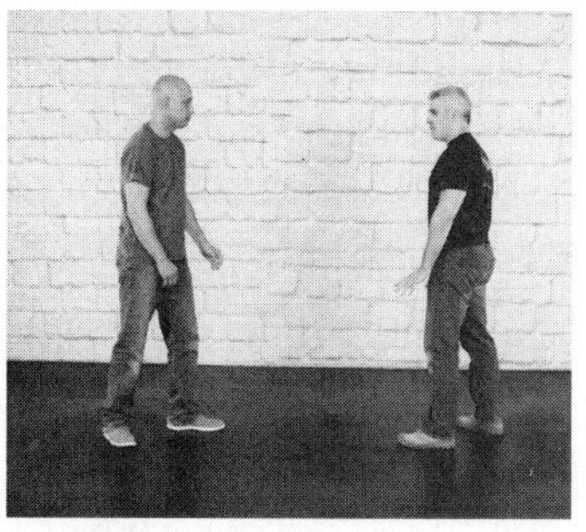
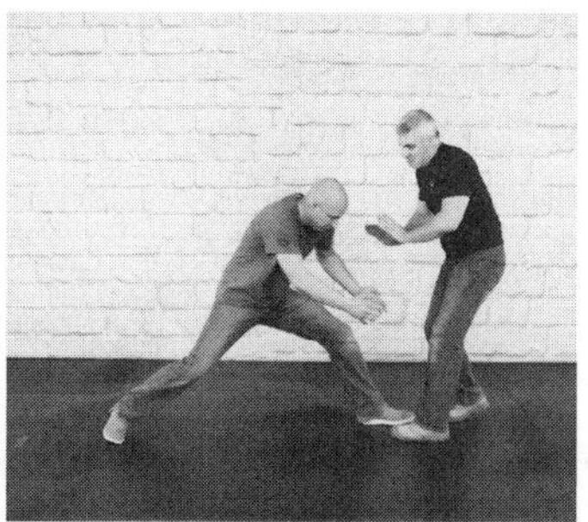
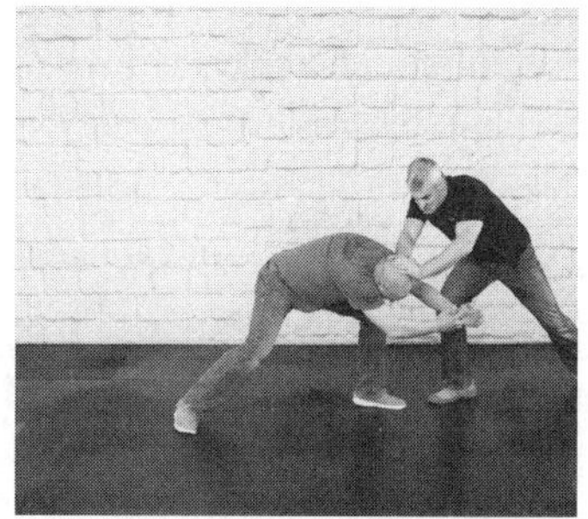
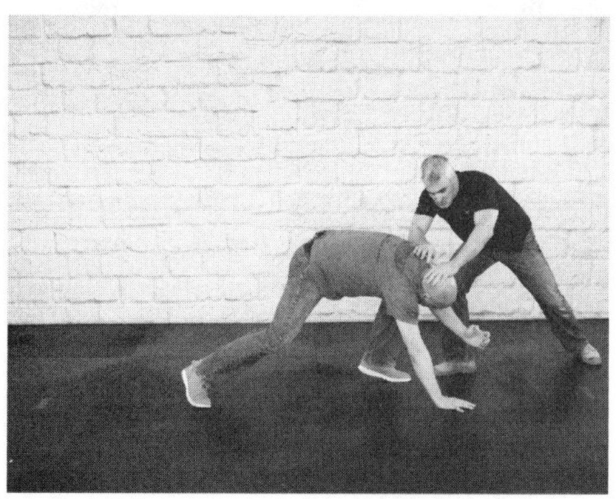
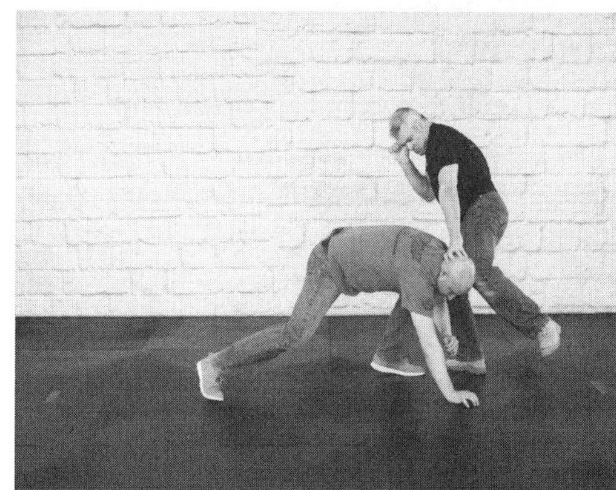
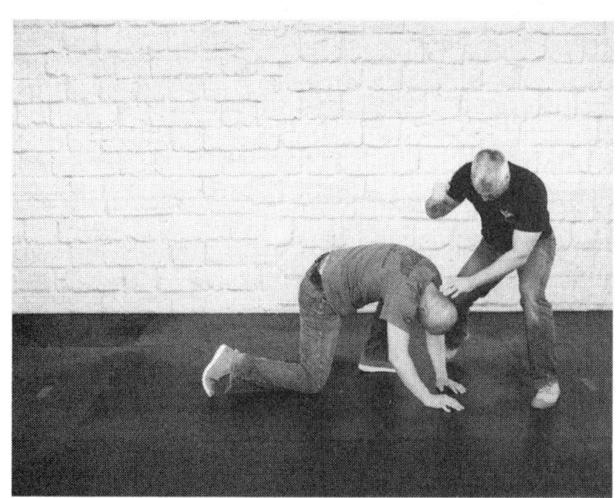
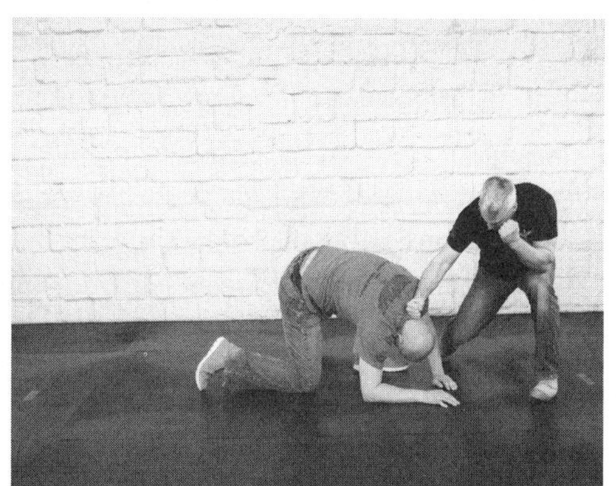

A popular takedown technique is a one leg grab where a grappler launches to grab your forward leg. Defensive tactical footwork by retracting your front leg to an opposite outlet stance removes your targeted leg and generates momentum for a counterattack such as a palm-heel strike to the ear followed by additional opportune combatives such as a kick or knee to the attacker's head.

Footwork and body positioning, whether standing or prone, allow you to simultaneously defend and attack, leading to the seamless combative transitions essential to retzev. It is self-evident that fight positioning determines your tactical advantage. Below are some essential footwork and positioning concepts:

- Footwork is crucial to defeating any attack. Correctly timed footwork *can* defeat any attack.
- Proper footwork requires gliding or sliding; do not use little jumps or hops or drag your feet. Balance must be achieved in your mobility. Fluid and fast footwork precede speed development in hands and legs combatives. The feet need to be a comfortable distance apart.
- Core footwork incorporates (1) the ability to easily and efficiently move the body while (2) maintaining the body's balance (3) as you maintain the ability to defend and attack at all times.
- Positioning yourself where you can counterattack your opponent more easily than he can attack you is most advantageous. Optimally, a skilled krav maga fighter will move quickly to a superior and dominant position relative to his opponent, known in krav maga parlance as the deadside. The deadside often provides you with a decisive tactical advantage. This strategy should revolve around your capabilities and preferred tactics involving long, medium, and short combatives combined with evasive maneuvers.
- The key to evasion is moving out of the "line of fire" or the path of an opponent's offensive combatives. A successful avoidance of an opponent's combative usually affords the opportunity for a debilitating counterattack.
- Protect the centerline of your head, vital internal organs, and groin (those targets you yourself would optimally counterattack).
- Use any object or environmental opportunity to aid in your self-defense.
- When engaged in a fight or hand-to-hand combat, keep moving in a correct bladed posture with sound tactical footwork. STAY ON THE BALLS OF YOUR FEET. It bears repeating: move always on the balls of your feet to facilitate movement and immediate reaction and to reduce inertia (which happens when you have both feet flat), while maintaining balance.
- As a stationary target you are much easier to "hit." If you move constantly, your opponent has a more difficult time judging distance. You should maintain a distance that keeps you just outside of your opponent's maximum range, understanding what your optimum closing strategy is when necessary. Note: Movement on the ground is different from standing movement. The nature of ground fighting can afford one attacker superior control and positioning; the other attacker cannot run or evade as he might while standing.
- If you keep moving, you facilitate the opportunity to attack. An object (you) in motion facilitates additional motion (combatives). If you are slow moving on your feet, your combatives will also be slow.

- In an ambush, your stance and position will be how you happen to be standing or positioned at the moment of attack. An ambusher chooses his timing and target. He will launch at you when he perceives you to be at your most vulnerable.
- Positioning becomes even more important when facing multiple assailants. Once superior position is achieved, the opponent will have minimal ability to defend or to counter your retzev attack.
- A crucial concept with weapon defenses is that an attacker usually expects you to naturally move away rather than close the distance to engage.

Tactical Retreating Combative Strategy

As part of your disengagement strategy, you may have decided simply to try to back away from a confrontational person, while still having eyes on the threat, until you create a safe distance. Your adversary may then decide to attack. Therefore, you must try to disengage while maintaining a strong counterattack capability, as the following methods show.

The Retreating Straight Kick

The retreating straight kick may be used when you attempt to de-escalate a situation by moving away from the conflict and yet the opponent follows you. Step back with your lead leg. As you step back, open up your hip by placing your lead leg (that now becomes your rear leg) foot at a 90-degree angle (the pivotal—pun intended—base-leg turn) for maximum reach and power.

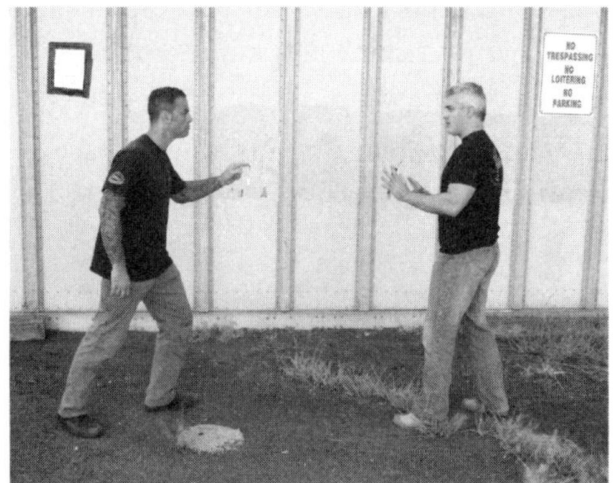
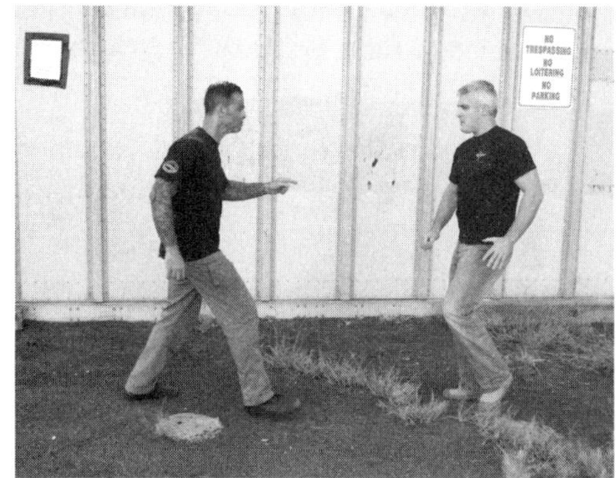
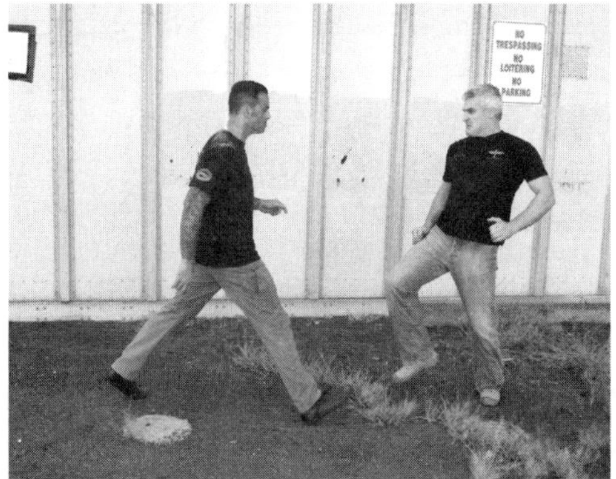
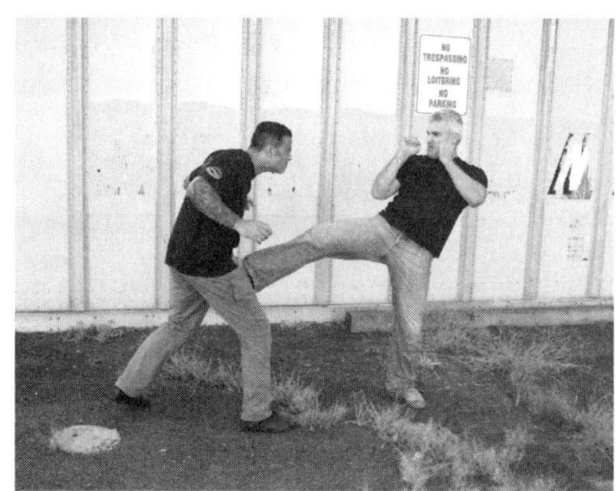

This series depicts a retreating straight kick when attempting to back away from confrontation.

Obviously, you cannot see what is behind you. This is especially true in a confrontation when your entire focus is fixated on the threat in front of you. It may be that you attempt to retreat as you try to reason with an aggressor only to back into an unseen obstacle. If you do not train for such an occurrence, the unexpected jolt might jar you and momentarily divert your attention from the aggressor. You cannot lose your focus as this moment of distraction might prompt the aggressor to close in on you. Therefore, in training you must practice such surprise occurrences (including other scenarios such as stumbling backward over an unseen curb) to not lose your composure and immediate ability to preempt or counterattack

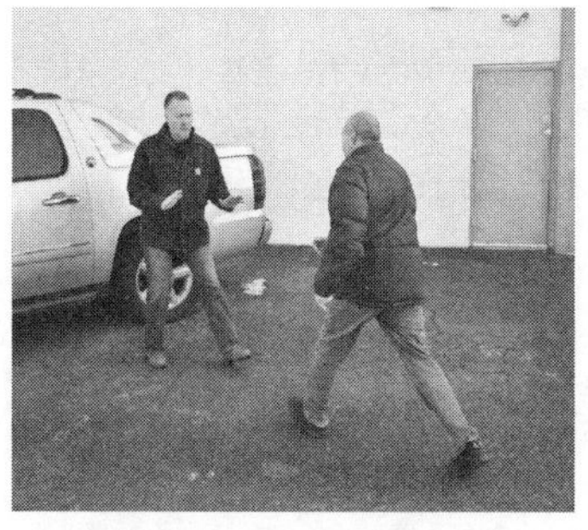
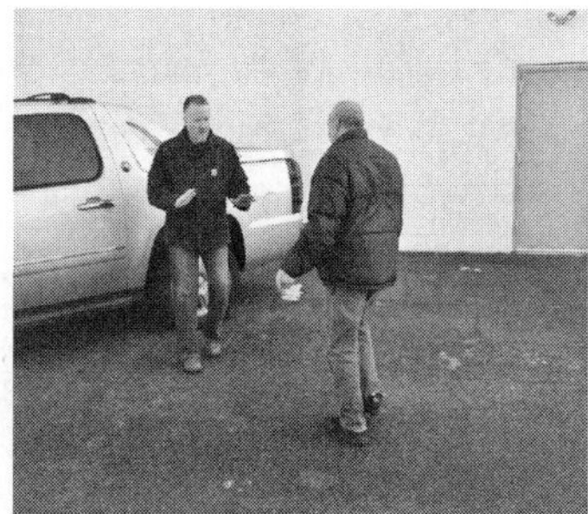
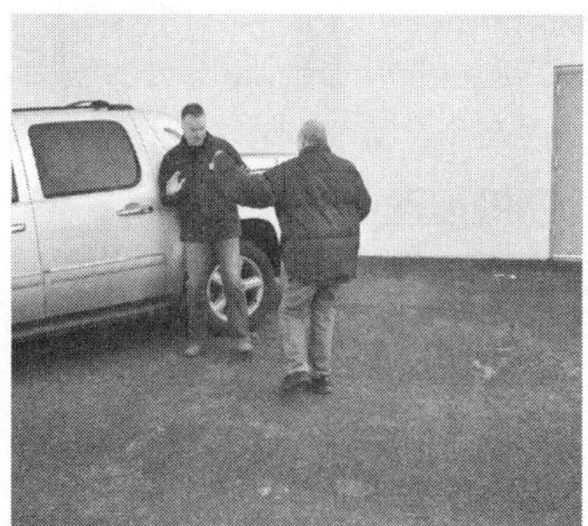
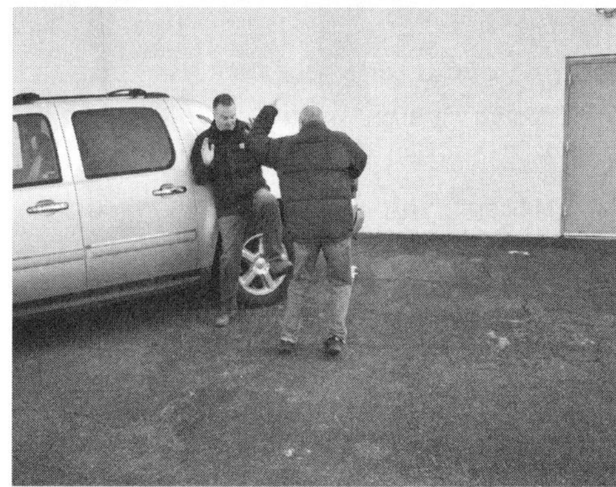
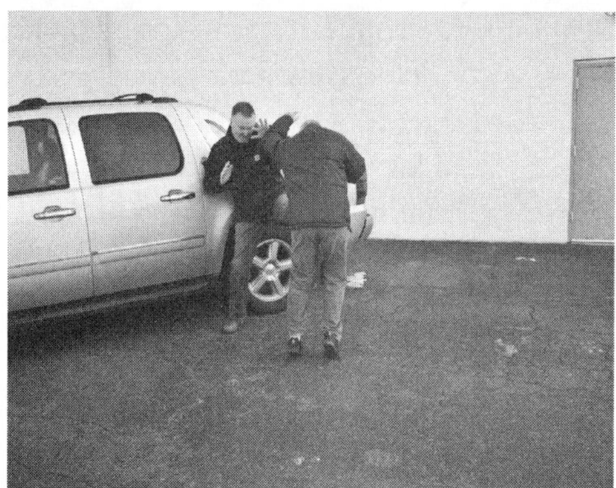
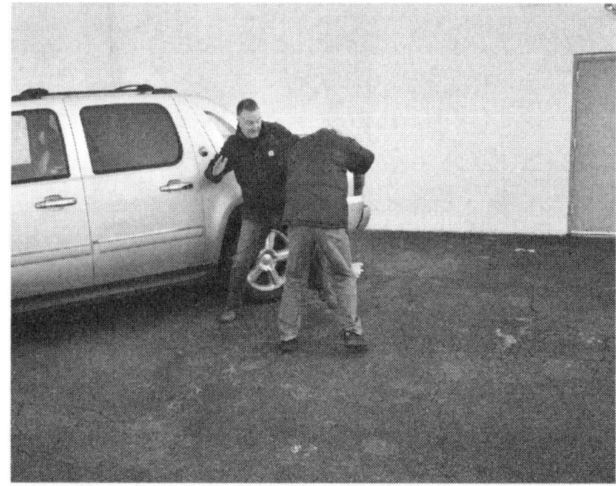
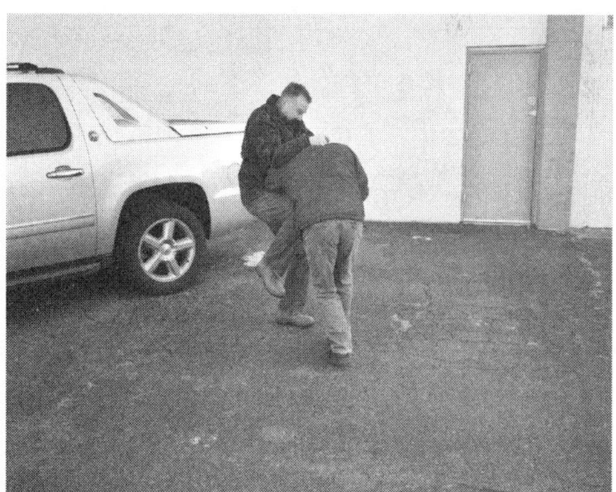

This series depicts an attempt to back away from a confrontation only to run into an unseen obstacle. As soon as you feel the abrupt impact of an obstacle, you must seamlessly transition from disengagement to engagement. Immediately launch a straight kick preemptive strike followed by additional combatives as necessary.

The Retreating Side Kick

While it is tactically unsound to turn your back your back on an opponent, the retreating side kick may be used when you try to walk away from a situation and yet the opponent follows you. Keep your head on a swivel as you attempt to disengage. As you walk away, you are well positioned to deliver a retreating side kick targeting your opponent's knee, thigh, or midsection. Be sure to kick with your heel and lean away with your upper body to keep your body away from any incoming strike (essentially a body defense) while you slide backward to deliver maximum reach and power. As you attempt to create distance, yet the attacker follows you, reverse your direction by initiating a rear crossover left step, while raising your right leg by drawing your knee up to your waist. As you deliver the right-side kick, pivot on the ball of the foot of your left leg. Drive your heel through the attacker's knee while leaning your upper-body defensively away from the attacker. Continue your counterattacks as necessary and disengage, moving to safety. Note: An opponent, even when skilled in delivering his attack, often leaves himself briefly open for counterattack. In this example, as the opponent delivers a straight punch, he shifts his weight forward, offering you the opportunity to deliver a side kick to damage his front knee.

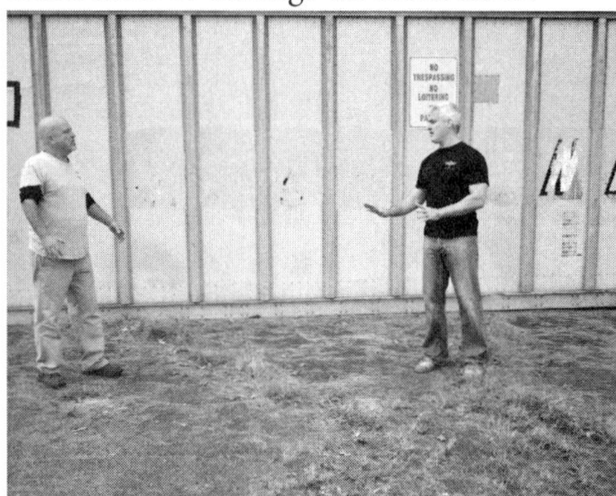

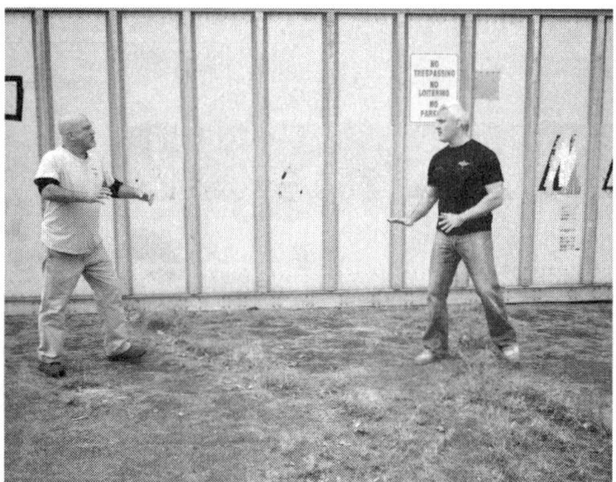

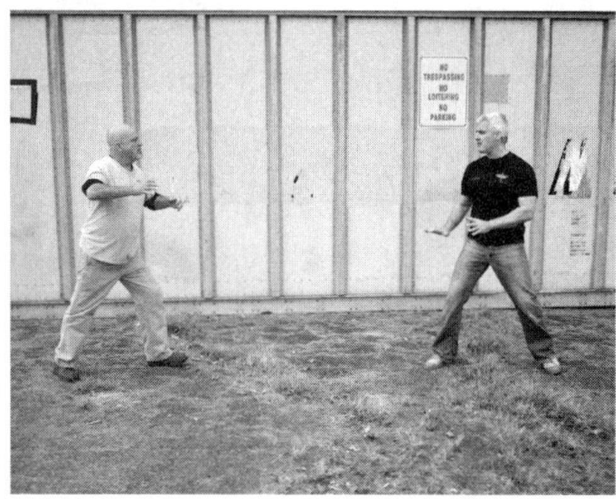

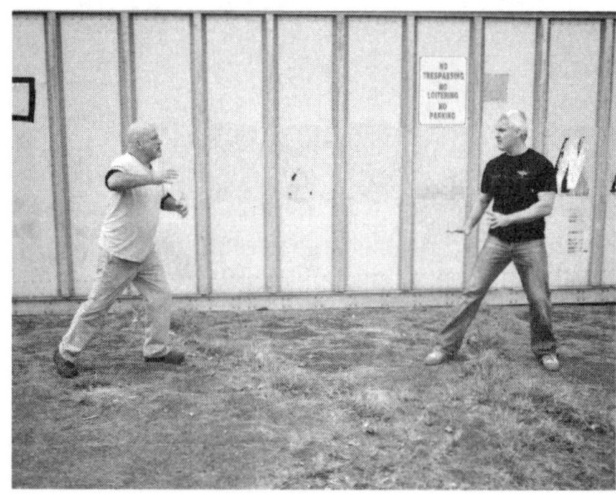

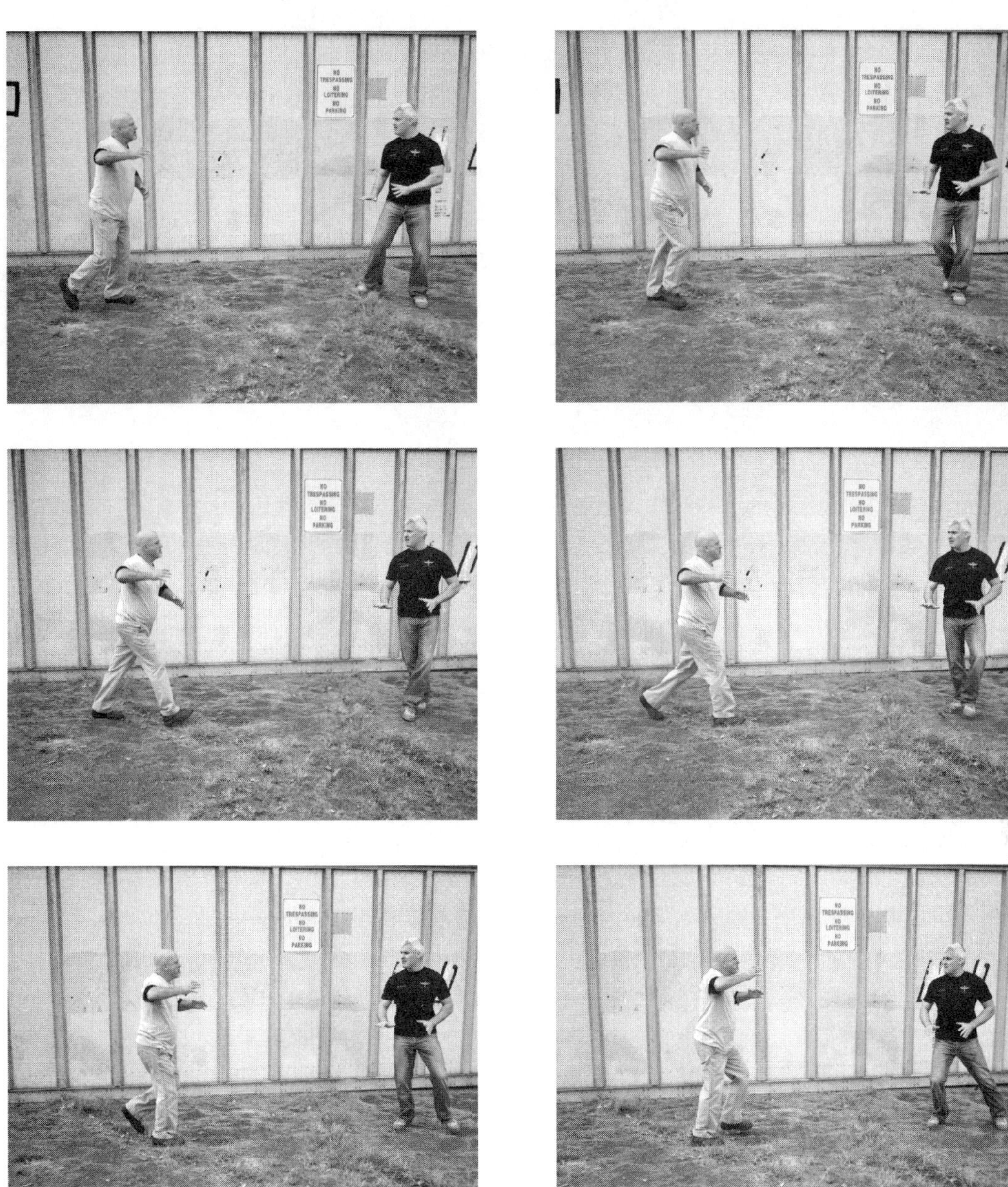

series continued on next page ...

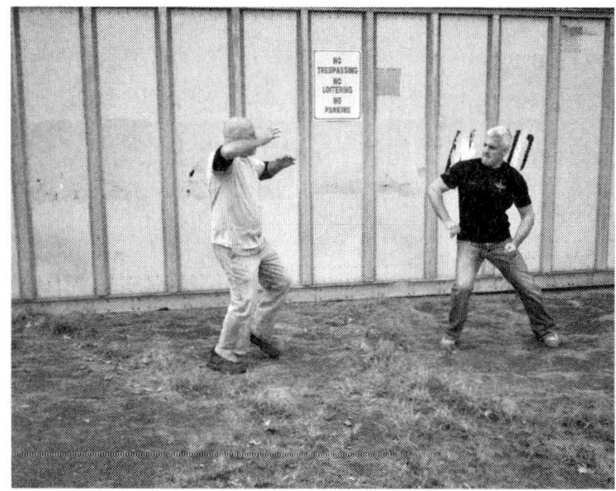

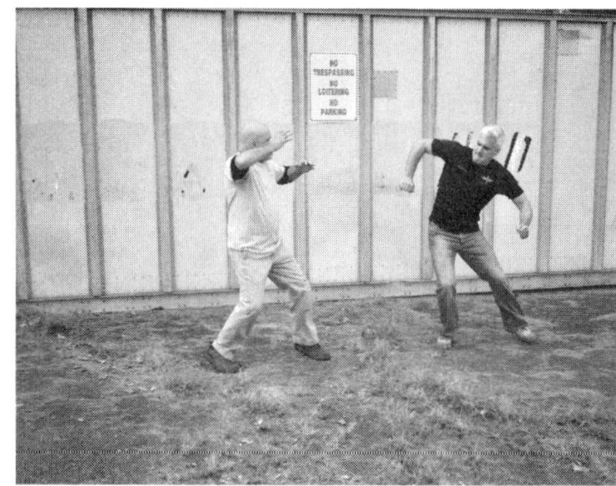

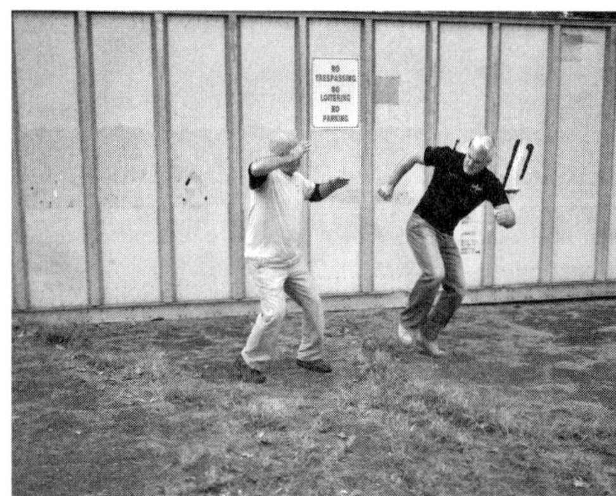

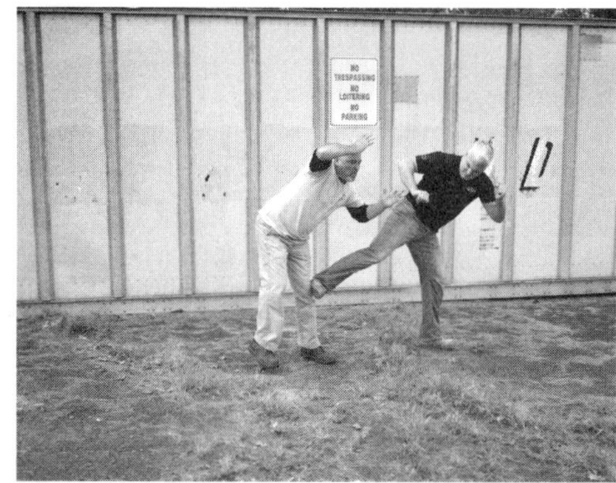

This series depicts an attempt to back away from a confrontation using shuffle steps only to have an aggressor come after you. A side kick from a retreating shuffle stance is highly advantageous, targeting the attacker's lead knee lead knee to quickly stop the attack and likely disable him.

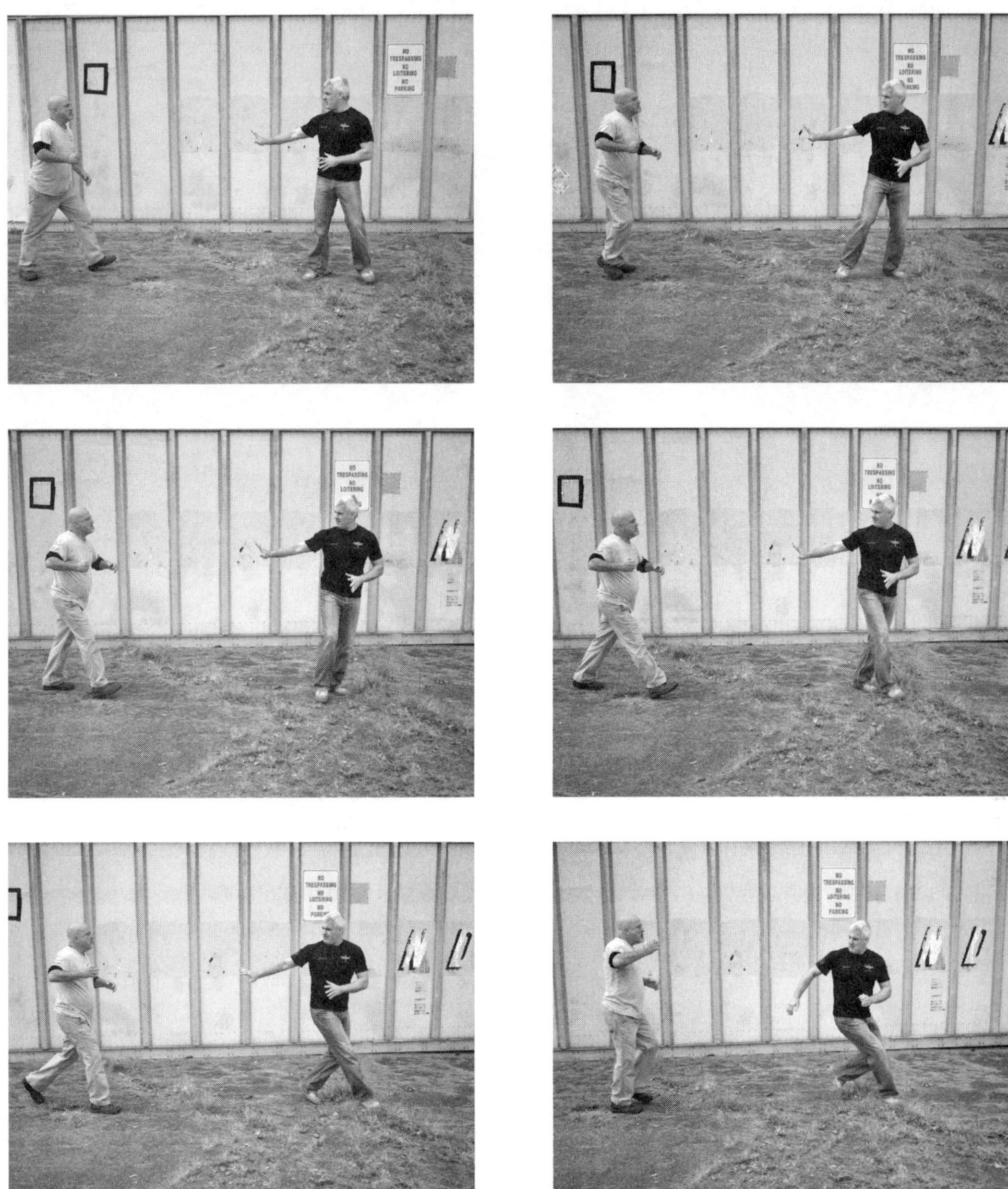

series continued on next page ...

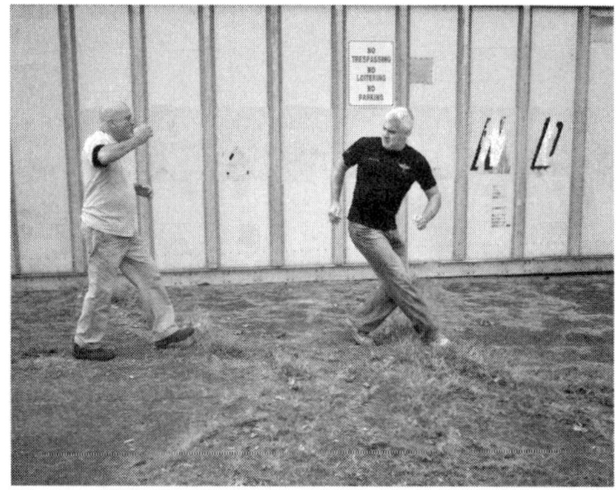

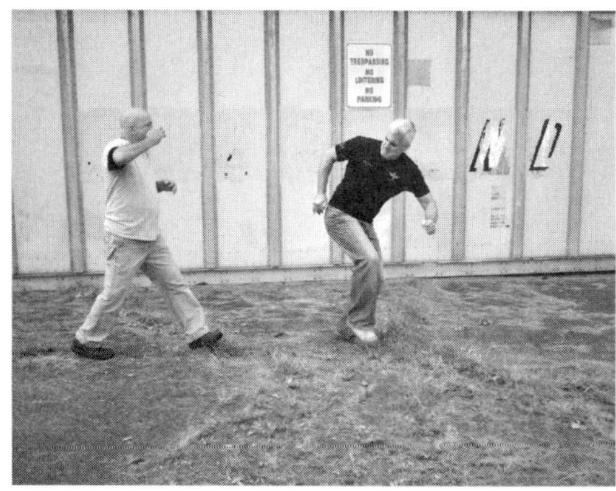

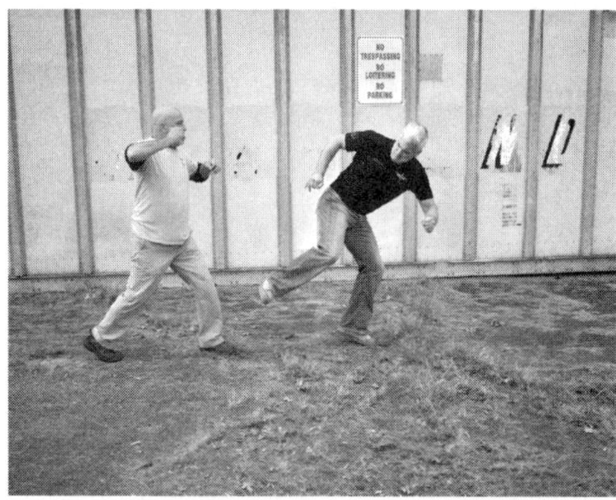

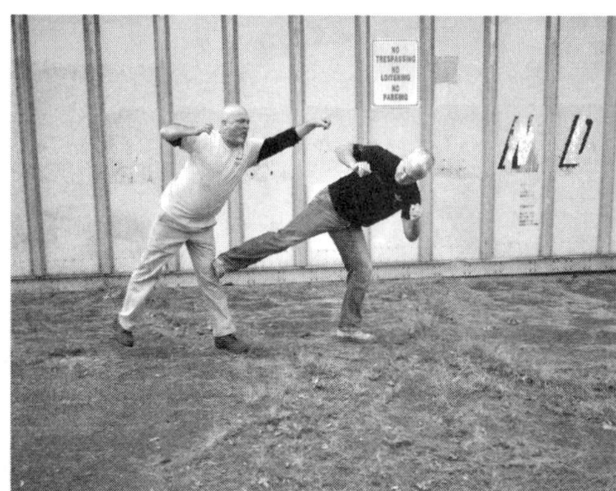

This series also depicts an attempt to turn and walk away from a confrontation only to have an aggressor come after you. Of course, never turn your back on an aggressor without keeping your head on a swivel to watch him as you try to create separation. This retreating cross-over step variation side kick targets the attacker's lead knee to quickly stop the attack and likely disable him.

Body Defense Strategies

Body defenses (often combined with parries against strikes) are integral to krav maga. A body defense is any movement that takes you off an attacker's line or plane of reach. Here are some essential body defense concepts and tactics:

- Slipping or moving your body off the line of a linear upper-body attack, a proven boxing tactic, requires exact timing and distance judgment so the defender barely escapes the attack. The slip allows for considerable surprise, and hence, superior counterattacks, as both of the defender's hands are free.
- Make the minimum movement when avoiding/redirecting the incoming blow. Minimum movement also accounts for a late instinctive reaction yet still allows for a successful defense.

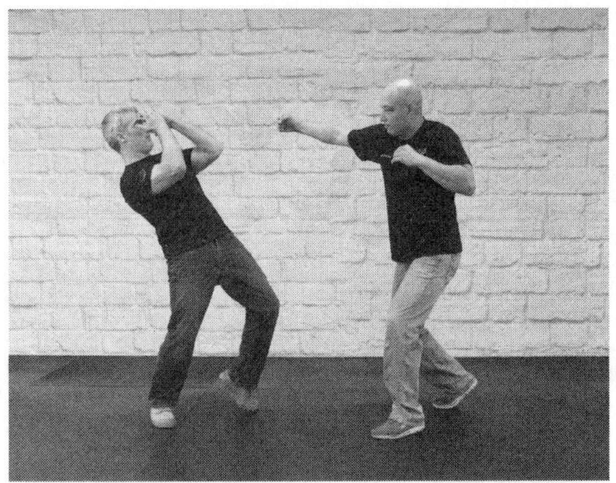
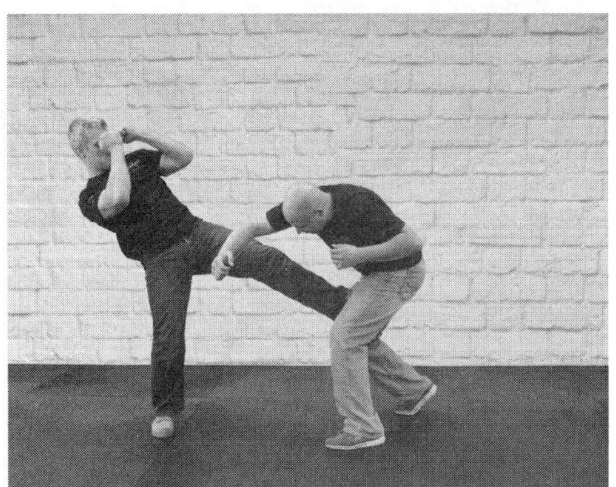

These two photos depict a pure body defense against a hook punch while using a straight kick counterattack.

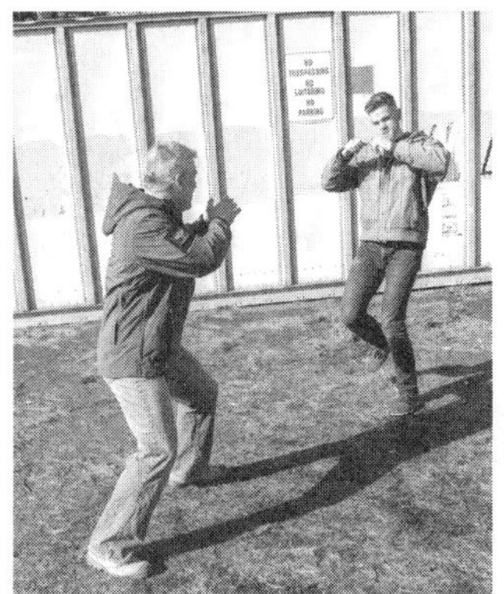
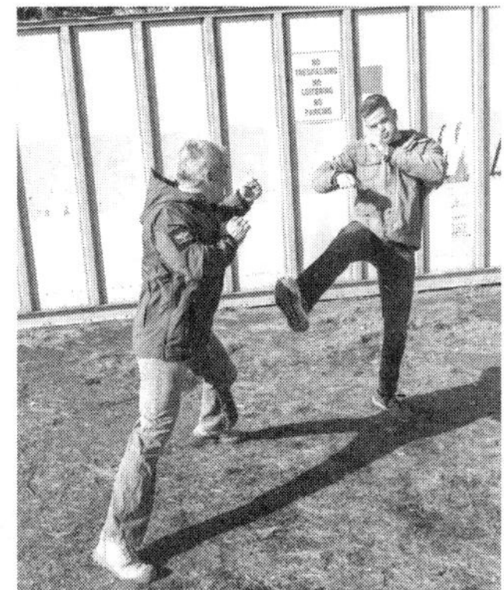
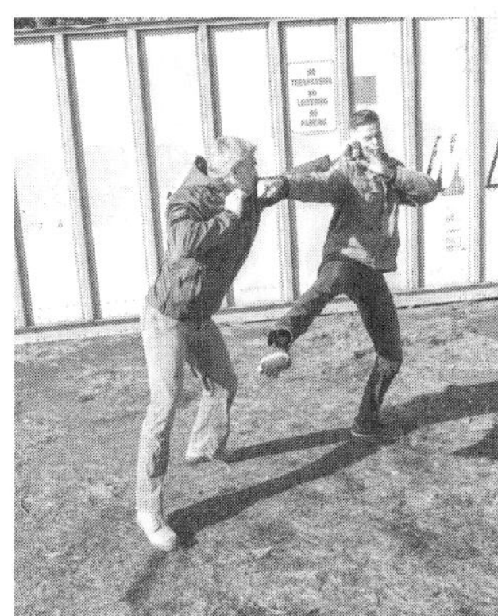

This series depicts a body pure defense stepping off the line combined with a counterpunch against a straight punch and kick combination attack.

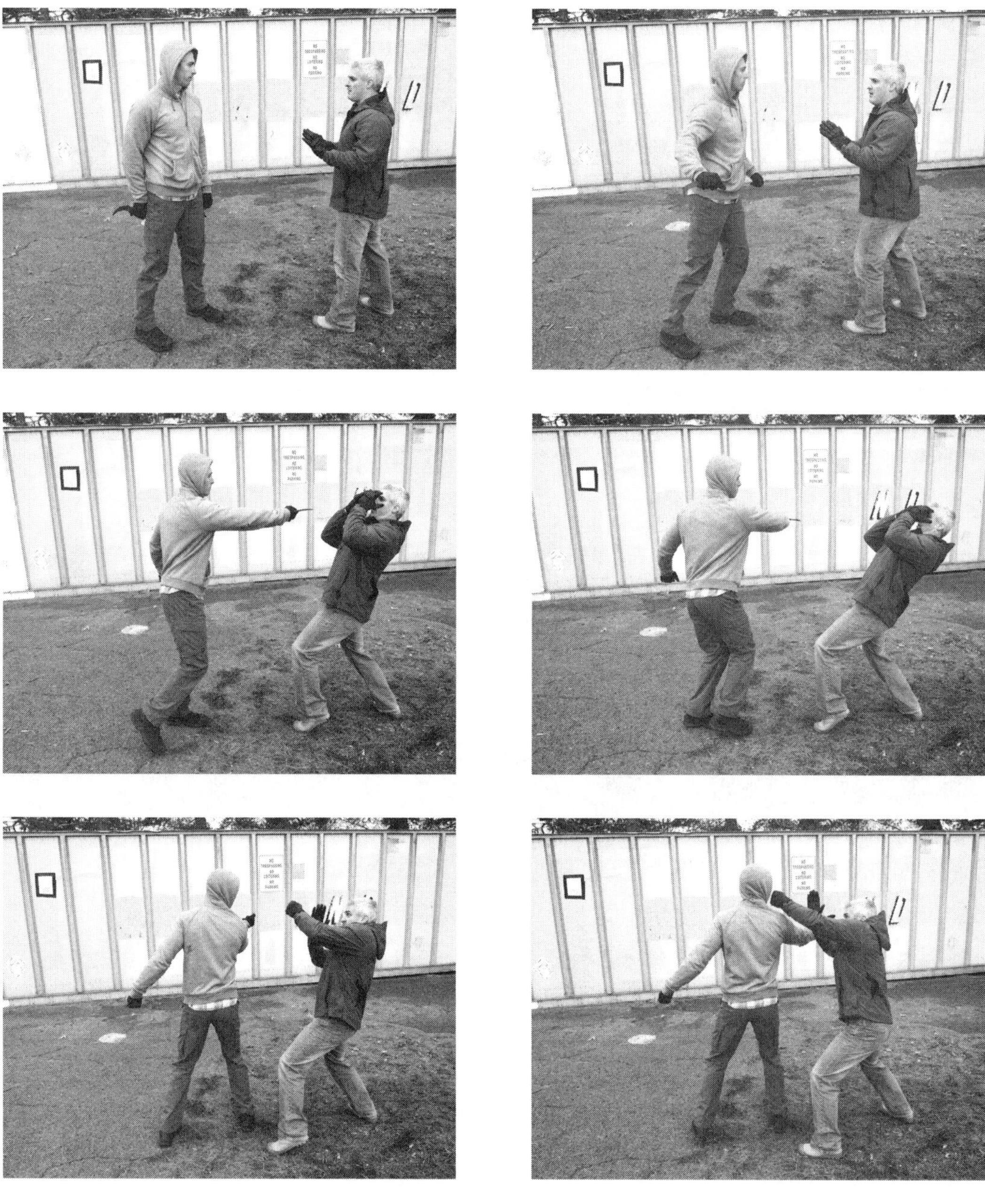

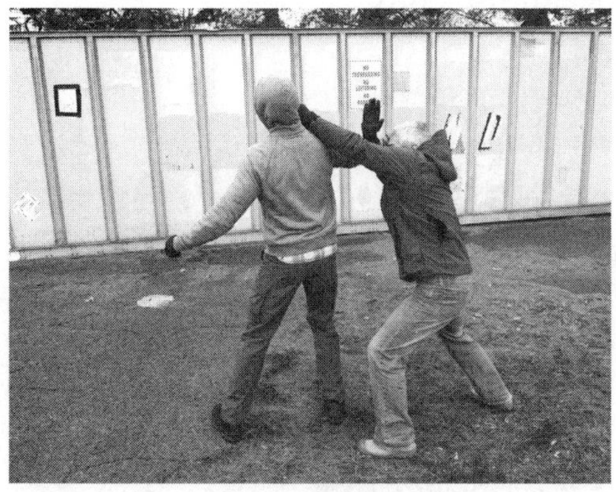

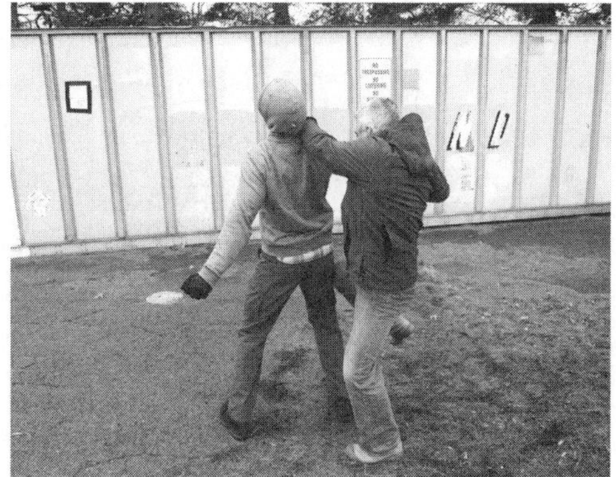

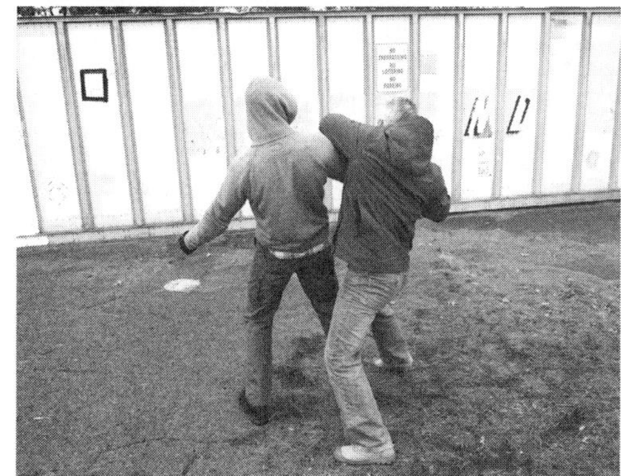

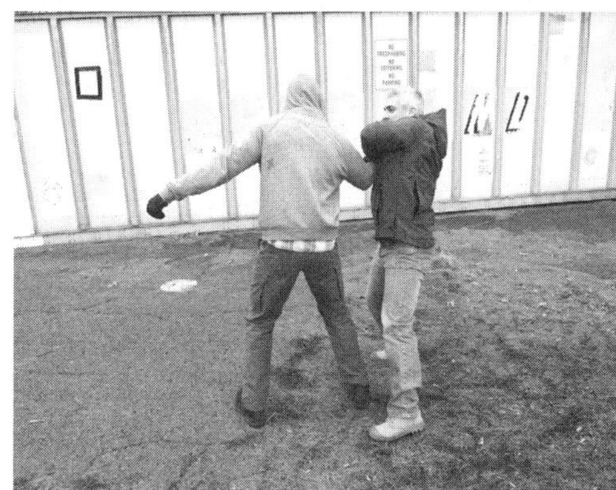

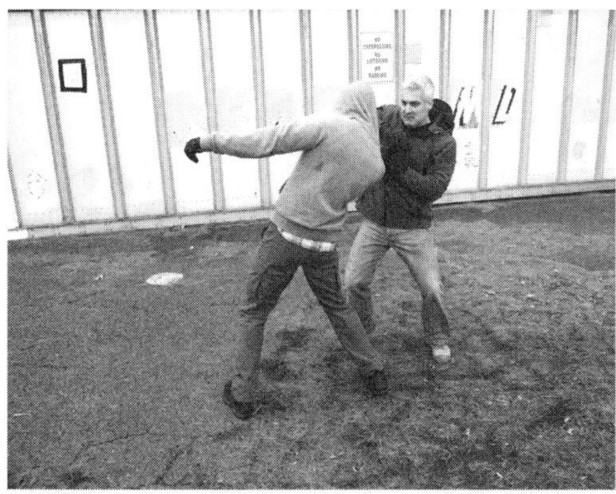

This series depicts a frontal forward slash and backslash defense targeting the neck. If you are taken by surprise, you must combine a body defense against a slash attempt by raising your arms defensively with your palms facing as you instantaneously shift your weight back by raising the ball of your front foot. You might also tactically decide that this initial retreat is a better method rather than immediately closing on the attacker to jam the slash. As soon as the blade passes by you, close to intercept and stop the arm, using a simultaneous over-the-top sliding counterpunch. Disable the attacker and confiscate the weapon using wrist cavalier #1.

Strategy for Intercepting an Attack: Parrying Versus Blocking

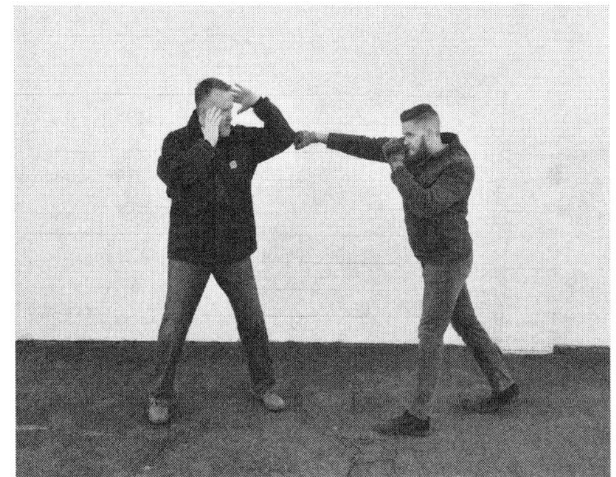

Blocking a straight punch.

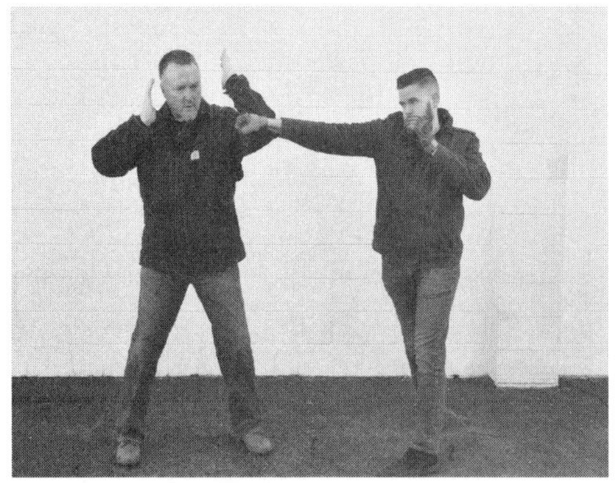

Parrying a straight punch.

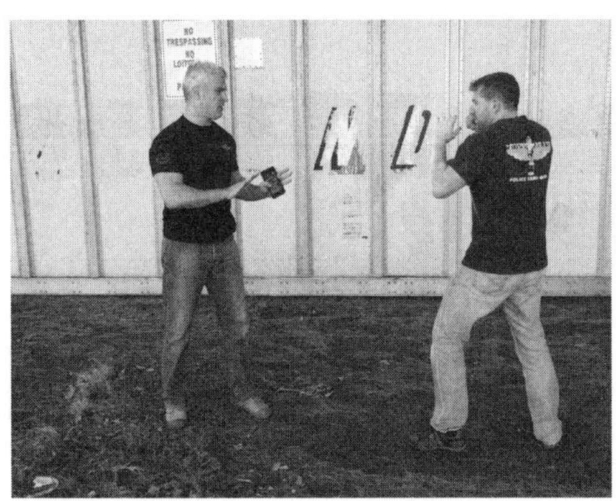

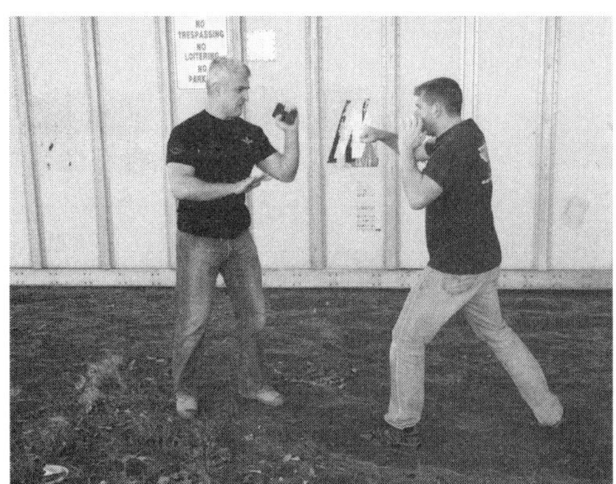

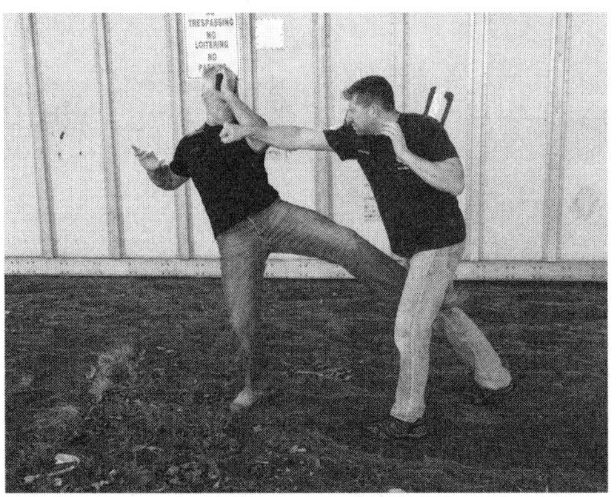

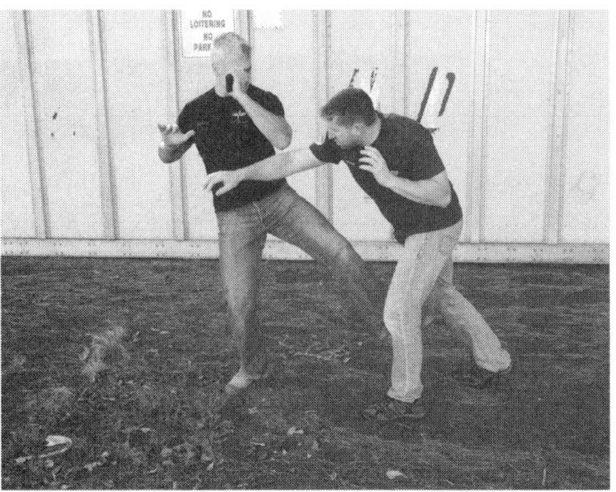

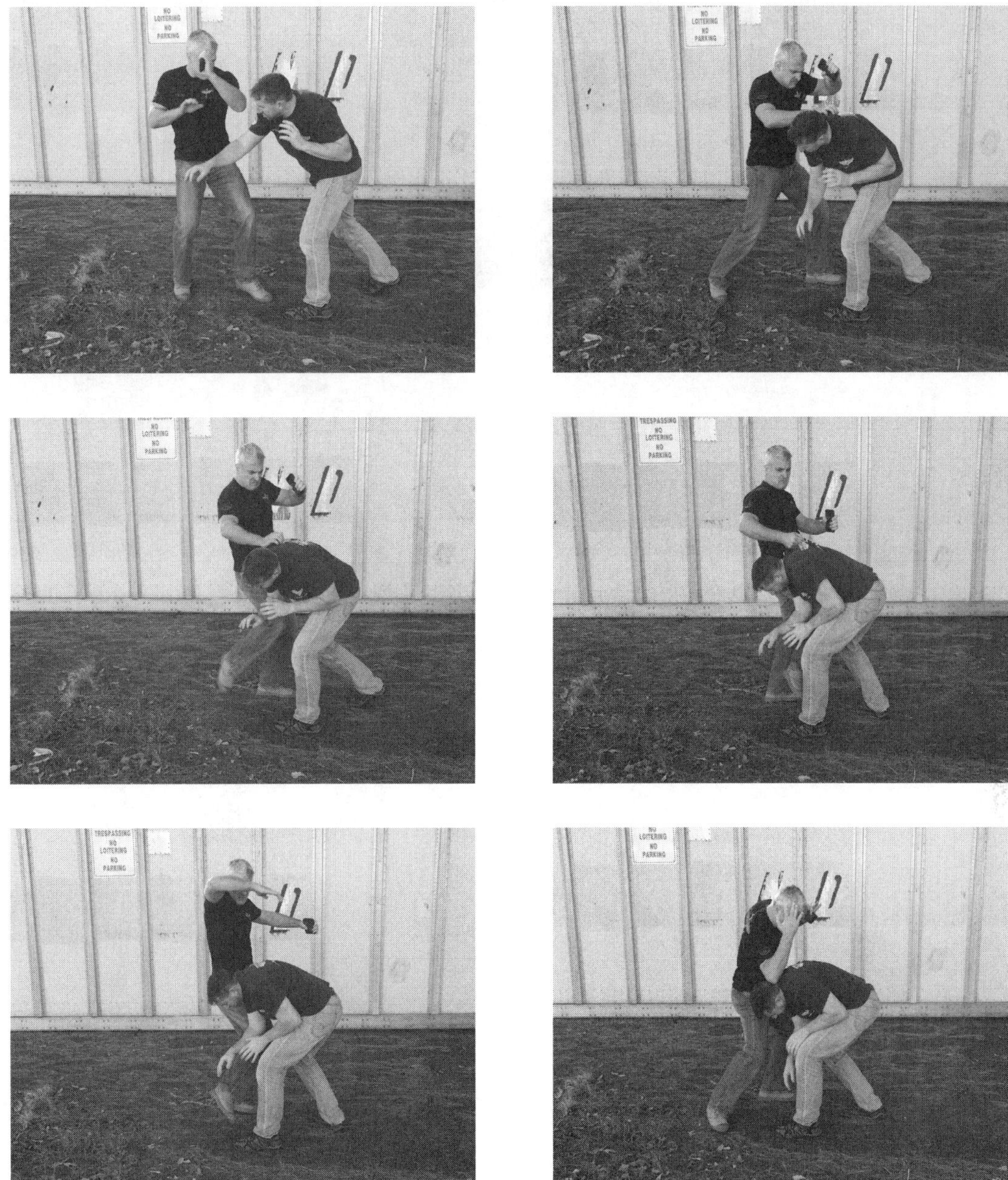

This series depicts a gunt defense against a straight punch with a mobile device in hand using a straight shin kick counterattack followed by a knee strike and drop-elbow strike combination.

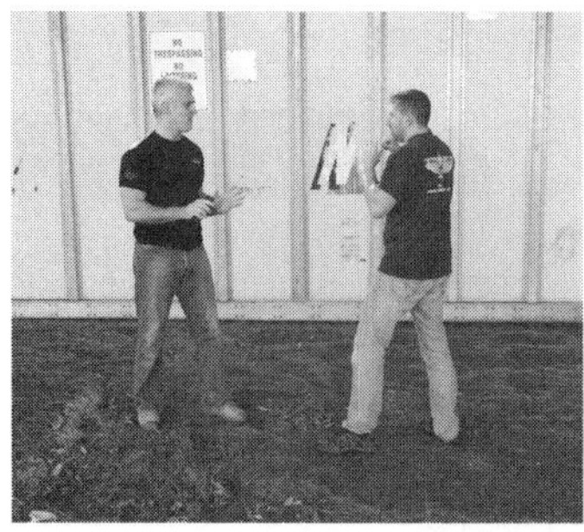
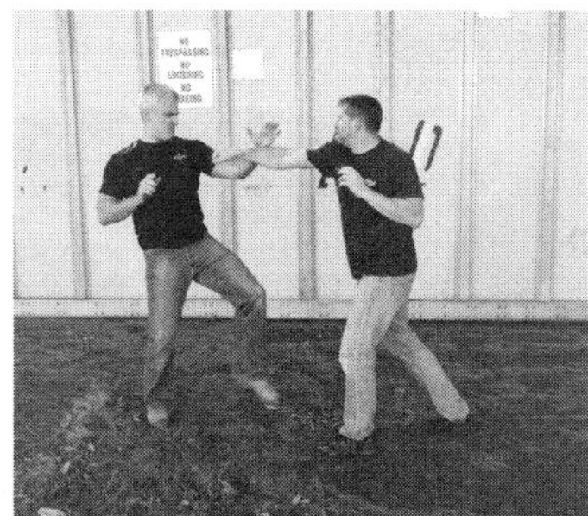
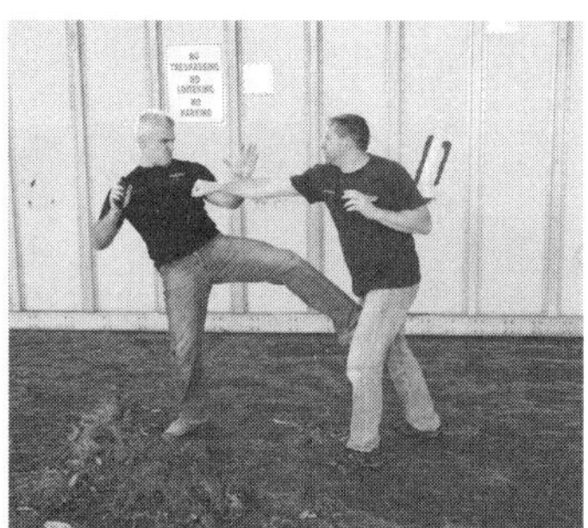

This series represents a parry defense against a straight punch with a mobile device in hand using a straight kick counterattack with the ball of the foot.

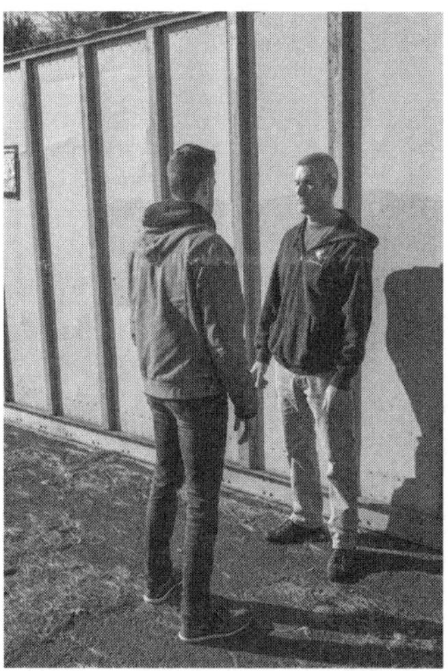
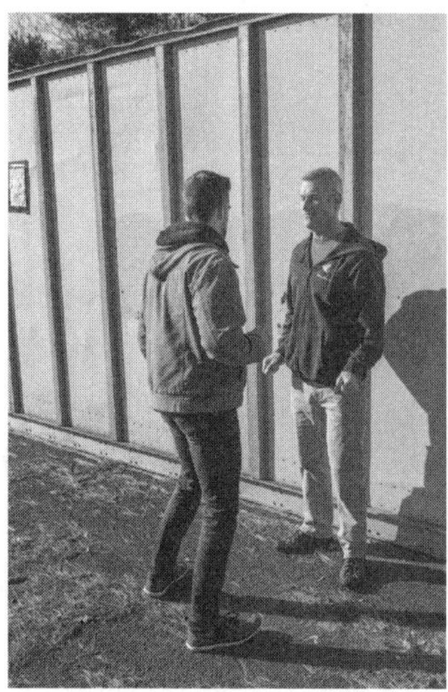
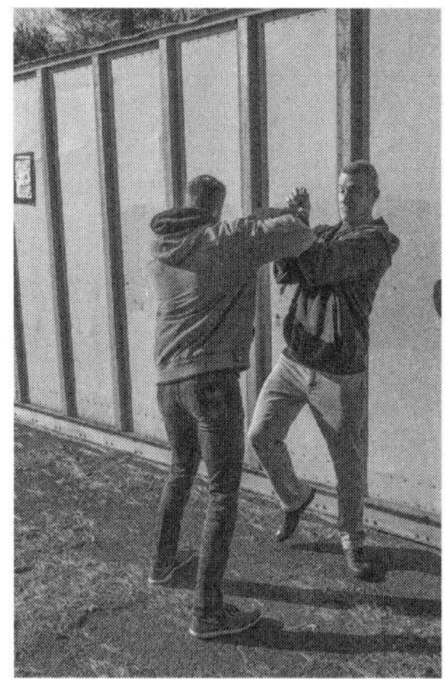
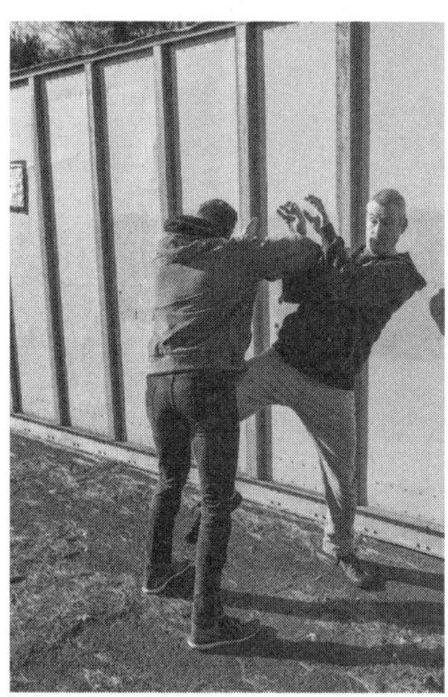

This series depicts a horizontal elbow strike defense using a double-arm absorption block combined with a simultaneous straight knee counterattack.

Remember, when possible, a preemptive linear or non-linear combative, sometimes coupled with an evasion, usually a sidestep, is optimally delivered when the opponent prepares to launch his attack. In other words, *eliminate his line of his attack before he can execute the assault.* Such a preemptive strike can then preclude the need to block or parry. An open-handed block is better referred to as a parry since the fist is not closed and the defender is not powering through the deflection.

Here are some essential blocking and parrying arm positioning insights:

- Parries and blocks must be shorter movements than attacks since the defender is "catching up to the attack." In other words, action (an attack) obviously precedes reaction (a defense). The defender must therefore compensate for this time in motion by making a shorter, economical intercepting movement. An efficient movement can overcome the fractions-of-a-second time delay required by a reaction. This concept applies to preemptive attacks as well. The defender must therefore compensate for this time in motion (action versus reaction/Colonel John Boyd's Observe Orient Decide Act [OODA] Loop) by making shorter, more economical and equally aggressive countering movements. Examples include:
  - gunting against a body blow
  - inside and outside arm rotations to attack the attacker's arm, intercepting and sending it off course
  - leg deflections/interceptions against straight and roundhouse kicks
  - linear straight punches against hook punches
  - linear kicks to the attacker's knee or thigh against rear roundhouse kicks (a straight motion versus a rounded motion).

- Blocking an attack must obviously be accomplished with correct timing: not too early and too late. Note: Blocking is the least efficient defense, as the method requires absorbing physical punishment. Importantly, krav maga does not rely on force versus force. Hence, krav maga emphasizes parrying (deflecting) when possible, as opposed to blocking (absorbing). See next paragraph.
- As with blocking, parrying an attack must obviously be accomplished with correct timing: not too early and too late. Parries should be used simultaneously with a change in distance forward (often a 45-degree forward step) or in a slight retreat, forcing the attack to be driven away or fall short. Importantly, the change in distance must not undermine your ability to counterattack; in other words, do not overextend. Be sure that your parries are well controlled, while at the same time forcefully attacking the attacker's arm.

- Parries, especially when combined with a body defense, are preferably used moving in a forward direction, providing strong stability and minimized exposure, while moving your feet equidistantly.
- For both parrying and blocking, keep your arms in a good defensive position with your hands in and in front of your face to allow the interception of all incoming strikes. For hand positioning in a comfortable fighting stance, I suggest dropping your hands to your sides and then simply raising them up to your eyebrows. Keep your elbows bent at about 70 degrees to extend your arm slightly away from your body. This is a natural position for your hands—not too close and not too far away from your head.
- In a fighting stance the arms should not be rigid and should be kept moving slightly to keep the opponent guessing your intent.
- An attacker who grabs you may be trying to stabilize your torso just before launching the attack rather than seeking social dominance by simply shaking or grabbing you.
- Attack the aggressor's incoming attacking limb with extreme prejudice. Parries and blocks should often be thought of as offensive not defensive, and as the beginning of your counterattack.
- Lastly, by presenting a vulnerable opening by retracting or dropping your arms to bait an opponent into attacking you and, thus, presenting an anatomical vulnerability for your counterattack, is proven fight strategy.

Absorbing and Moving with an Attack

It is not always possible to completely avoid a strike; however, the goal is to avoid receiving a blow at full force. It may be that an ambush type of attack happens so quickly you can neither parry nor block, in which case you might have to absorb a blow. In the event you must absorb a blow to the head, you should move away from the incoming combative, or, explained differently, with its direction. If you are struck, it is best to be struck by a glancing blow resulting from your movement. If you are struck, you also want to move with the strike to better absorb it and dissipate its impact; do not resist it. In other words, you are not strengthening or tightening up your neck muscles to absorb the blow.

Mobility and stability are key to your ability to defend, but not mutually supportive. A compromise is required. The ability to maintain balance while constantly shifting body weight is an ability, or an art, that requires training to master. When struck, move your head to not take the full jolt, as demonstrated in the photos. You must counterattack as soon as possible to halt any further attacks.

Absorbing a Combative's Energy

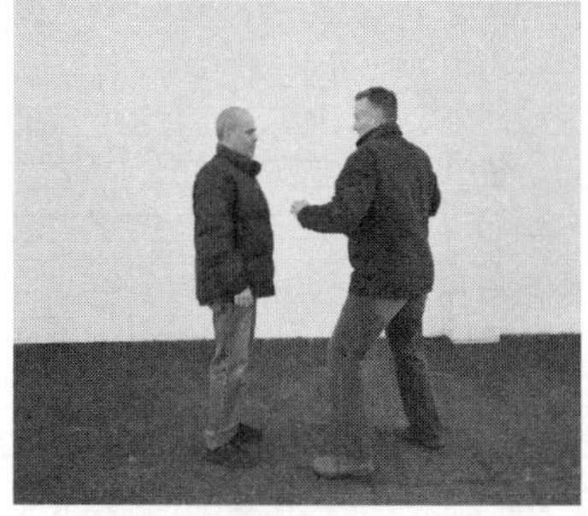
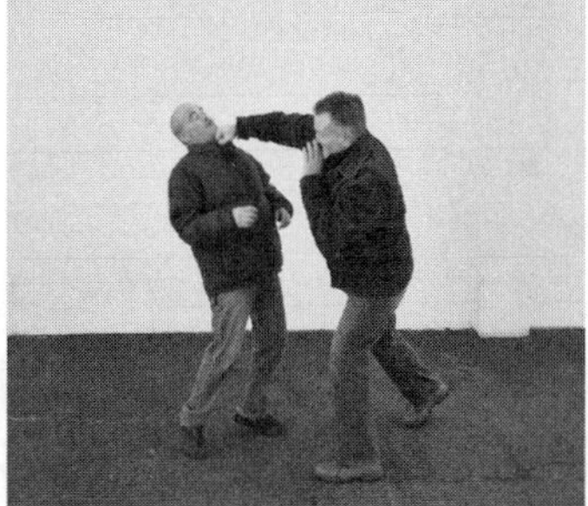
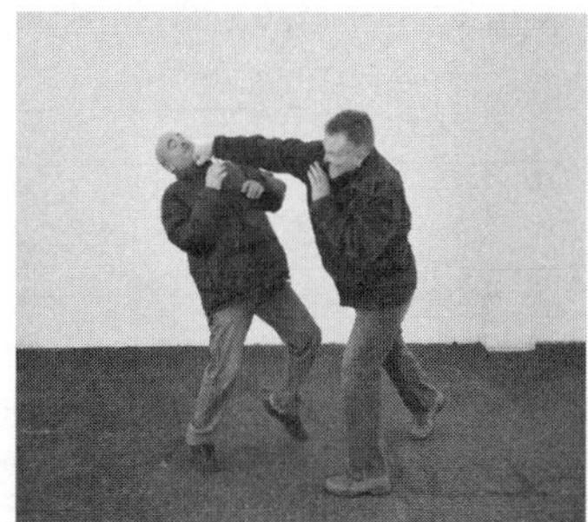
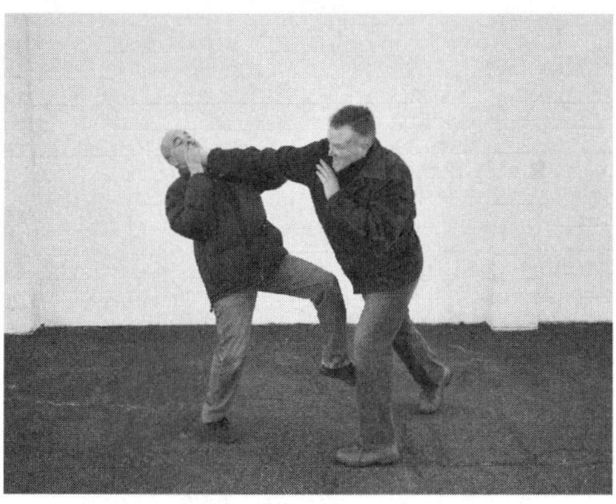
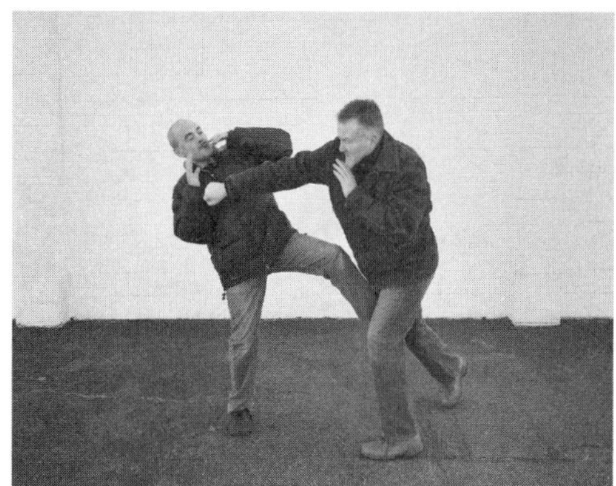

This series represents getting hit and moving with a punch while launching a near-simultaneous counterattack straight kick with the shin.

Harnessing an Attacker's Momentum

It may also be that an ambush takedown attempt from the rear happens so quickly you have no choice but to move with it. It is a logical strategy that you harness the attacker's forward momentum and use it against him as you can.

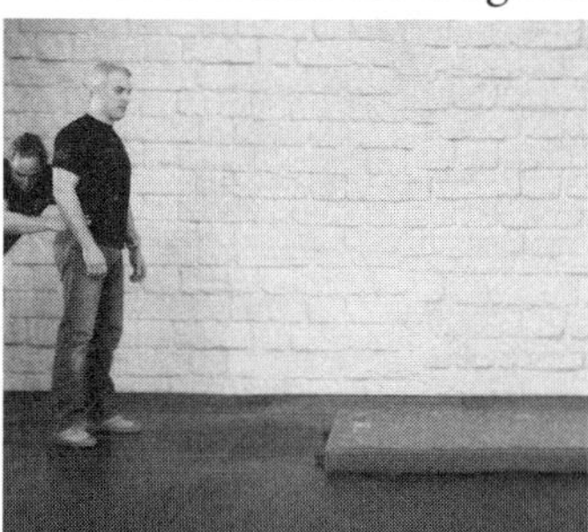
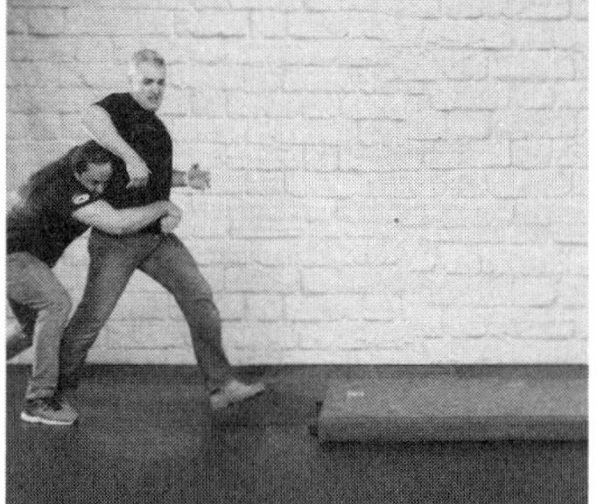
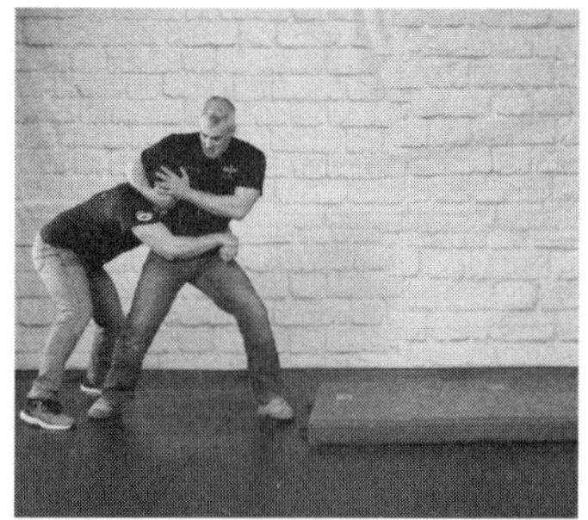

series continued on next page ...

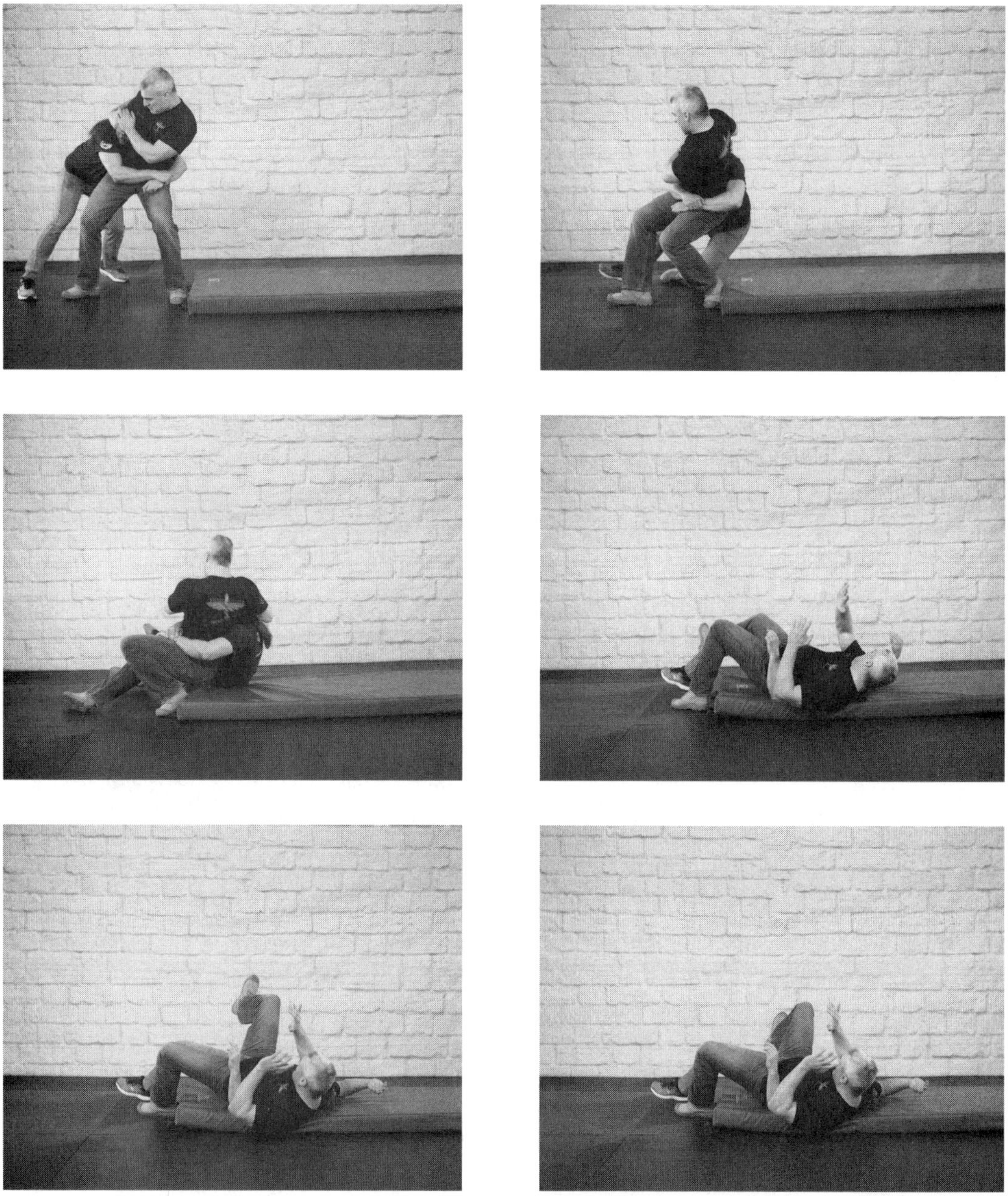

This series depicts defending against a rear takedown ambush where the attacker builds up momentum. When he jolts you forward, you must move with the attack by instinctively stepping forward. Usually, the attacker will place his head to the side, allowing you to clamp down on it. As you are forced forward, tai-sabaki footwork allows you to harness his momentum by taking a 180-degree step to create a controlled descent for you. Land with your body weight on top of the attacker and administer additional combatives as necessary.

Fighting Range Strategies

In an impending fight, begin to dominate by controlling the attacker's distance and position, along with drawing on your ability to engage in tactical targeting. When the opportunity arises, utilize what is known as the combat circle: let the opponent move wildly around you while you use economy of motion, footwork, and energy conservation. Keep in mind that verbal exchanges and fusillades begin often within leg or hand range.

A few general points to incorporate into your self-defense strategy:

- Most attacks and fights take place at close range.
- Fights are frenetic and unpredictable.
- Attacks can commence without warning.
- Verbal aggression or subterfuge may precede the physical attack.
- Against an opponent whose arms and legs give him a longer reach, if you are forced to fight, you must get inside his reach or stay just outside of it, and when he commits to an attack, you must meet him with your momentum against his momentum to inflict maximum damage.

The angle between you and your attacker dictates offensive and defensive capabilities for both of you. Superior positioning reduces your need to rely on speed. Your stance facilitates speed and timing by allowing you to orchestrate linear punches and kicks that are much more difficult to intercept than circular attacks. A good stance allows you to defend against all types of attacks. It is crucial to have each of your limbs positioned so they can defend linear and circular strikes, grabs, throws, and takedowns. Once again, you must be comfortably on the balls of your feet to facilitate movement and spring into action.

If you cannot overwhelm the attacker and end up temporarily disengaged while facing him, you should keep moving to prevent becoming a static target. Controlled movement also allows you to camouflage any additional attacks you may unleash as you launch into retzev. In short, movement from movement is more difficult to discern then movement from a stationary position.

Here are some essential fight-range concepts and tactics:

- Fights involve different phases that are best categorized by the distance or proximity combatants maintain as the fight progresses.
- From a long or medium range, fighters can use unhindered movement to batter one another, usually involving long kicks, medium punches, and other hand strikes.
- From a short range, knees, elbows, headbutts, shoulder butts, and biting become options. Also available are a variety of standing entanglements involving medium and short strikes, trapping, clinching, throws, takedowns, and standing joint locks combined for "close retzev."
- The final ground phase occurs when both fighters lock up to unbalance one another to the ground, involving medium and short combatives combined with locks and chokes.

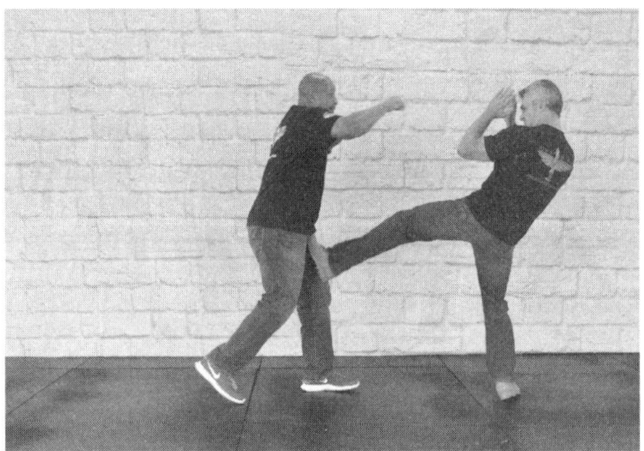

Long-range engagement kick.

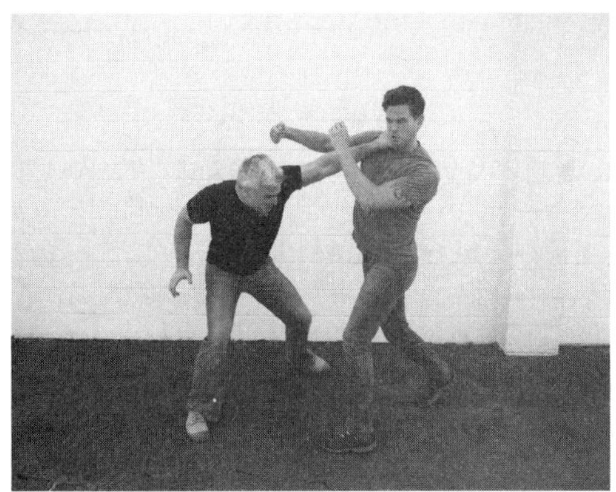

Medium-range engagement using a linear arm strike.

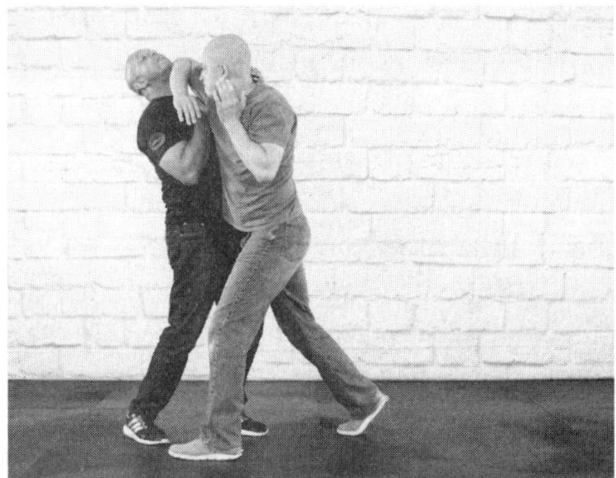

Short-range engagement using an elbow strike.

Grappling Range Engagement—Bites

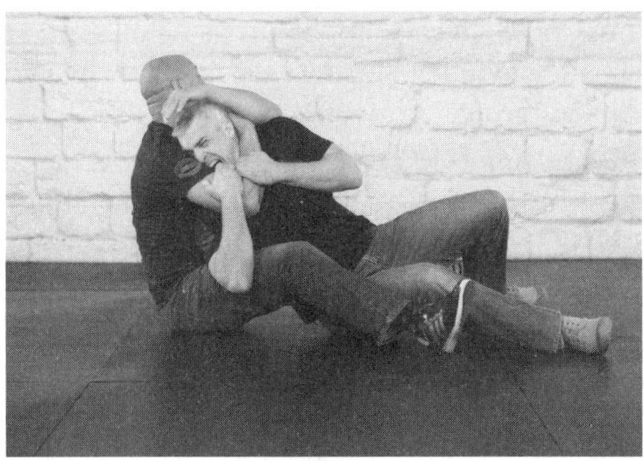

Intimate-range biting.

Sample Defense Strategies against a Skilled Fighter

In grappling, it is key that you be able to control your own body, and particularly your balance, while preventing your adversary from controlling his. The center of gravity is generally just below the navel. To disrupt an adversary's balance, you must force the opponent's center of gravity away from his centerline.

Krav maga teaches simple and effective takedowns that usually flow naturally from other techniques to put an opponent on the ground. Think of these techniques as extensions of a previously completed combative technique, such as a gouge to the eyes to disorient an opponent as you perform an outside reverse sweep (osoto gari) as described in this book. Advanced hip-throws and other takedowns are integral parts of advanced krav maga training.

As noted, selecting a takedown or a throw is generally determined by body positioning and the dynamics of the entry to the throw. As with all krav maga strategy, the goal with throws and takedowns is to have the greatest effect with the least effort. Your aim with any type or throw or takedown is to disrupt the opponent's balance while hastening his impact with the ground. In other words, undercut your adversary's balance by collapsing his structure. Tactically, this could include crippling one of his knees, sweeping his feet from under him, or picking him up and dropping him pointedly on a specific part of his anatomy. You can disrupt an opponent's base by (1) severing the connection of his feet with the ground; (2) moving him to the edge of his base so his center of gravity falls outside of it; or (3) demolishing his stance, forcing his center of gravity beyond his base. Keep in mind that the center of gravity of a moving or non-static threat constantly moves as his base changes.

In short, krav maga takedowns and throws principally distill into two aforementioned methods: (1) removing the opponent's base (his legs), destroying his balance or (2) forcing his center of gravity (just below the navel for most people) beyond a stable base (his two balanced legs).

This type of combative that forces the opponent to drop unassisted or pounds him into the ground is designed to inflict serious damage such as neck or spinal injury, skull fracture, wrist fracture, elbow or coccyx fracture, a damaged shoulder, or a concussion. So, obviously use this type of combative only when necessary. (Keep in mind that if you trip or throw someone to the ground, a jury will probably conclude that you intended to inflict serious injury.)

Clearly, in a life-and-death violent encounter, you may wish to make the throw as damaging as possible. With a throw or takedown, physics allows you to heighten an impact's velocity by approximately 50 percent by undercutting both of the opponent's legs instead of just one. While you can also maximize impact by adding your body weight if you fall on top of the opponent, krav maga emphasizes remaining standing and mobile whenever possible.

In summary, infighting incorporates many different martial skills including how to tie up, clinch, take down, apply joint/body locks, bludgeon, choke, and strangle an opponent. Accordingly, infighting requires all the skills to be interwoven and used interchangeably. Understand, too, that clinching is a position rather than a specific tactic.

Mixed Martial Arts (MMA) fighters, wrestlers, judoka, and other multi-disciplined skilled fighters with strong takedown and ground tactics excel at controlling an opponent's body movement when grappling, and, ultimately, locked up. Generally, the average person and, sometimes, martial artist alike are untutored in grappling and ground survival. Krav maga teaches you to close on an opponent to disable him. Conversely, he may also attempt to close in on you. This may well lead to a clinching and grappling scenario which, in turn, may lead to a ground survival scenario. Of course, not going to the ground is best, so one's long- and medium-range combatives should be optimized to obviate locking up with anyone. MMA practitioners are skilled at accurately assessing distances and how to measure distance with time and time with distance. Accordingly, a skilled MMA practitioner will patiently wait for the optimum moment to close when you or he (often through a feint) put yourself in a vulnerable position.

Many escalations and stare-downs bring two hostile parties within bad breath range of each other—ideal clinch range. Many MMA fighters excel at clinching for punishing knee strikes along with throws and takedowns. Therefore, counter-clinch tactics are instrumental in avoiding these potentially debilitating entanglements and, equally important, in avoiding being taken to the ground. Notably, for two unskilled combatants, the progression of a violent encounter often results in some sort of clinch. Keep in mind that takedowns most often result from:

1. A skilled practitioner's design or strategy.
2. Instinct to tie up an adversary when the defender is at a disadvantage.
3. Misstep or mistake by either or both of the combatants.

To best defend a takedown, you need to match the adversary's stance height. He will have to initiate to take you down, so exploit his entry. UFC former champion Chuck Liddell excelled in this type of counter-takedown strategy. Keep in mind that he may feint a strike, so you must be prepared to defend a strike followed by a seamless takedown tactic.

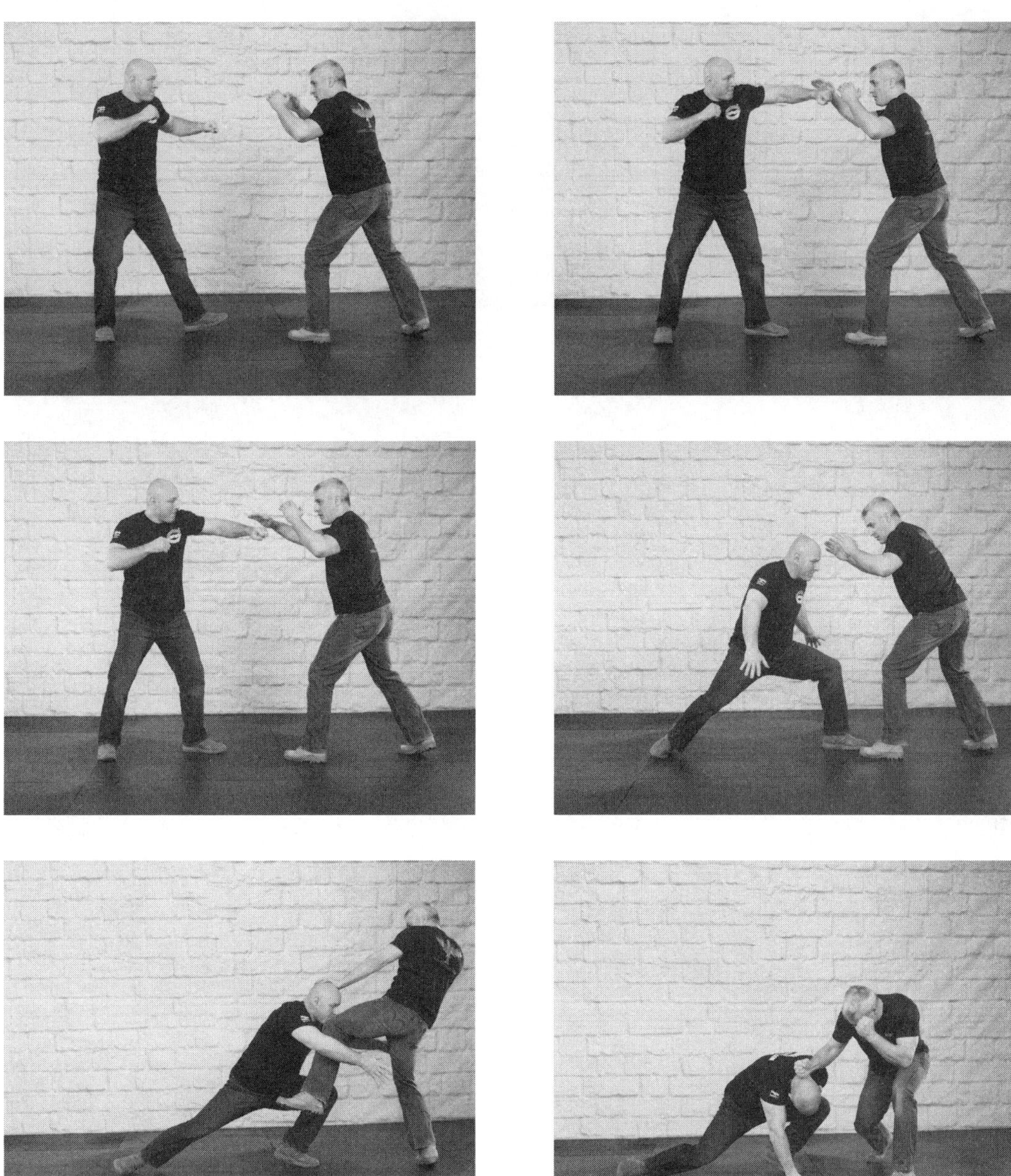

This series depicts an adversary who feigns or delivers a straight punch and drops his level to attempt a takedown. While you must honor the punch by staying on the balls of your feet, you can react by delivering a quick front leg shuffle straight knee to the attacker's face, using the strategy of the closest weapon to the closest target.

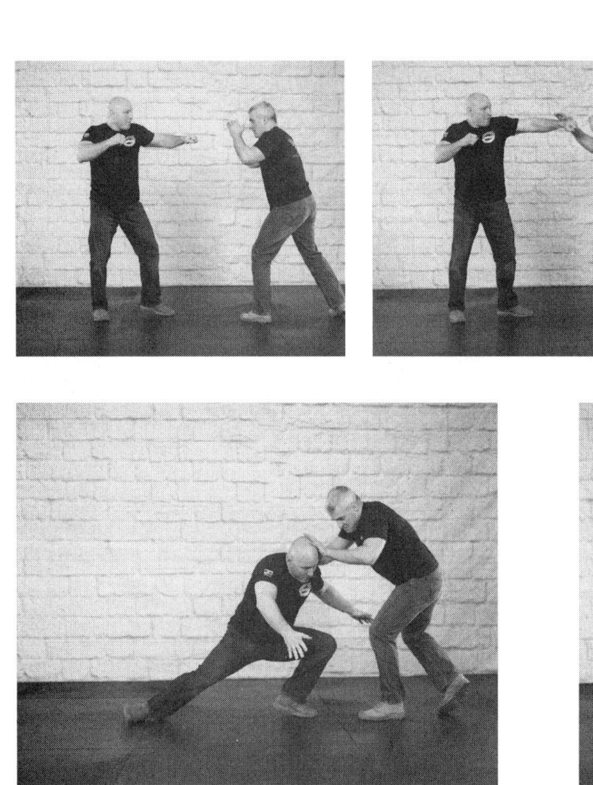
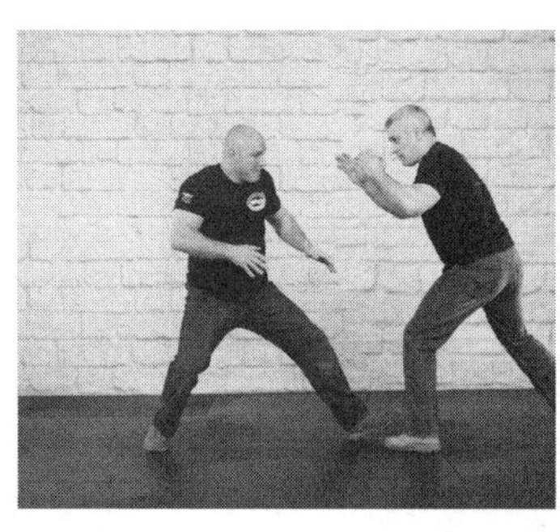
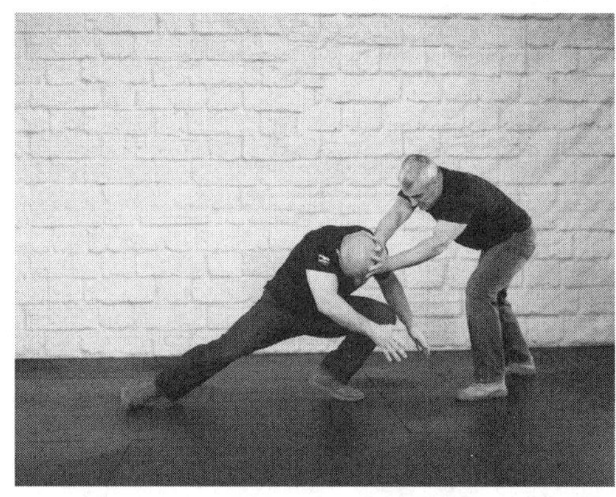
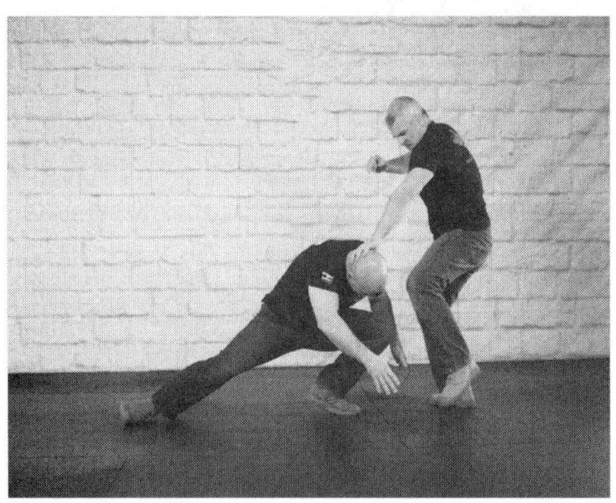
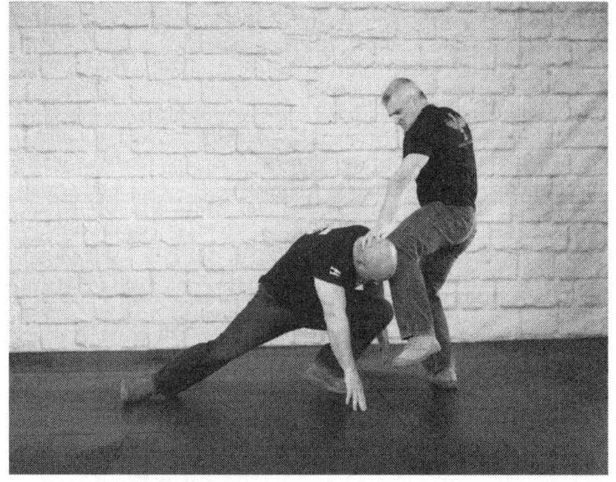

This series depicts an adversary who feigns or delivers a punch and then drops his level to attempt a takedown. Once again, while you must honor the punch by staying on the balls of your feet, you can react by delivering a strong double palm-heel jam to the attacker's face, followed by an immediate shuffle straight knee to his face.

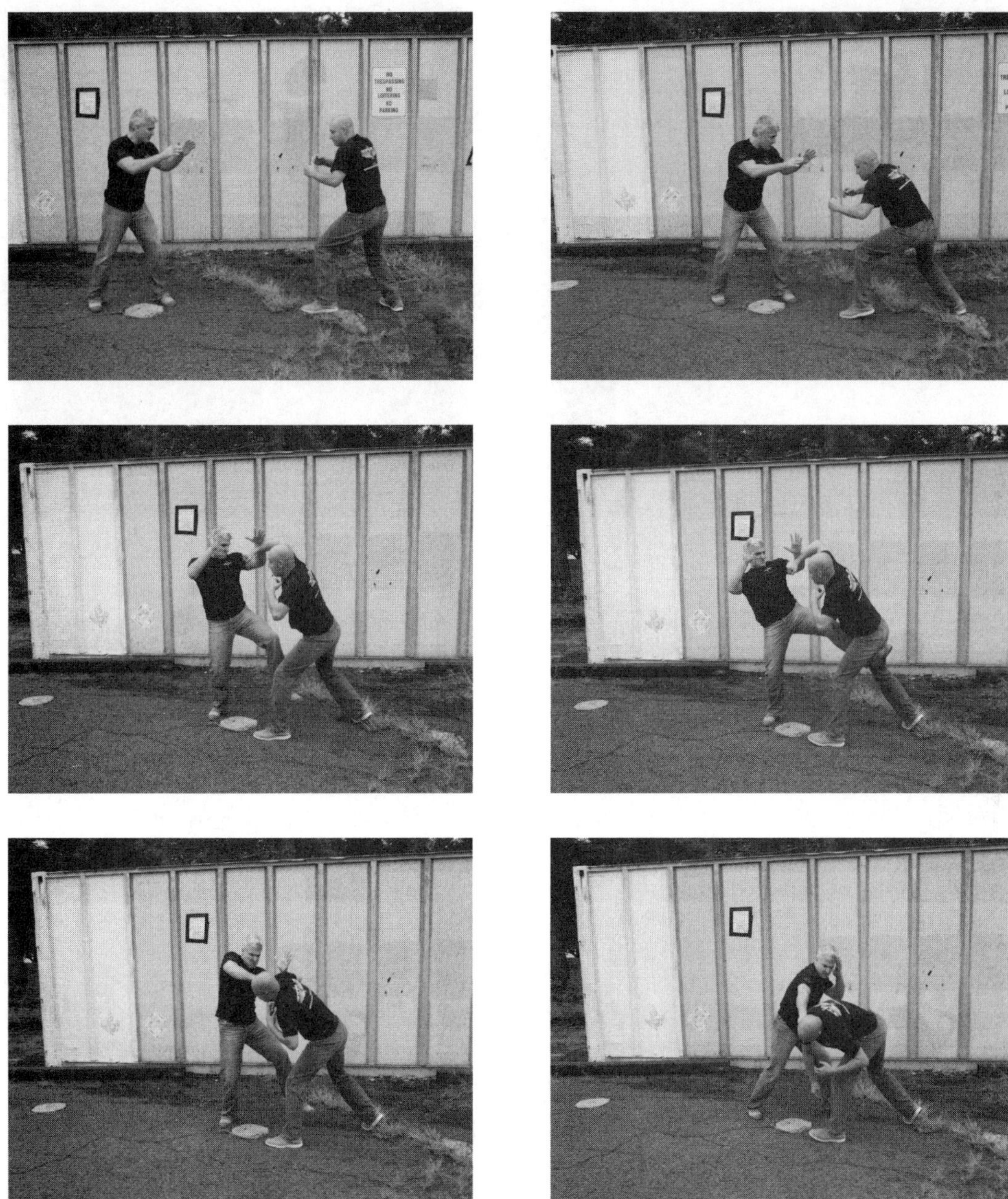

This series depicts a skilled adversary who may dip his body to feign a tackle takedown only to rise up at the last second to punch you in the face. Once again, you must always remain on the balls of your feet prepared for any eventuality—in this case honoring the takedown threat while intercepting, parrying, and countering the straight punch attack.

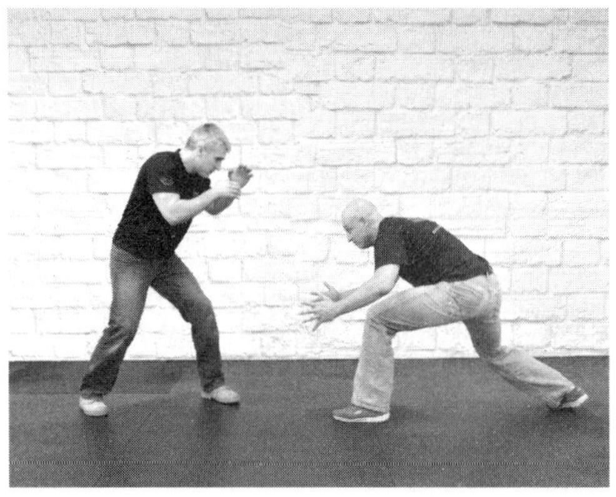

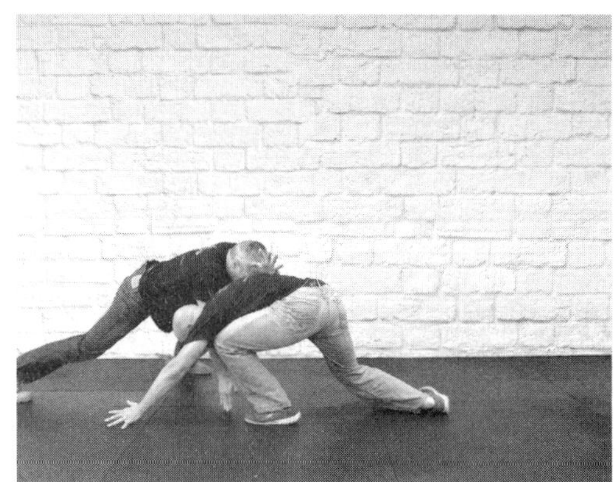

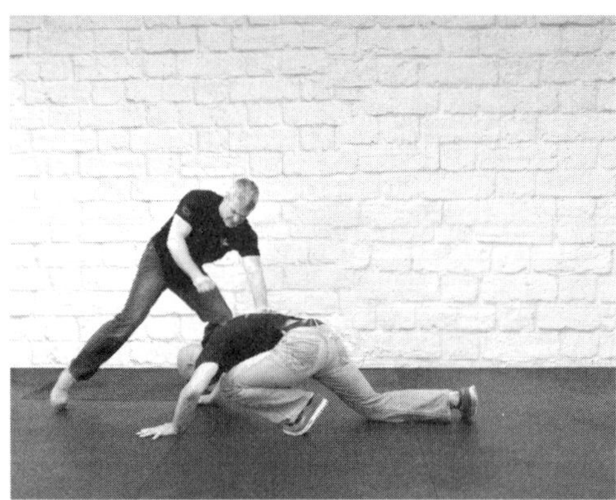

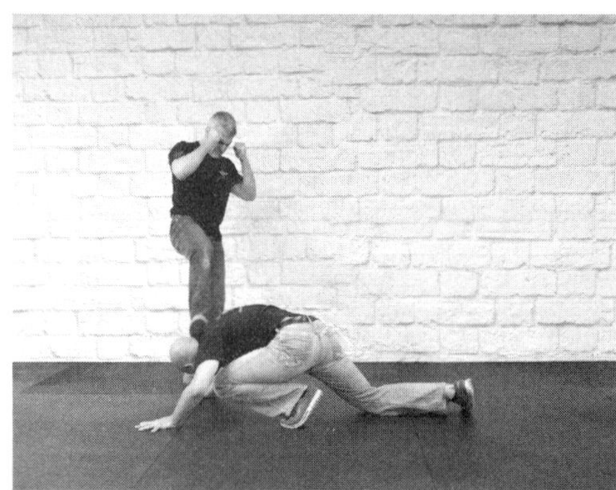

An inside sprawl option (defined as placement of the right arm against the attacker's inside shoulder) is depicted against an opponent who succeeds in catching you off guard or who slips underneath your defenses. When defending, keep your weight on the balls of your feet. Shoot your hips back while simultaneously dropping your nearside arm to the ground to intercept and block the takedown attempt. Your torso is slightly off-angle from the attacker's torse. Place your body weight on the attacker's head and upper torso. This defensive footwork allows you to get up immediately and use a power heel kick to debilitate the attacker.

Defending against a One-Hand Clinch and Punch to the Head

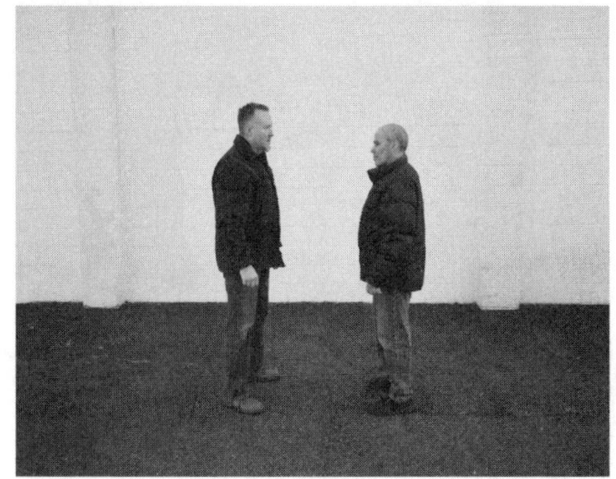

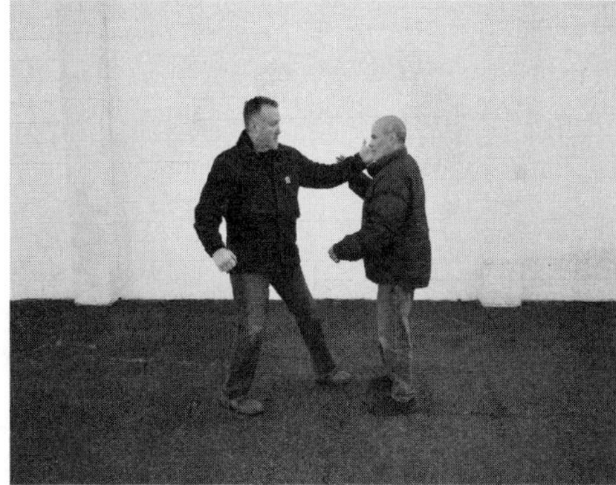

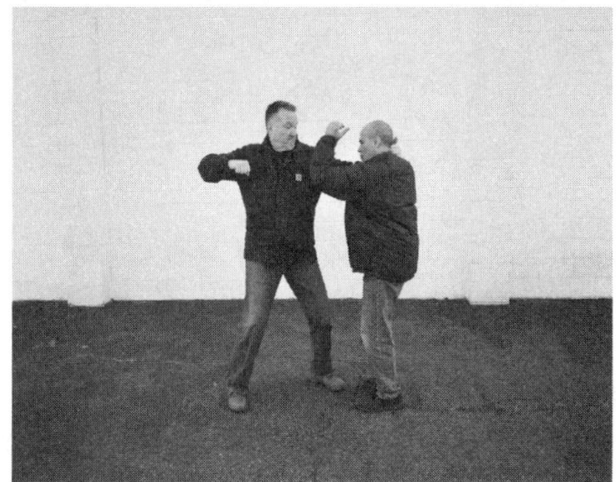

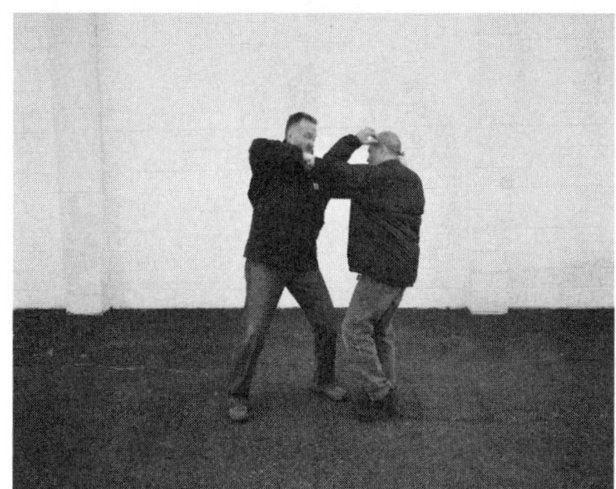

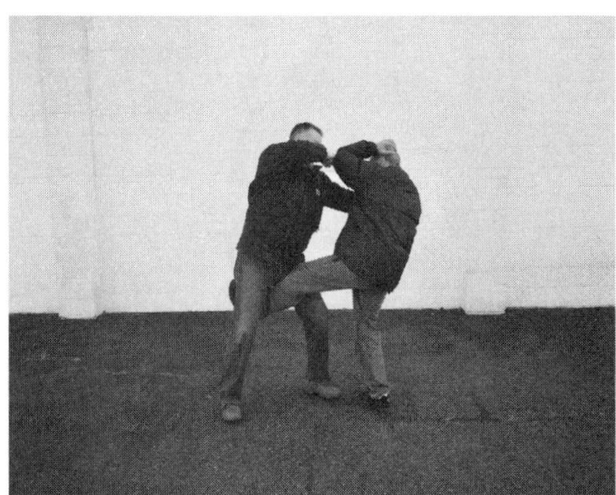

This series depicts an adversary who attempts to secure your head with a one-hand clinch and punch you in the face. Use a gunt deflection defense combined with a straight shin kick to the attacker's groin.

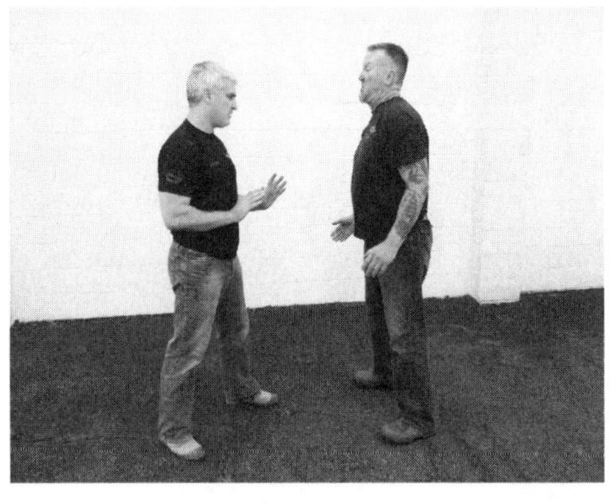
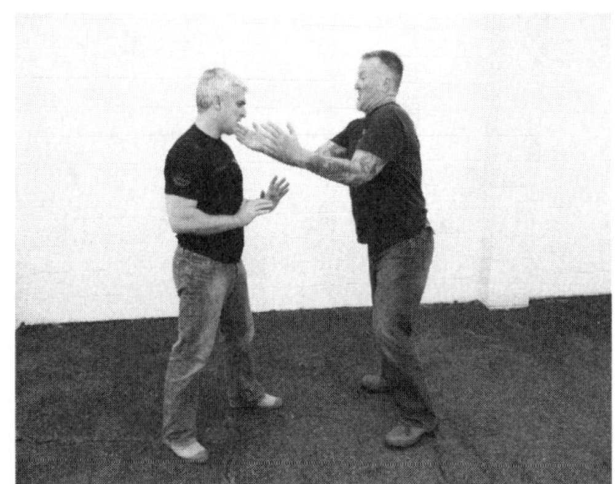
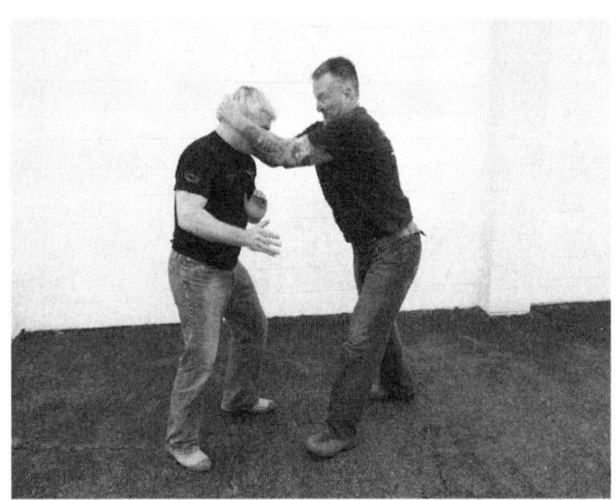
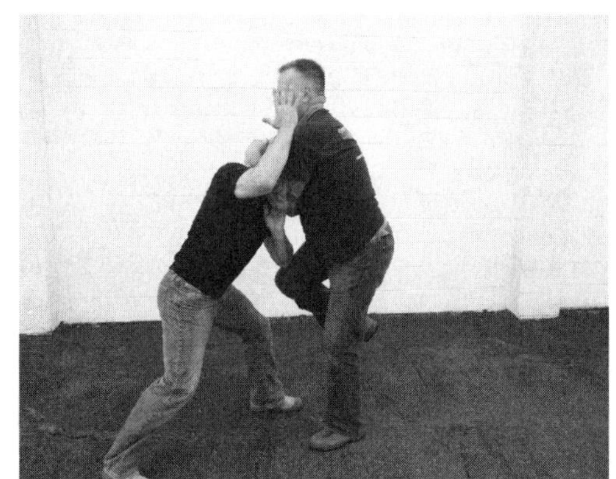
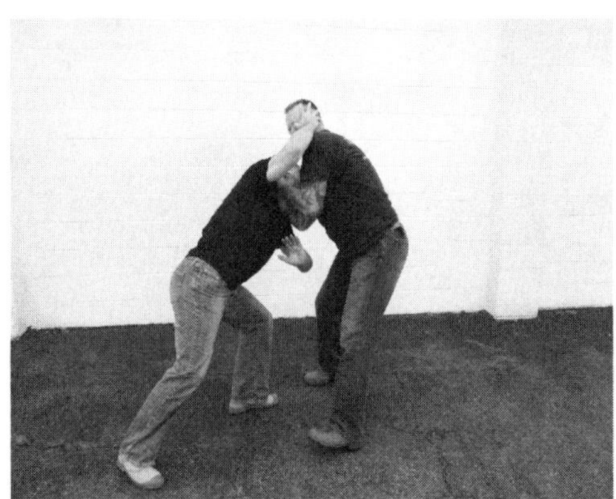
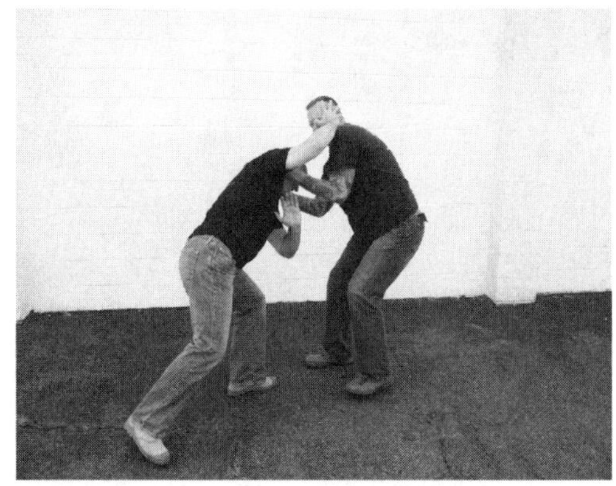

This series depicts an adversary who attempts to clinch your head and knee you. Defend with an elbow gunt deflection against either his right or left knee with a simultaneous eye gouge using this rule of thumb: find the cheek bone and you will find the lower eyelid in which to screw-drive your thumb.

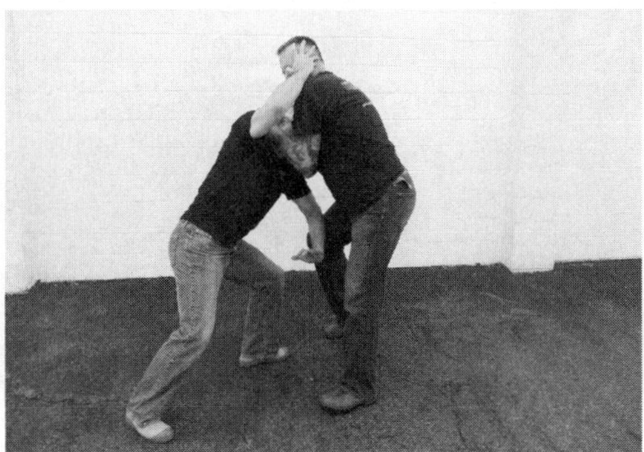

Here is an alternative forearm block against an adversary who attempts to secure your head with a one-handed clinch and knee you.

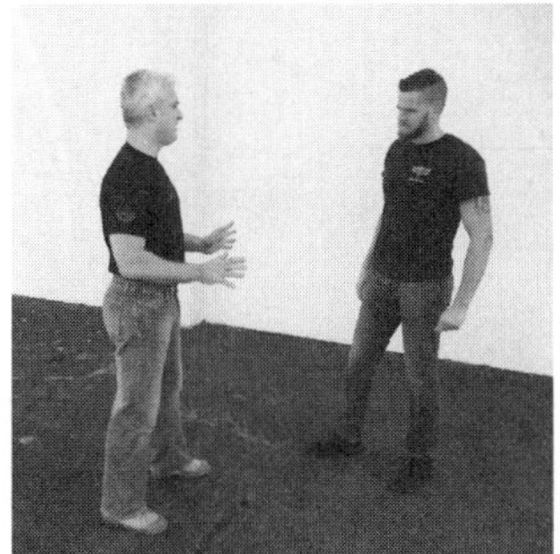

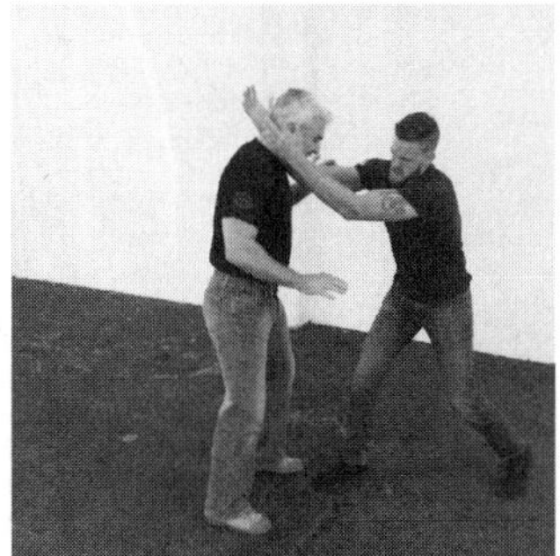

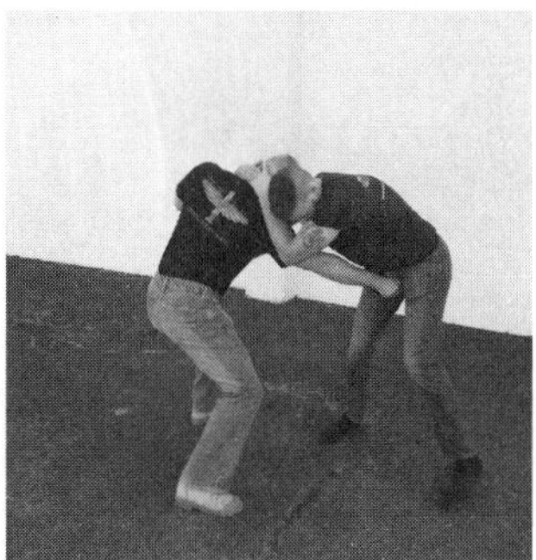

This series depicts an adversary who succeeds in clinching you head. To prevent any further attacks, you can use an instantaneous hammerfist strike to the groin.

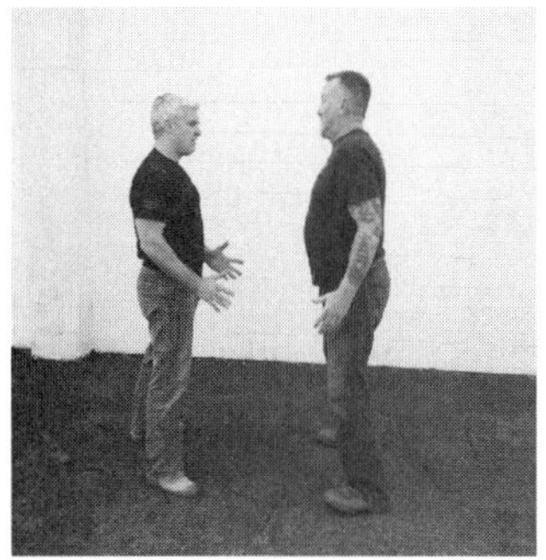

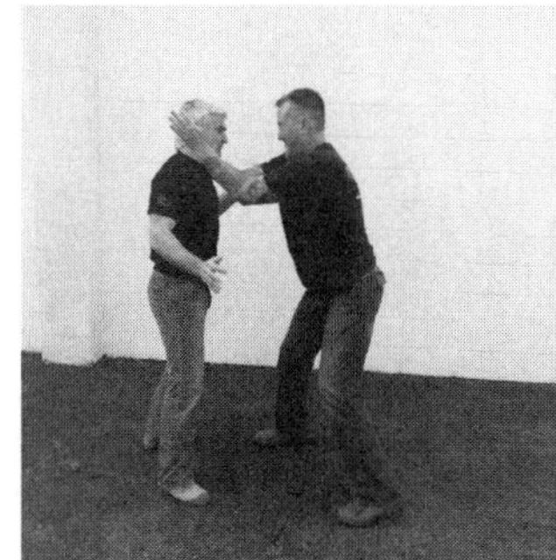

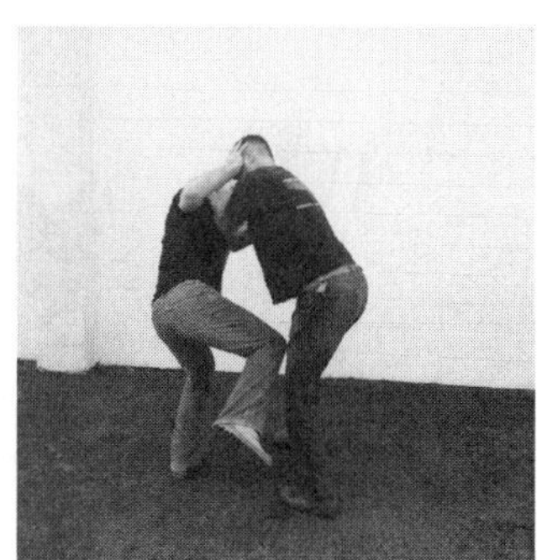

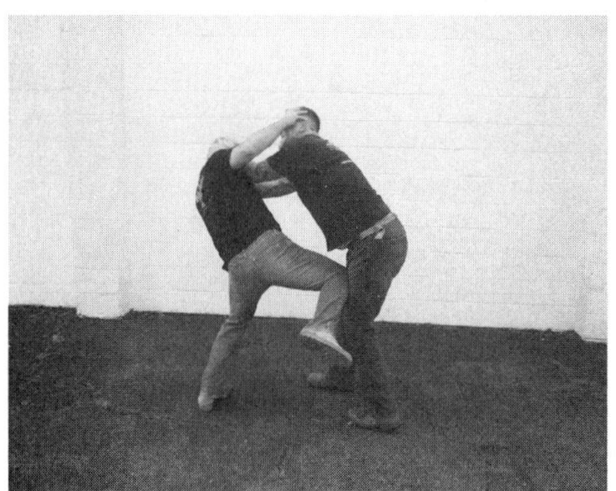

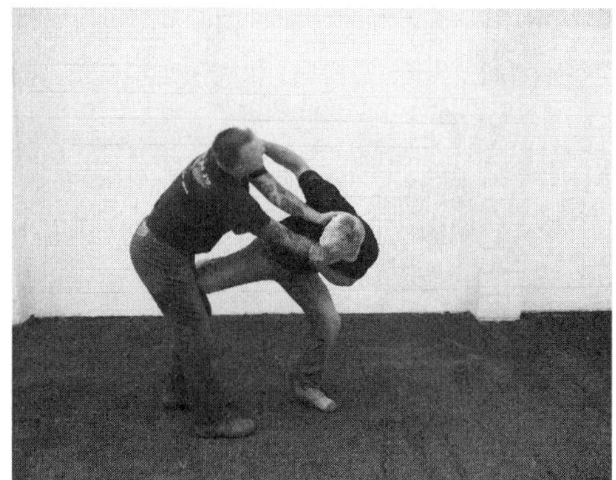

This series depicts a clinch defense using a foreleg counterstrike and brace and simultaneous rule-of-thumb eye gouge.

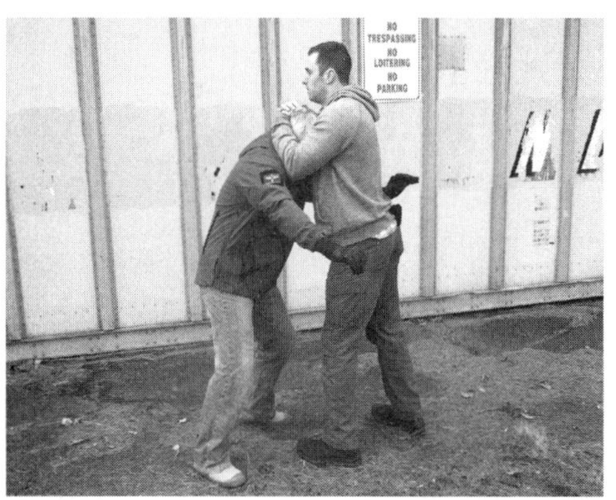

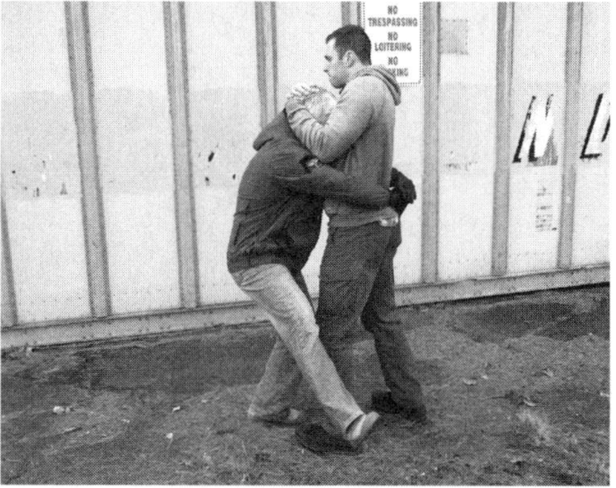

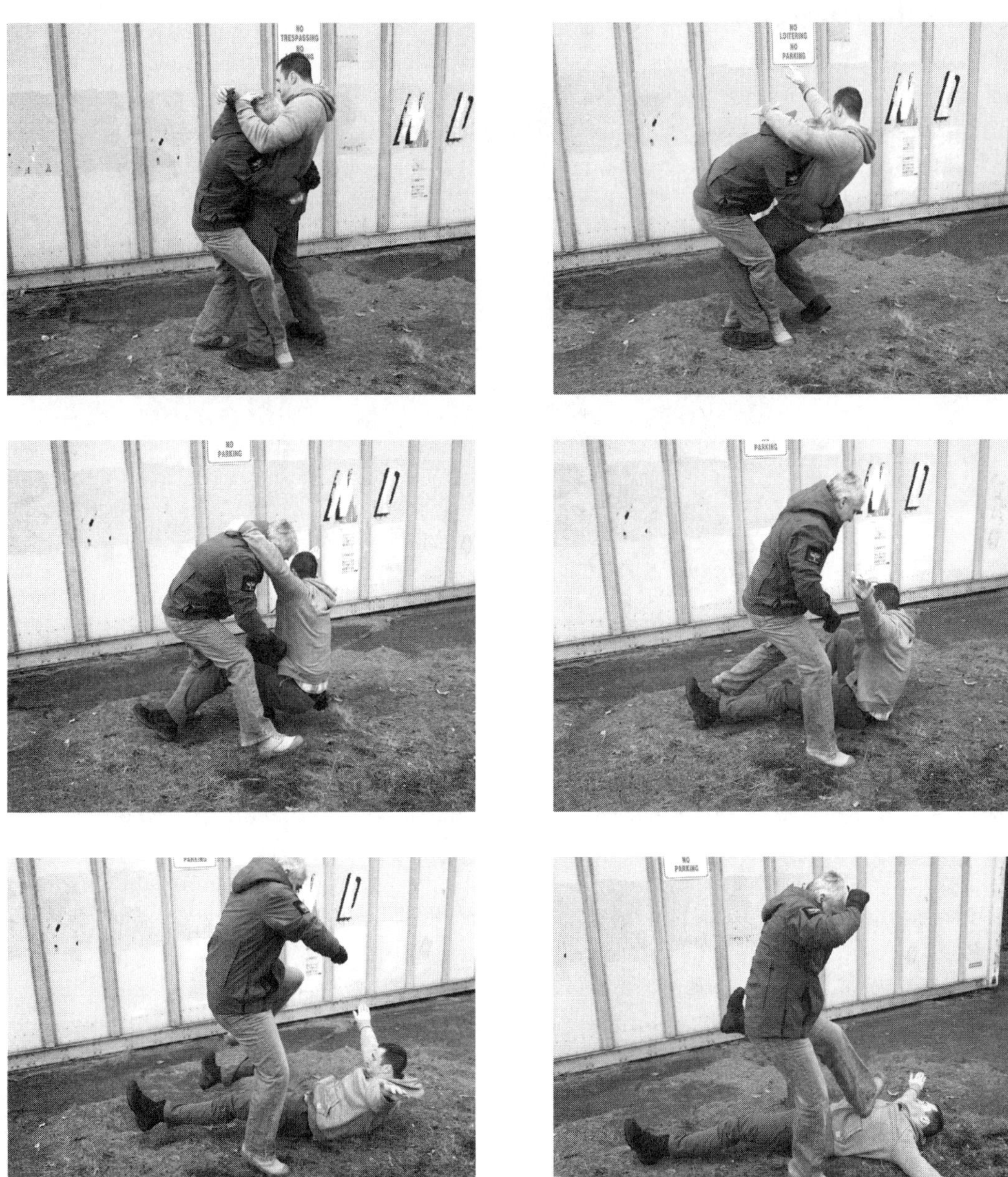

This series depicts a two-handed head clinch defense where you close the distance to secure your adversary's torso briefly against yours. As soon as you secure his torso, utilize a kosoto gake takedown and follow-up kick. Note that your footwork strategy is not to step over the fallen opponent. Rather, step to his side to deliver a stomp and protect yourself from being kicked in the groin.

Ground Survival Strategic Insights

As stated earlier, krav maga ground survival may best defined as "when possible, what we do up, we do down," with additional specific ground-fighting capabilities. First, try to remain upright. Going to the ground hampers your ability to recognize a weapon being deployed and the grave danger of multiple opponents descending on you. Try not to allow or give the opponent the opportunity to get behind you or "take your back" in either a standing or ground position.

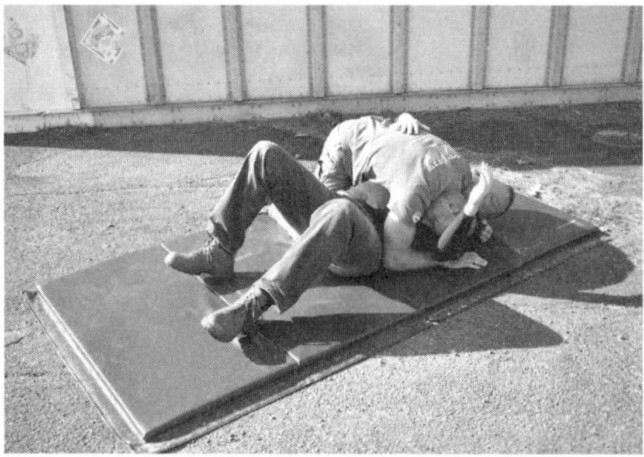

A trained ground specialist understands how to use his body weight best without necessarily using a great deal of strength or explosiveness while exerting draining, uncomfortable body pressure on his opponent—until he decides to decisively attack, choosing a ground and pound, armbar, shoulder lock, leg lock, or choke to damage and submit the opponent.

Going to the ground can induce panic, especially if a skilled fighter has you mounted and is pounding you with strikes ("ground and pound"), has taken your back, or has you pancaked against the ground to exert draining, uncomfortable body weight pressure on you. Trained ground specialists understand how to use their body weight best against you without necessarily using a great deal of strength or explosiveness—until they decide to decisively attack using a rear naked choke, armbar, shoulder, or leg lock, etc.

Training against skilled ground fighters is necessary so that you can feel and understand, at least somewhat, sustained body weight pressure and what it means to be placed in a compromised –5 position. You must learn the required patience not to panic and expend all of your defensive energy while learning positioning. In short, when training with a skilled opponent, particularly when you find yourself in a bad position, you'll learn how to maneuver and not panic.

As a krav maga instructor under Grandmaster Haim Gidon, I am a big proponent of having a diverse understanding of grappling, BJJ (Brazilian jiu-jitsu), and judo. Key elements of these formidable fighting systems are built into Gidon Krav Maga training. One needs to keep in mind that krav maga founder Imi Lichtenfeld was a European wrestling champion, while Haim excelled in Greco-Roman wrestling. In addition, the Arab armies specialized in judo training as their primary hand-to-hand combat method. Accordingly, krav maga, to provide effective counter-tactics, focused on the most effective judo throws and counter-throws. In the early 1990s, Haim, with Imi's approval, began to incorporate the core tactics of BJJ and sambo.

Another important consideration is how and why krav maga evolved. Imi was constantly confronted by multiple assailants often armed with cold weapons (edged and impact). As a wrestler and later a judoka, Imi recognized the constraints and dangers that a grappling-centric strategy would impose. Therefore, a kravist must be well rounded in all aspects of a fight.

- Legitimate krav maga trains you against skilled, determined adversaries who also know the dirty tricks of the trade. What you can do, they can do. Anatomical targeting works both ways, but it is incredibly hard to do so when someone has your back or has you in a compromised (–5) ground position. Lastly, it is important to emphasize that hot (firearms) and cold (edged, impact) weapons are integral to training and are used seamlessly both while standing and on the ground. Remember that compliance with the aggressor's demands may be the best strategy when you are threatened with a weapon.
- With proper body positioning on your part, an adversary on the ground can be pummeled severely, while you give him little defensive recourse. The same of course can be done to you. In both standing and ground fights it becomes difficult for an adversary to fight effectively if his hands or limbs are broken. Obviously, rendering an adversary unconscious quickly ends a fight.
- While we teach certain core, arm, shoulder, and knee joint locks along with chokes to civilians, once you have an understanding of basic biomechanics, you can apply the principles to many situations. This is especially important in the fluidity of a fight. Every type of lock requires moving the joint against its natural articulation with breaking pressure. Optimally, you will use the entire force and weight of your body to apply such force against an adversary's joint. This is the key principle for joint locks. Remember that a joint lock, however decisive and quick, still ties you up momentarily, potentially exposing you to your adversary drawing a weapon on you or a second adversary—or multiple adversaries—attacking you.
- Your training should include learning how to apply a myriad of locks and chokes in quick succession just like a trained grappler. This will become a form of ground retzev. By learning which locks apply in which positions, you will comprehend the dangers should you find yourself slipping into such a situation or if an opponent attempts to maneuver you into such a position.
- The optimum defense against any type of choke or joint lock is obviously to prevent it from being applied in the first place. For example, do not dangle an arm thereby inviting an armbar. Don't let an attacker take your back (keep your back to the

ground unless you are sure you can disengage to get up). Don't expose your neck by letting an attacker wrap his arm around it.

- Remember, whether you are standing, clinched, or on the ground, krav maga is designed for everyone. A smaller opponent can defeat a larger, stronger, and perhaps more athletic opponent by using tactical leverage. A well-trained kravist will possess core defensive-tactics training in any position. In a rapidly unfolding, desperate fight, the best way to defend against an offensive technique is to first know the offensive technique yourself. Knowing an array of attack techniques solidifies your ability to defend against such techniques when they are used against you.
- If you cannot go one way to escape a hold, then you must find another escape route. Most importantly, you cannot spend time debating what to do next. If your initial defensive movement does not work, instantaneously switch to another. Finally, however, keep in mind that some ground tactics may require patience and incremental movements that underscore the need for resilience, confidence, and patience.
- Should you choose to use a choke or stranglehold in an actual fight, it is advisable that you do not entangle your legs or hook them into your opponent as it is difficult to disengage from such a position quickly, and multiple assailants can take advantage of the this. Also, if you attempt a choke or other type of control hold, you must remember that the opponent could have a weapon sequestered on his person. If you commit both of your arms to the choke hold while he is still conscious, he could pull out a weapon such as a knife or gun and cause you egregious bodily harm.

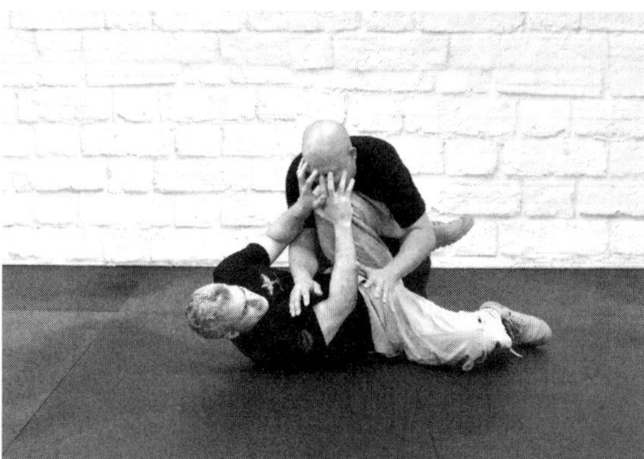

Topside knee positioning is vital when you are the ground to create a brace or barrier between yourself and the opponent. A knee barrier allows you to use your strongest muscles (your lower body) to create separation and not allow the attacker to mount you or pin you. Pull your nearside knee into the assailant to create a barrier. Use your fingers to rake his eyes to facilitate separation to allow additional kicks, secondary weapon deployment, and to get up off the ground.

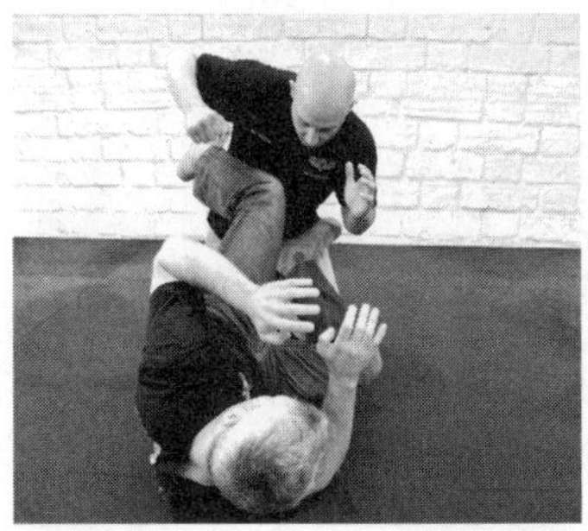
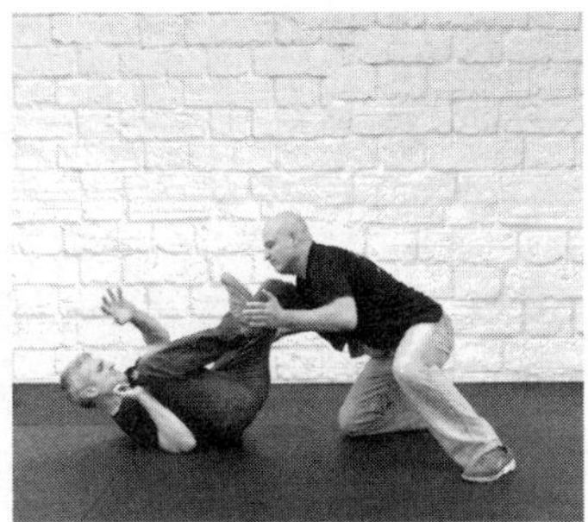
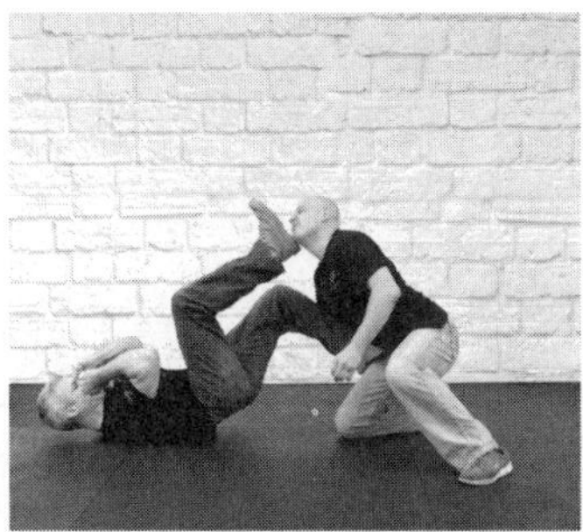
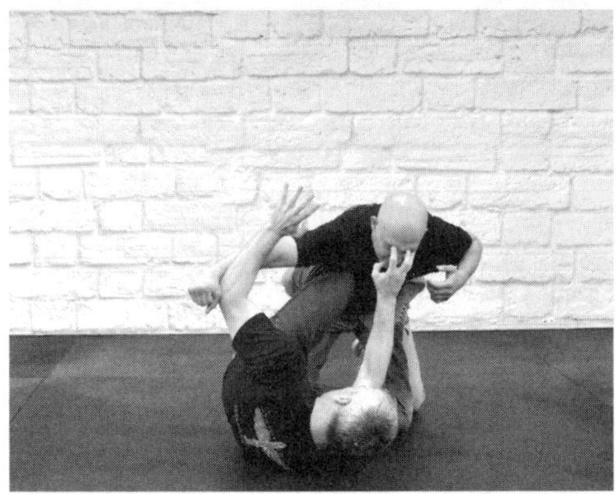
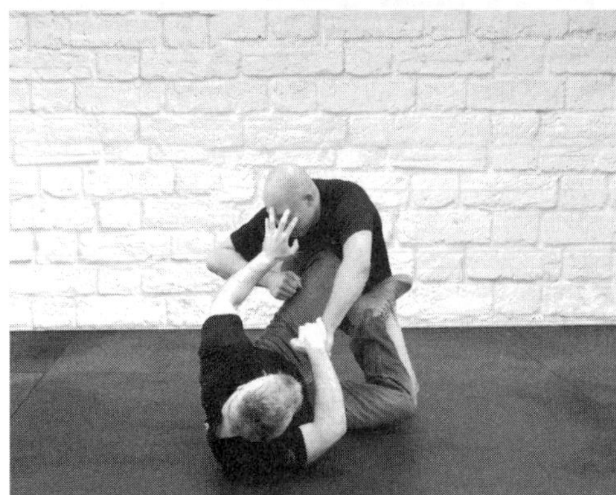

The all-important foreleg brace position (on your side with your top foreleg/knee braced across the attacker's torso and your lower heel against his hip) allows you to defend against upper-body attacks using the same simultaneous defense and attacker principles you learned in your standing defenses, including kicks and upper-body strikes with a few modifications.

The following photo series show a few select ground survival tactics against popular types of attacks. As always, the best defensive strategy is to not to allow yourself to be put in this specific situation.

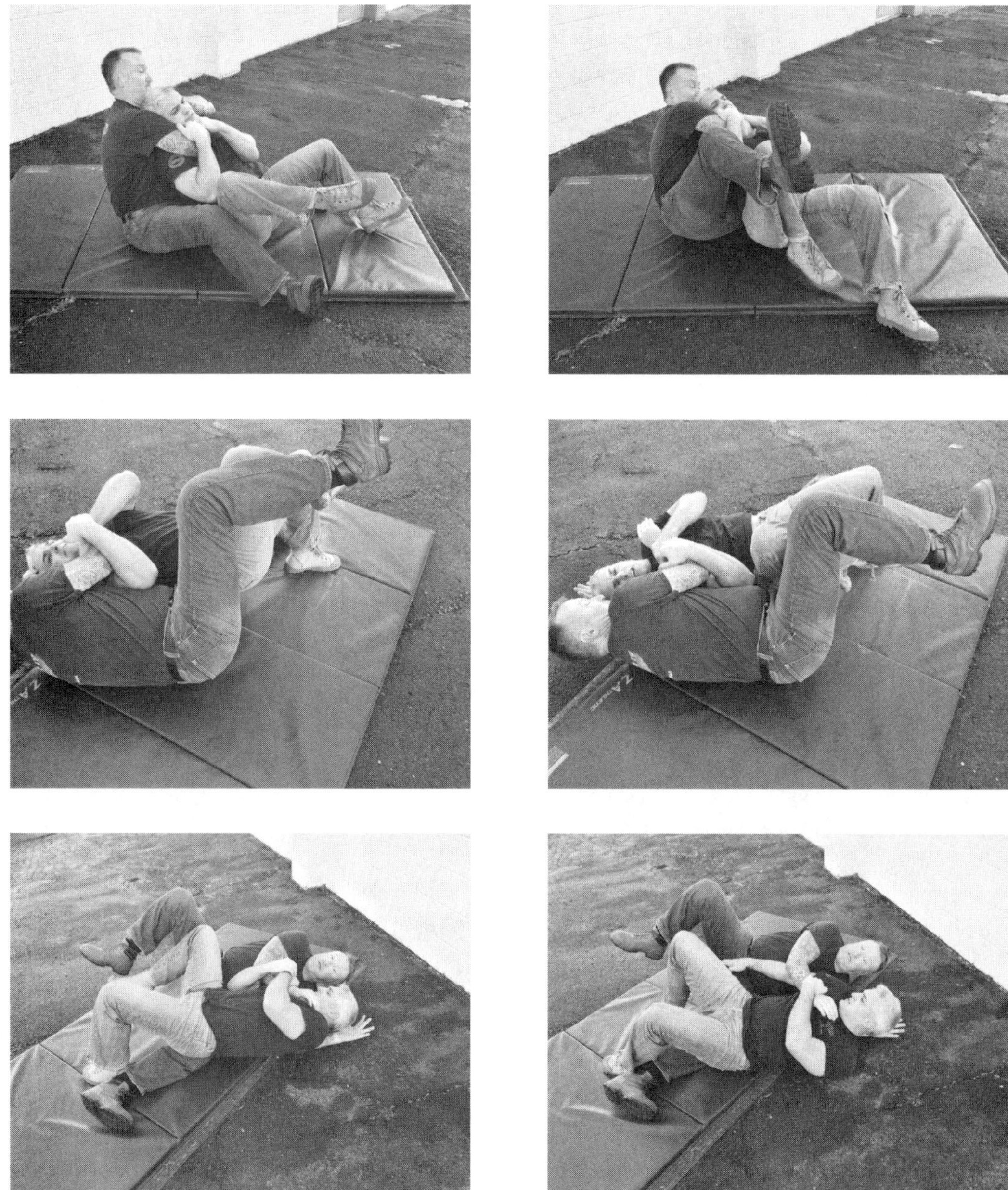

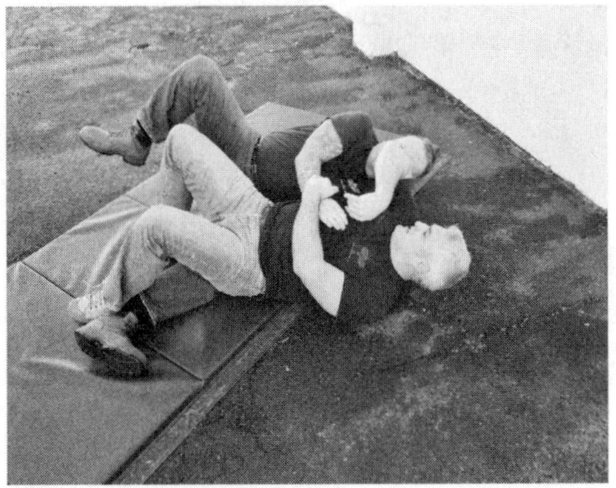

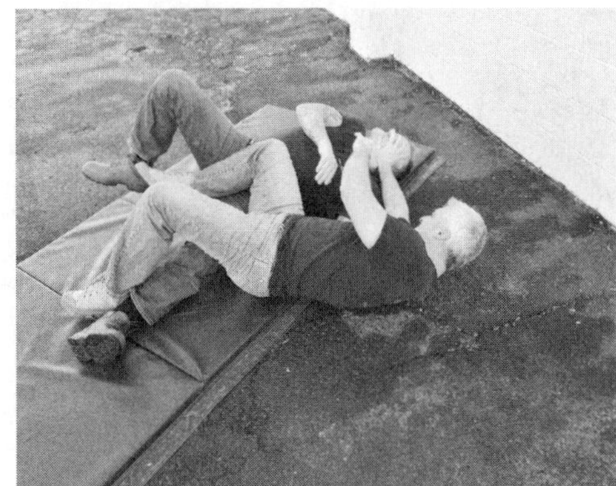

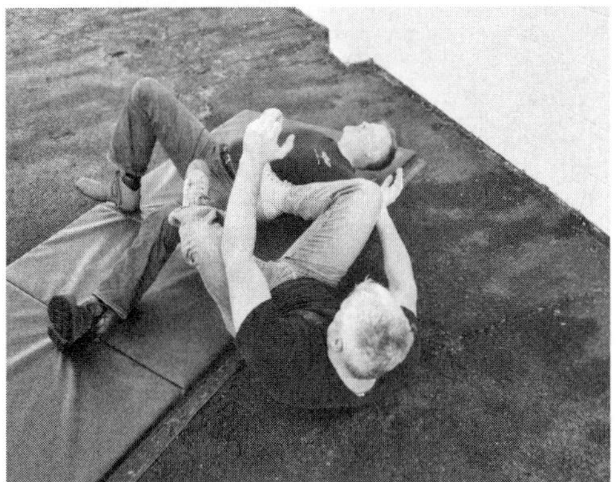

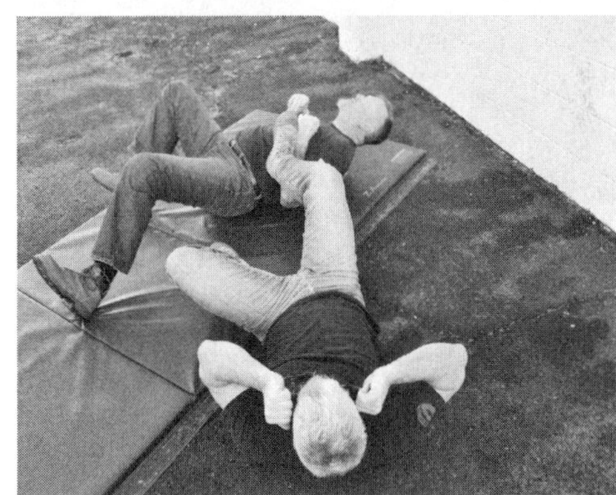

This series depicts a rear naked choke defense on the ground. The key is that you recognize the choke danger early, sink your hips down and away, and do not allow the attacker to sink his leg hooks (wrap his legs around you). Note that you must turn into the attacker's elbow crook similar to krav maga's standing defense, underscoring the strategy of learning a tactic that can be used in multiple situations with variations.

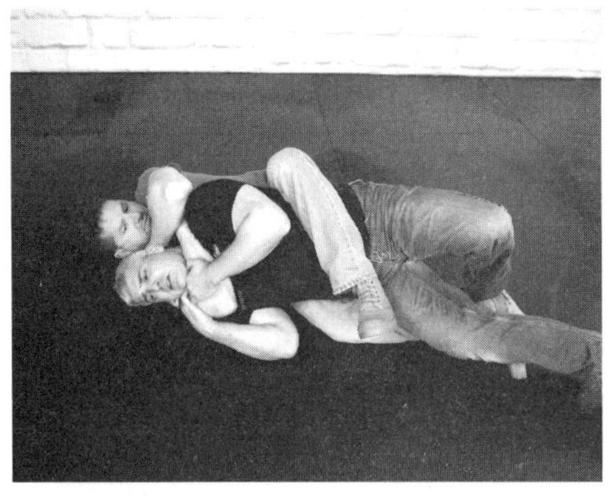

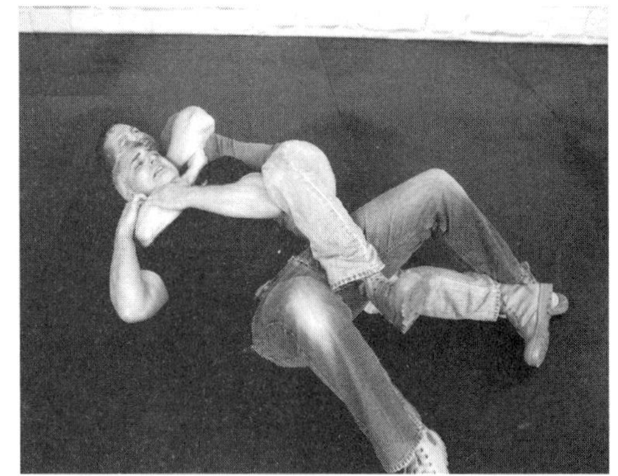

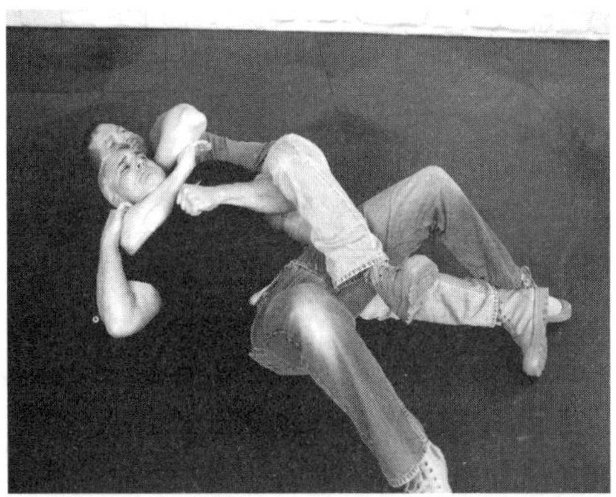

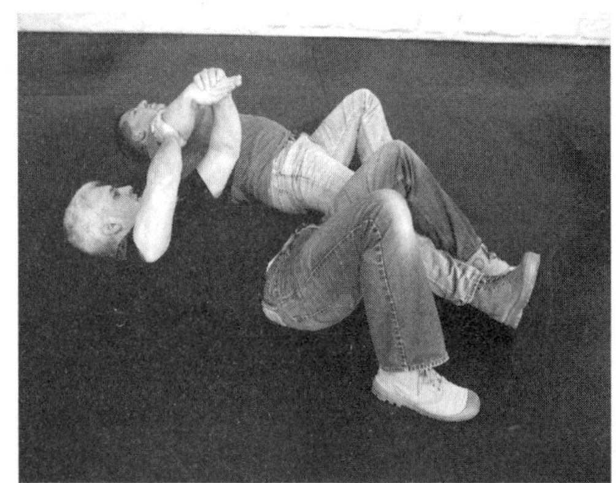

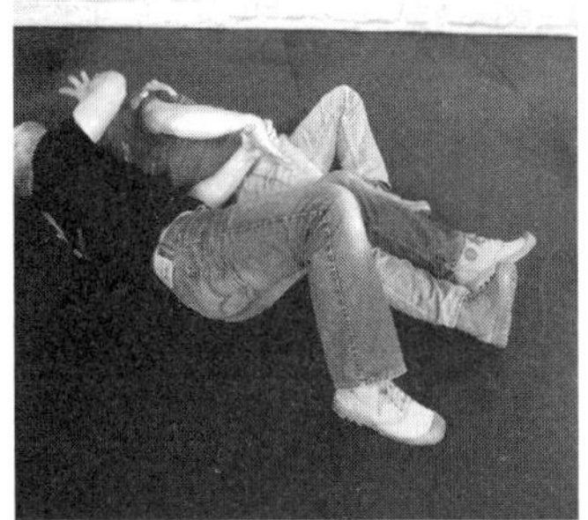

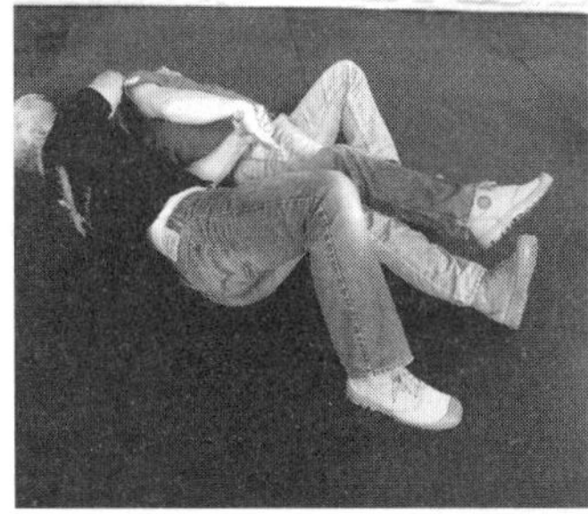

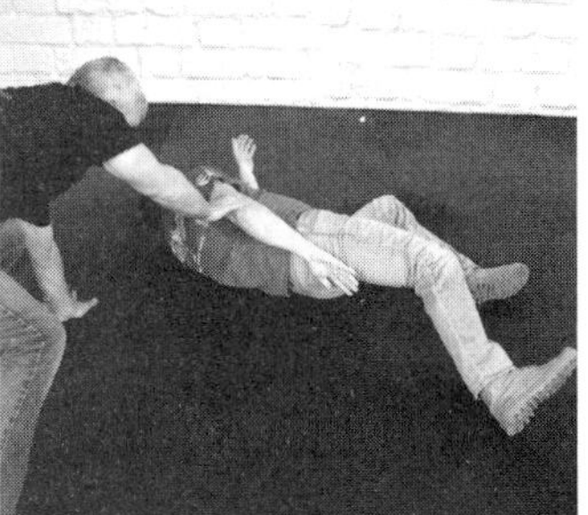

This series depicts another rear naked choke ground defense option where an attacker has sunk one leg hook (his top leg is wrapped around your top leg). Rather than turning into the attacker's elbow crook, instead you must turn *away* from his elbow crook. This underpins the strategy of learning an adaptable tactic.

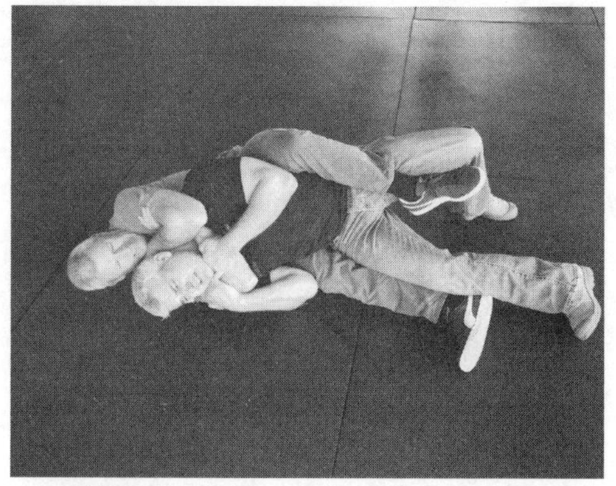

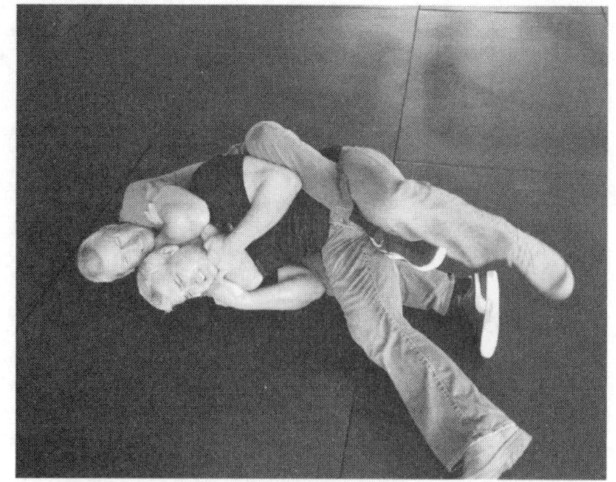

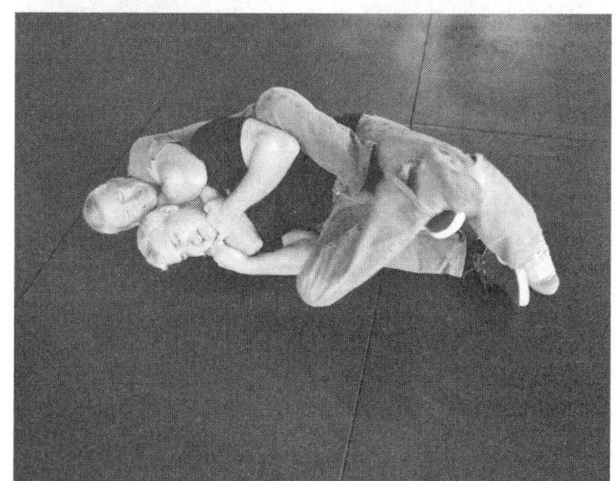

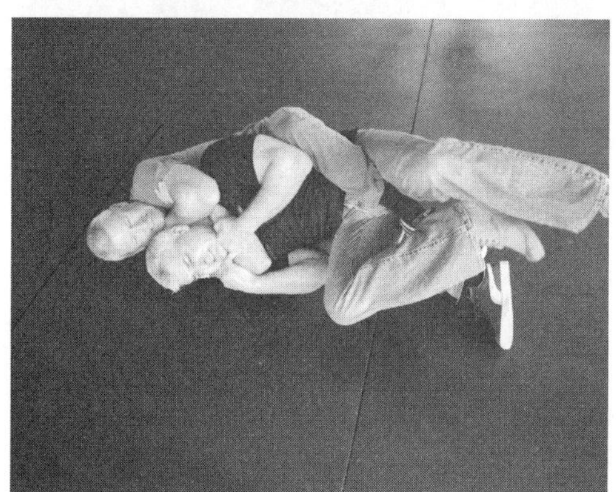

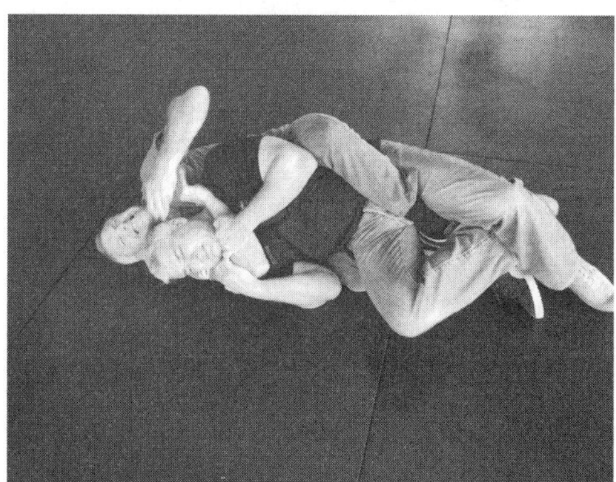

This series depicts another rear naked choke defense solution when on the ground and the attacker sinks one leg hook (his top leg is wrapped around your top leg). In this situation you cannot escape and pivot onto your back to defend (as the previous example depicts), because his leg hook anchors him to you. Therefore, you must attack whatever vulnerable target you can. In this case, the defense incorporates an ankle lock with breaking pressure, once again underpinning the key strategy of technique adaptability. Follow up with additional attacks as necessary.

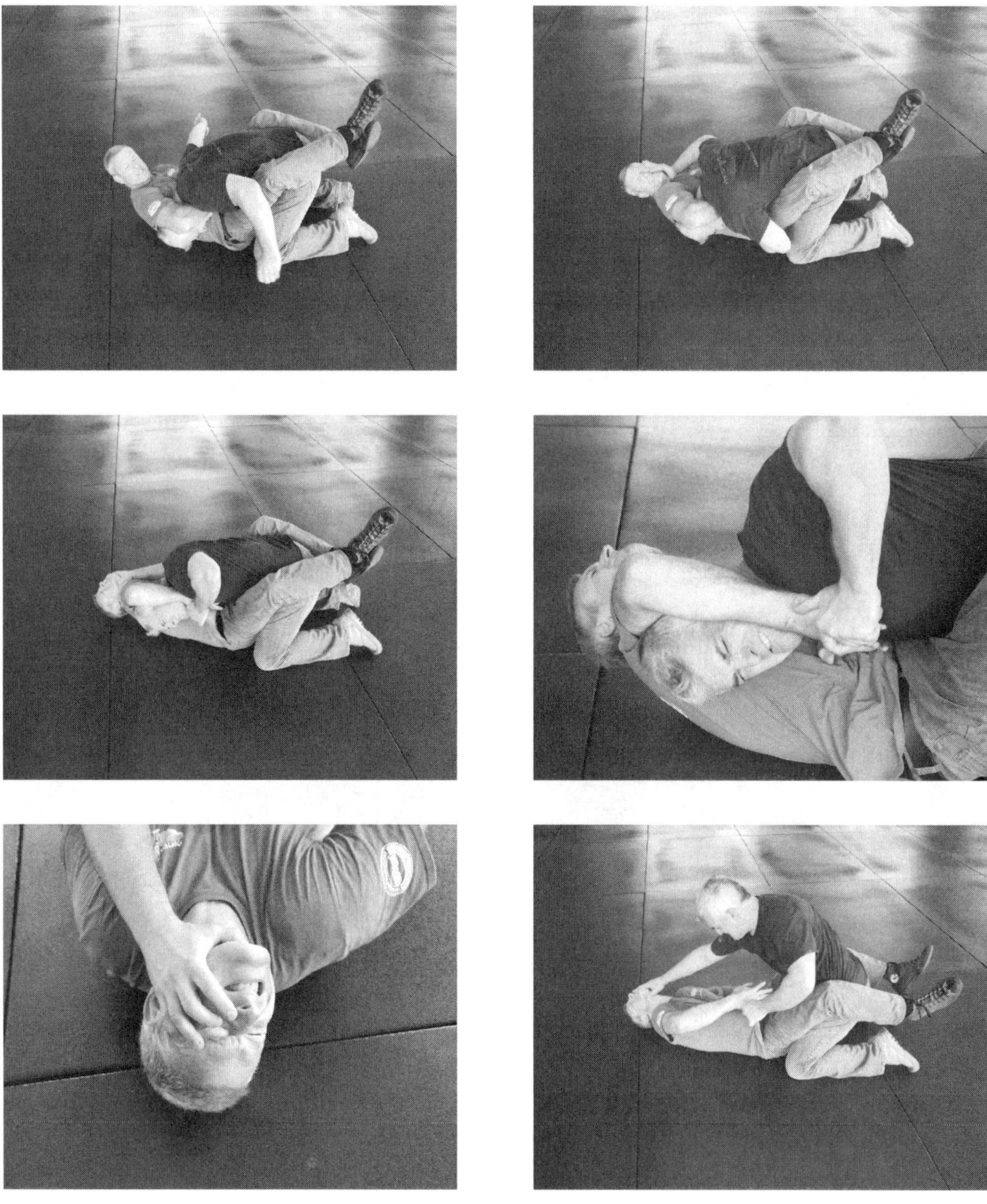

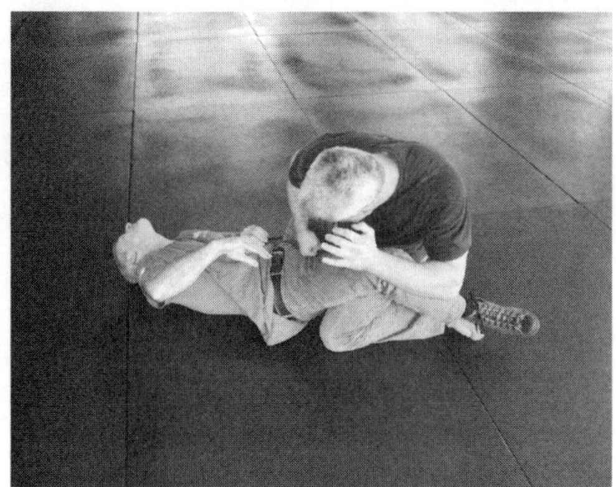

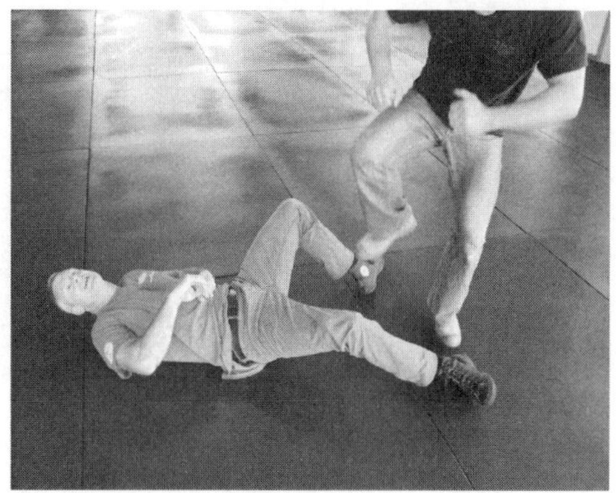

This series depicts a highly dangerous guillotine defense against a choke that is administered from the guard position. Similar to all choke defenses, you must react immediately by placing maximum counterpressure against the choking arm while attacking anatomical vulnerabilities. Try to break or jam the attacker's fingers to release the hold, while also embedding a finger of your opposite hand deep into the eye orbit entering from the lower lid. Follow up with additional attacks as necessary.

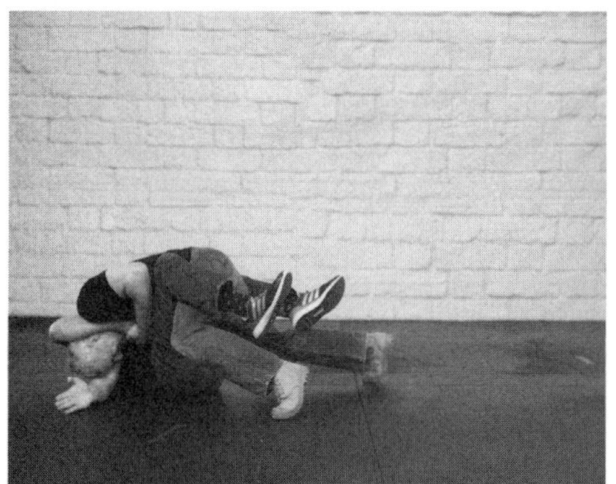

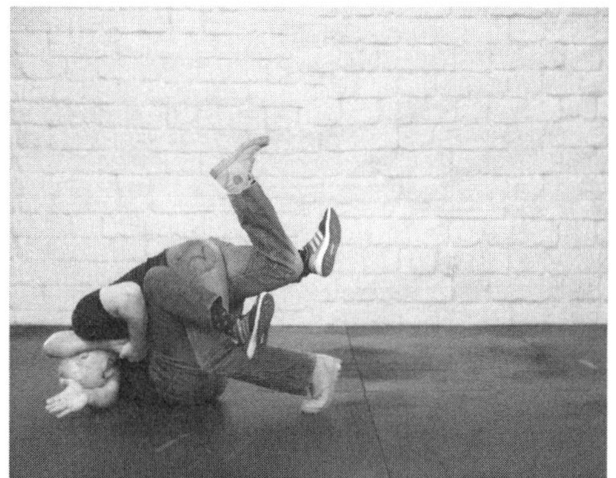

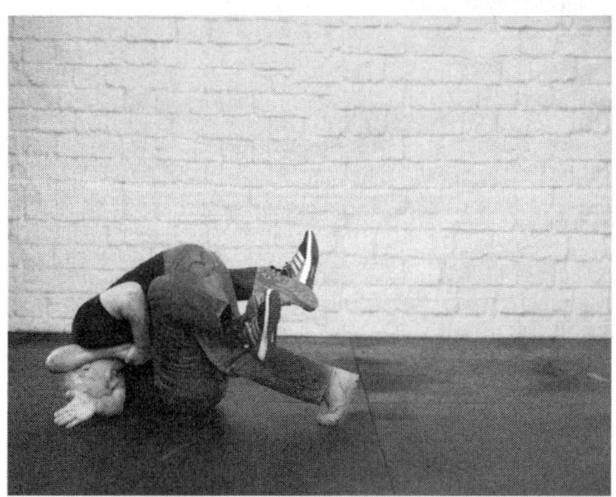

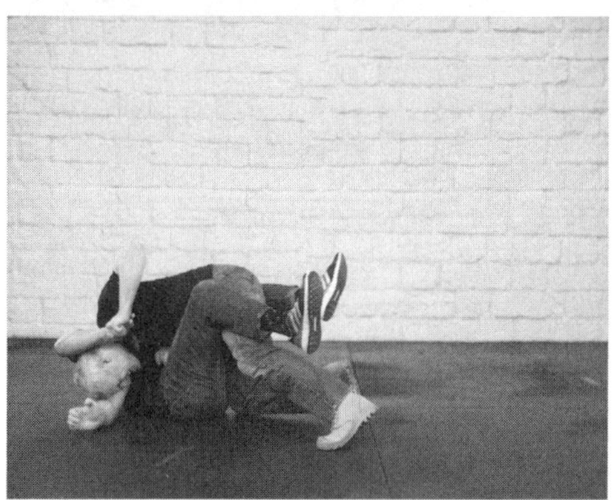

series continued on next page ...

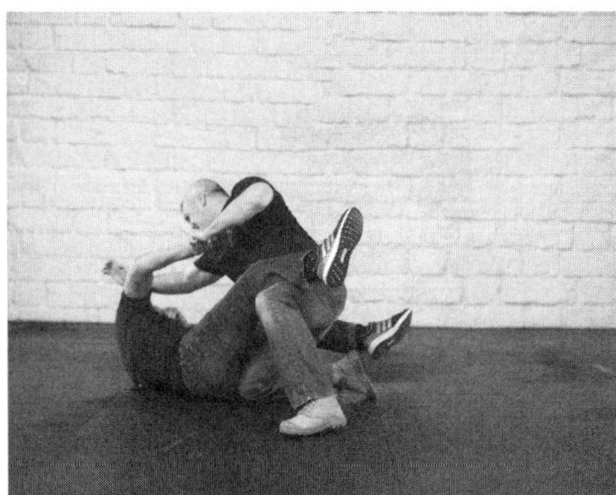

This series depicts a guillotine choke variation defense against a choke that is administered from the guard position where your arm is trapped. Similar to all chokes, you must react immediately by placing maximum counterpressure against the choking arm, while attacking anatomical vulnerabilities. As with the previous defense, try to break the attacker's fingers to release the hold. Because your other arm is immobilized, use a knee strike to the attacker's groin and coccyx. Note that this knee strike tactic can also be combined with the previous guillotine defense. Follow up with additional attacks as necessary.

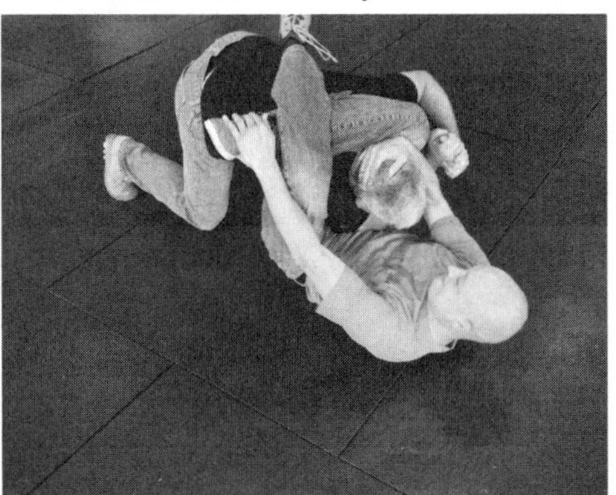

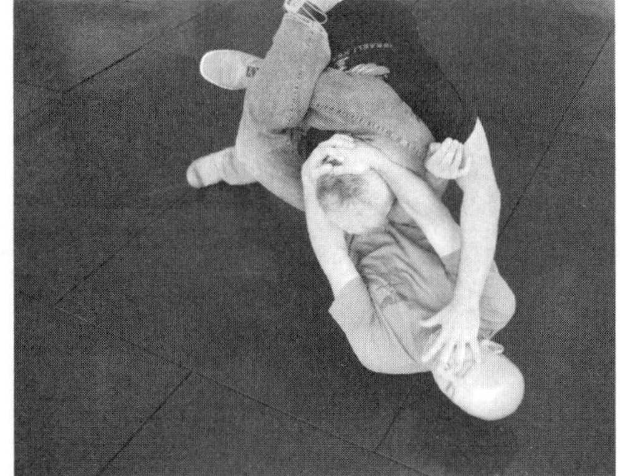

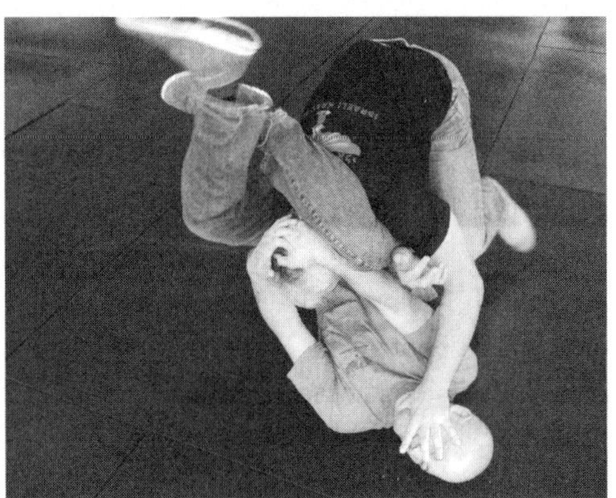

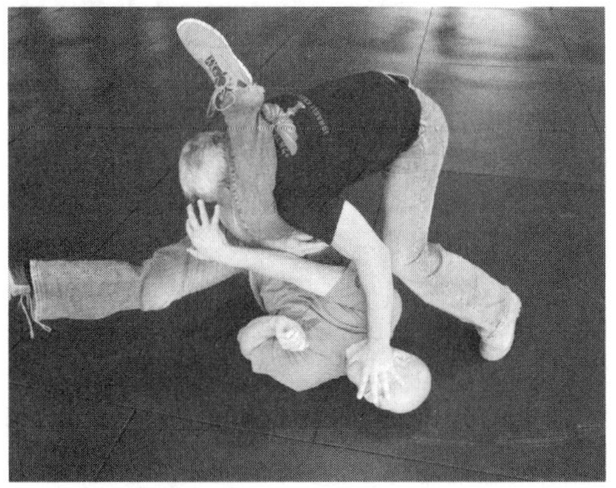

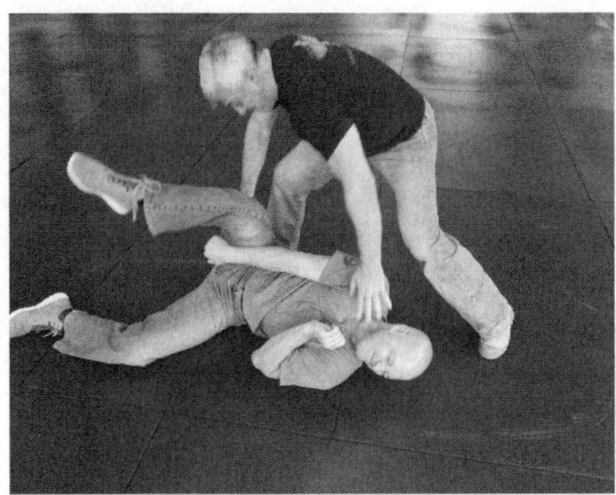

This series portrays a highly dangerous triangle choke defense from the guard. You must counter this attack as soon as you feel it coming as the attacker pulls you in and begins to maneuver his legs atop your shoulders. (Remember the important concept of tactile feel defense.) Similar to the stacked armbar defense, turn in the direction of your trapped arm to break the angle of attack (here, a choke) and immediately attack exposed anatomical vulnerabilities, the eye orbit in this case. Follow up with additional combatives as necessary.

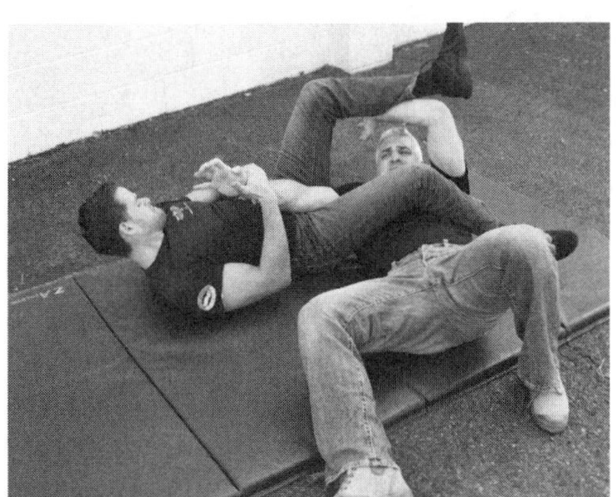

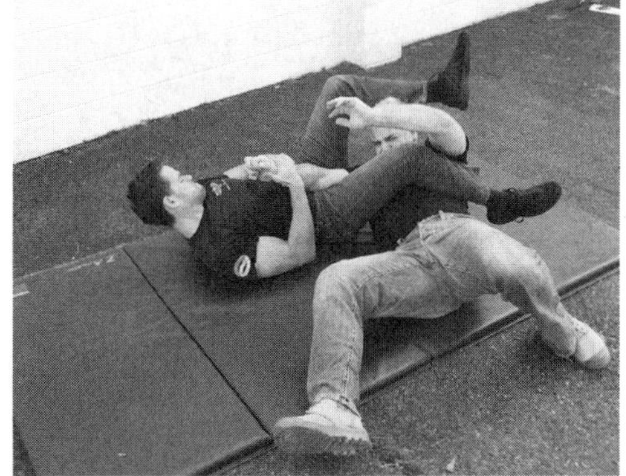

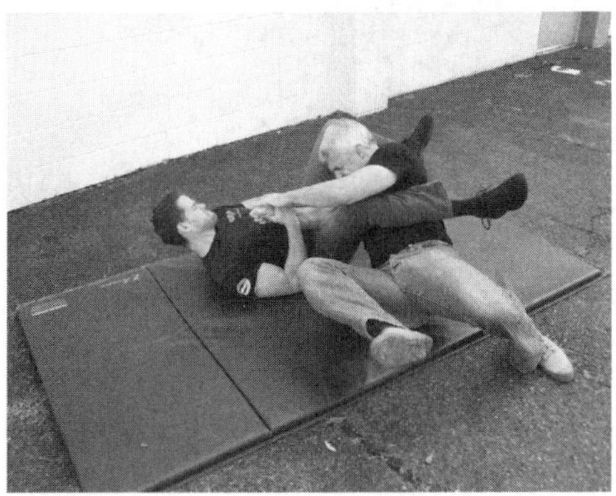

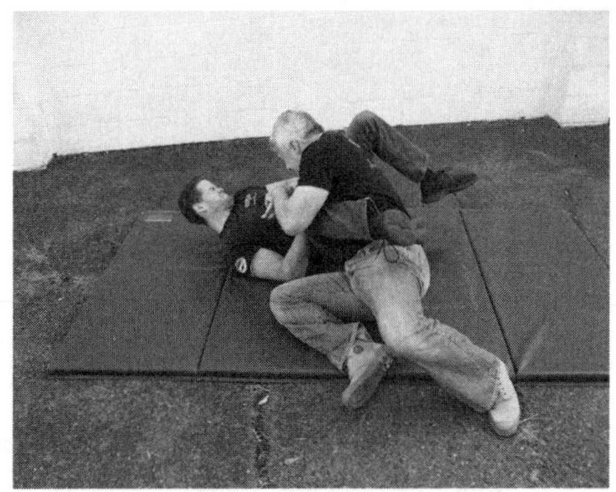

series continued on next page ...

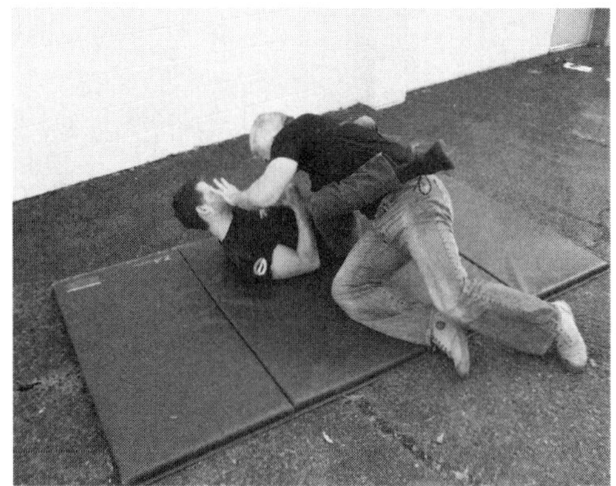

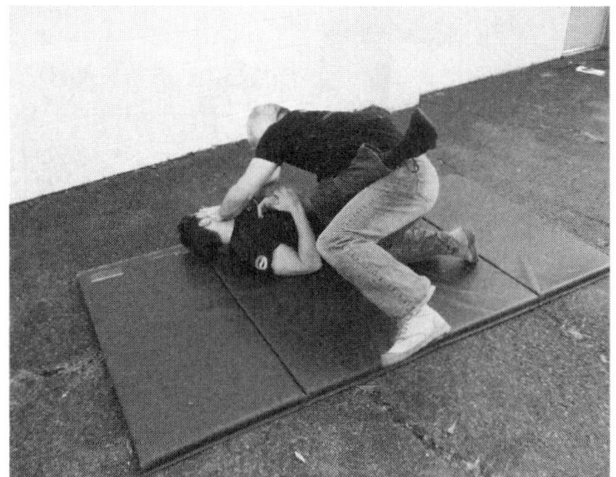

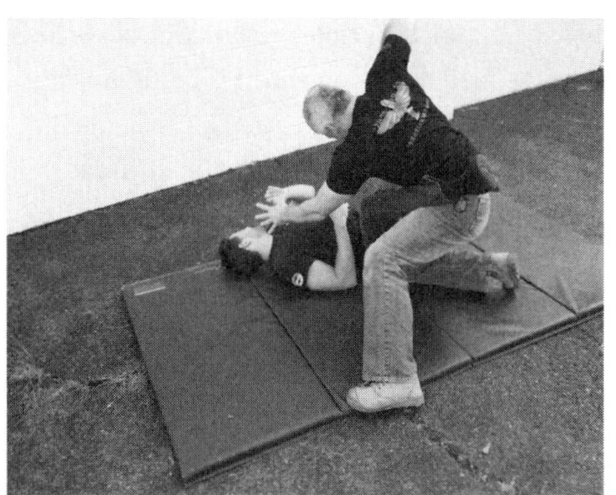

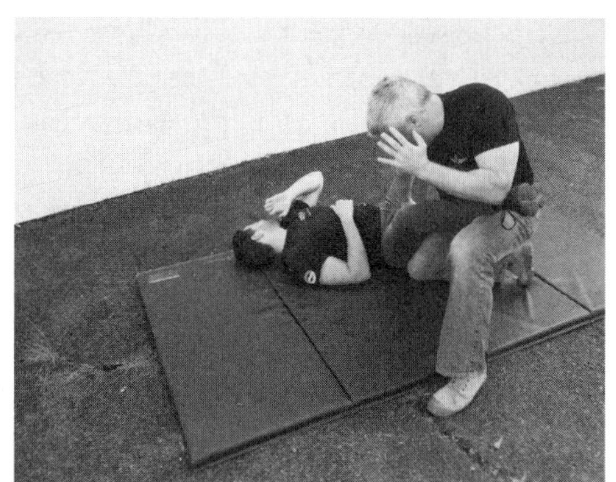

This series depicts the defense of a straight armbar attempt where the attacker has not yet pincered both of his legs over you. You cannot allow the attacker to drape both of his legs over your torso and head. Use your forearm to block the attacker's topside leg maneuver. Immediately turn into the attacker to prevent the armbar while immediately attacking vital anatomy.

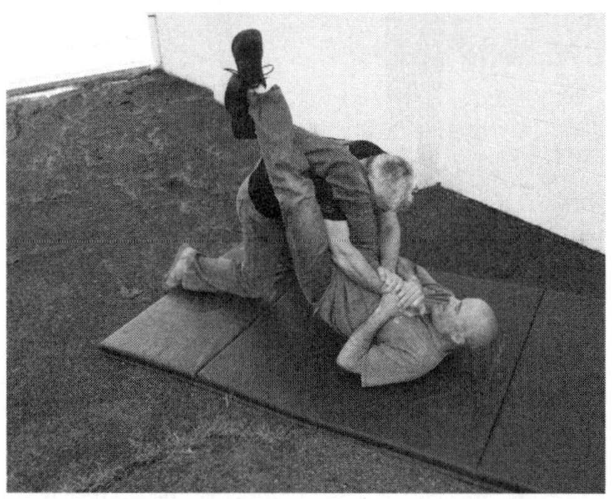

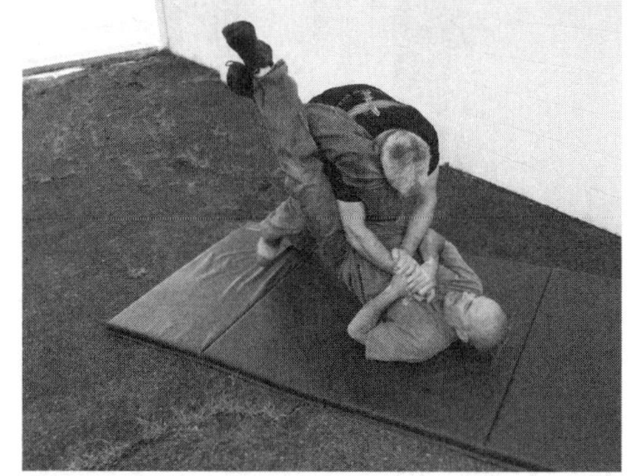

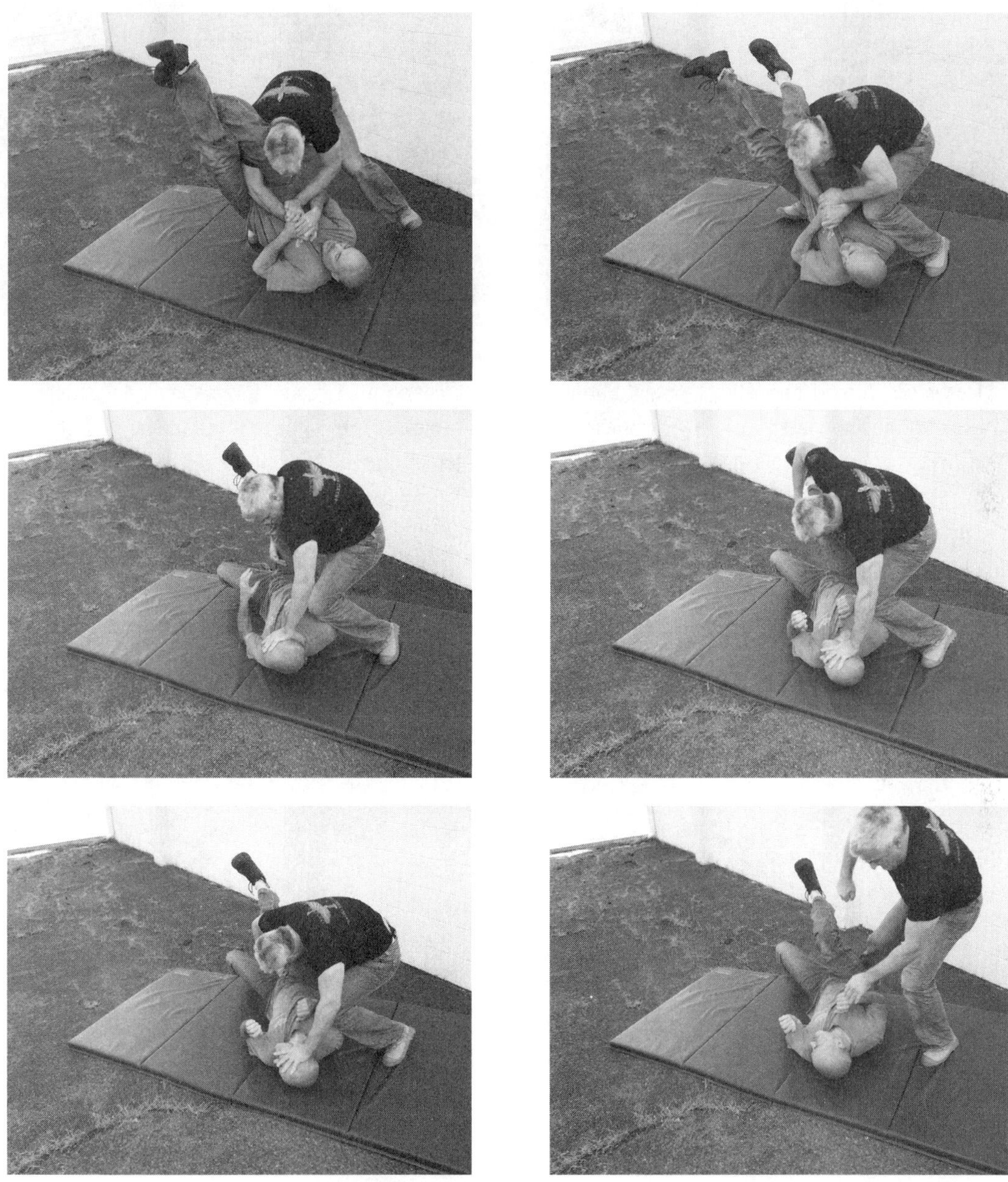

series continued on next page ...

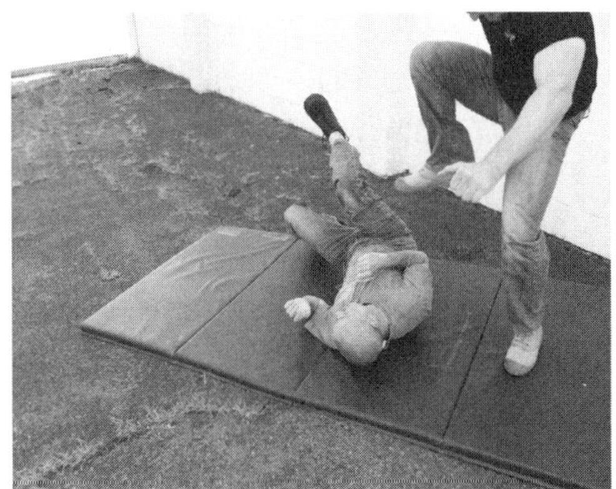

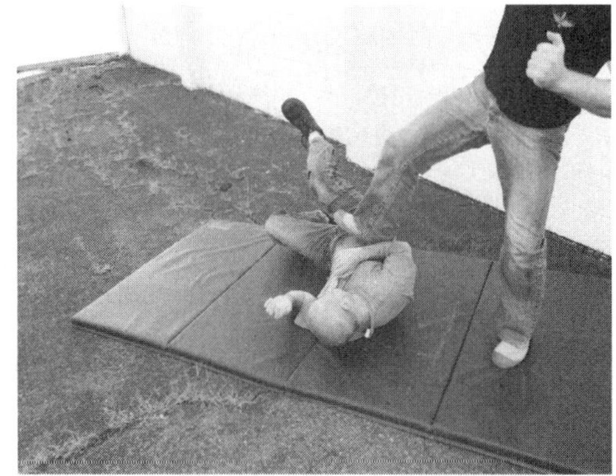

This series depicts defending a straight armbar attempt when you are caught in a kneeling position. Exert as much counterpressure as you can against the attack by leaning your mass forward into the attacker to compress his legs. Against a right armbar attempt, immediately break the angle of attack by rotating your whole body clockwise to prevent the elbow lock. As soon as you have safeguarded your arm, counterattack using an eye gouge with your free arm. Follow up with additional combatives as necessary.

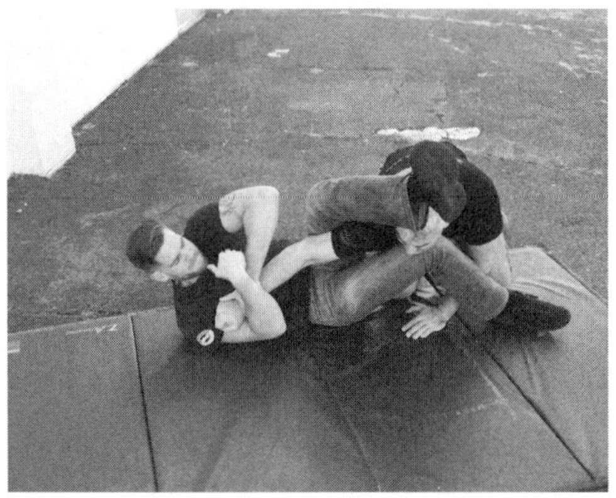

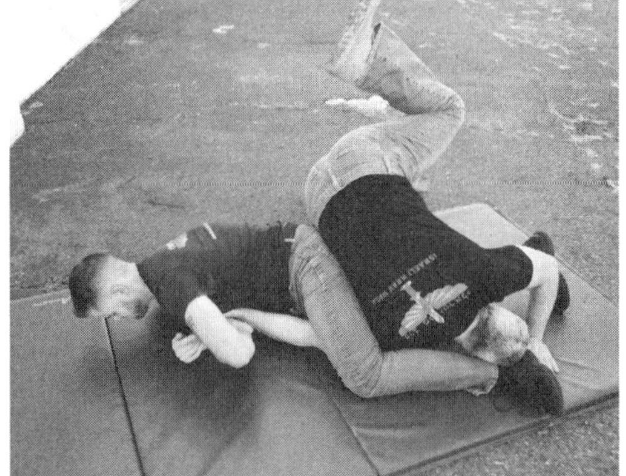

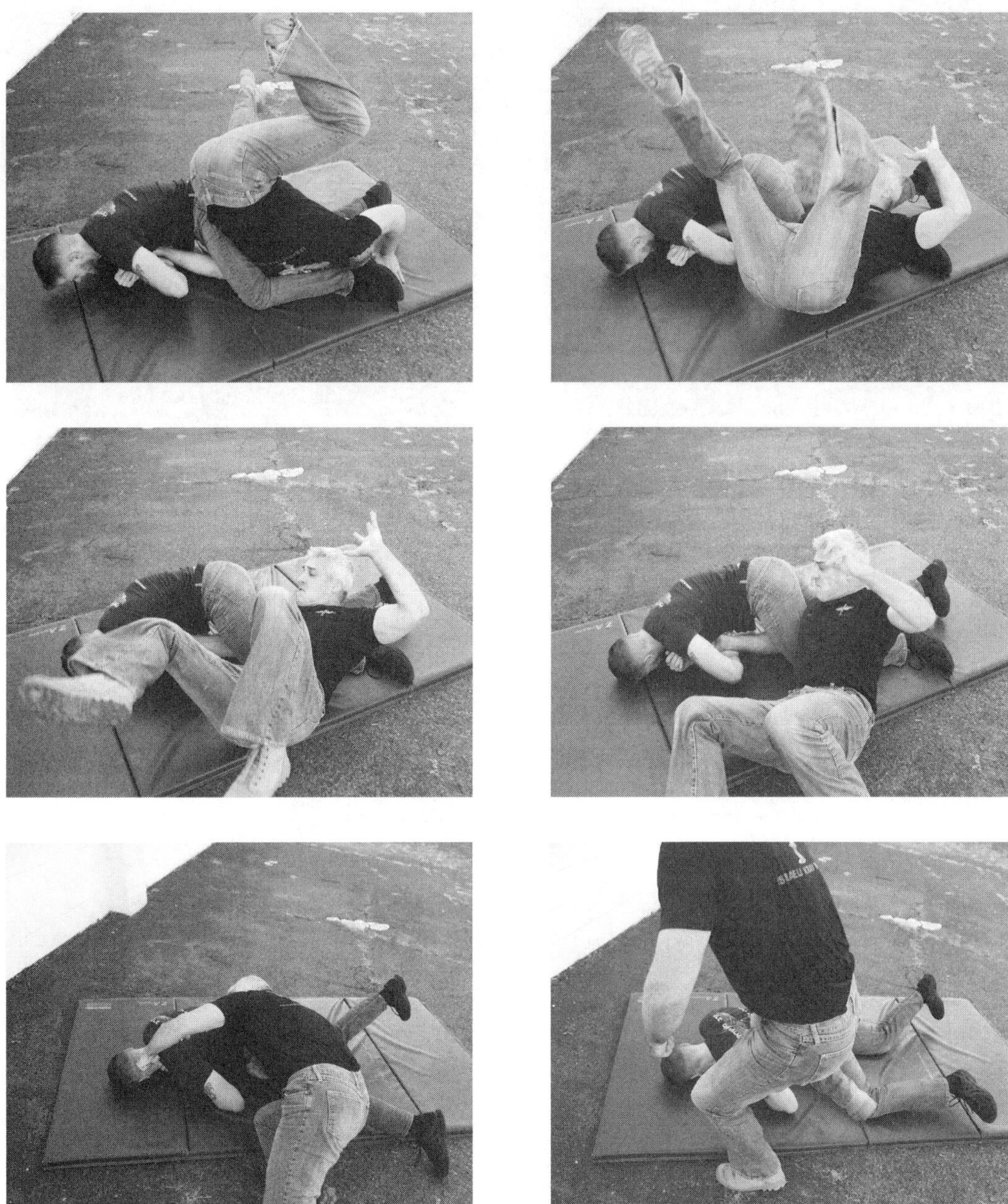

This series depicts an attacker attempting to turn face down to catch you in a straight armbar. Similar to other preceding krav maga defensive techniques, you must move with and not resist his momentum. In this case you must roll in the direction he intends to catch you to sink an armbar. Complete a full roll to break his angle of attack, counterattack, and disengage.

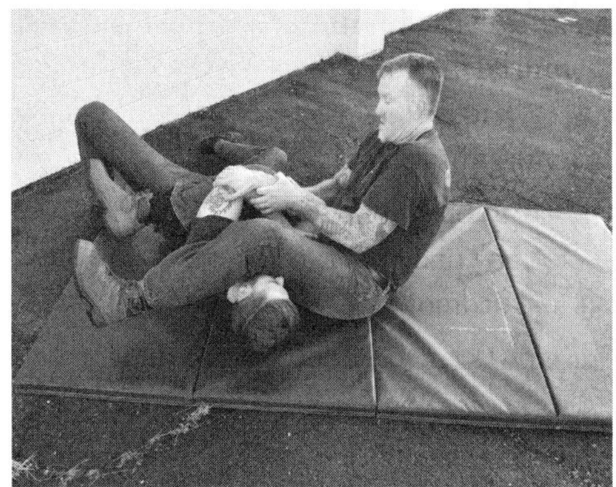
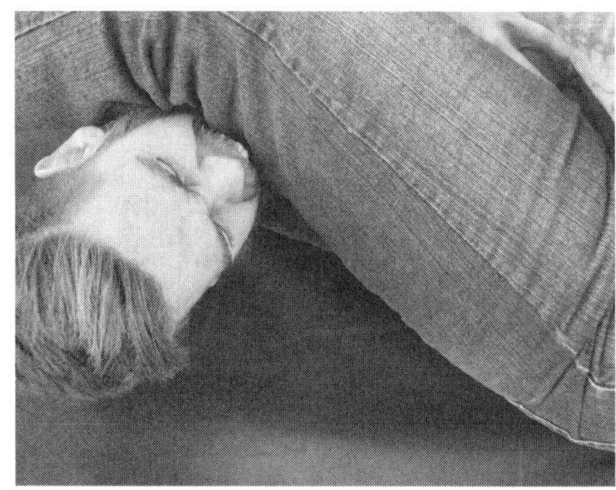

This series depicts the danger of an attacker securing your arm with both of his legs pinning you to the ground while he is also anchoring himself to you, a –5 situation. Obviously, by design, this places you in a position highly vulnerable to having your elbow dislocated. Should this (or any other type of mayhem) happen, primeval self-defense must always be the default strategy. As the attacker places his legs over your head and you feel or see the imminent armbar attempt, you are likely to instinctively (and through training) clutch both of your arms together as a stop-gap to prevent the armbar. Immediately counterattack by sinking your teeth deep into the attacker's hamstring and tearing away at it. In close-quarter fighting, biting is always an option. Remember that, strategically speaking, *what you can do he can do.* So watch out if you have the advantage over a desperate person—he may try to bite you.

Combatives Power and Balance

Developing power and balance is crucial for any self-defense tactic. Regardless of what type of combative strike you deliver, shifting your body weight forward combined with correct pivoting will allow you to place all of your body mass behind a combative to connect with the greatest velocity and subsequent force. A point that Grandmaster Gidon constantly reinforces is that without the proper execution—optimum execution—of krav maga's essential combatives, krav maga may not always be effective. Whatever you weigh, however tall or short you are, and whatever strength you possess must all be single-focused into driving your body through an opponent's vulnerable anatomy to end his attack.

Here are some essential power and balance concepts and tactics:

- Momentum = mass x velocity
- Force = mass x acceleration

- For maximum-effect striking combatives, don't simply *strike at* the target, *blast through* it. Retract your striking limb immediately along its original path into an optimum position (not a large windup) to deliver the next instantaneous optimized strike. For kicks, land in an opposite fighting stance when necessary to make yourself ready to deliver the next optimal combative.
- For successful combative execution, use your whole body in such a way that all its parts move in concert in a balanced, semi-relaxed manner just prior to delivering an impact. Importantly, an overly tense body leads to short, staccato, sub-optimal coordination along with telegraphing. Grandmaster Gidon emphasizes that the hand must lead the body for a punch while the foot leads any kick. If delivered properly, both strikes harness the body's mass behind them. Note that, though the attacking limb and body move in concert, this does not mean they move at the same speed. As we observed earlier, to deliver optimum combative strikes your striking limb should move or lead your body. Initiating with the limb enables maximum reach, speed, and weight transfer through a combative strike. Beginning a combative with a designated foot, hand, elbow, or knee (depending on your selected strike) minimizes any telegraphing of your intention. It is important to bear in mind that even though your striking limb has started to move or lead, in reality your entire body has already initiated a chain of motion. For optimum power, the limb and body stop moving simultaneously, concentrating all the energy through the combative.
- While on its way to deliver an impact, a limb should not be tense. Of course, on impact the limb should be strong and tight to deliver maximum force and prevent it from becoming a shock absorber, decreasing the combative's effectiveness. Improper limb preparedness will result in the loss of considerable energy and, hence, effectiveness.
- Do not draw your arm back prior to delivery of a combative or raise your leg up and pause prior to kicking; you will telegraph your intent.
- When excess motion is removed from a strike, its pre-launch signature disappears, with the result that there is no telegraphing that an opponent can recognize early. Telegraphing may be thought of as not revealing any clues, tells, or any other tips about what you intend to do. Accordingly, when you stop telegraphing you become fast, and fast generates momentum to inflict maximum damage.
- You must not just defend particular combatives but also how the accompanying energy that propels and accompanies attacks will affect your balance, posture, and overall structure.

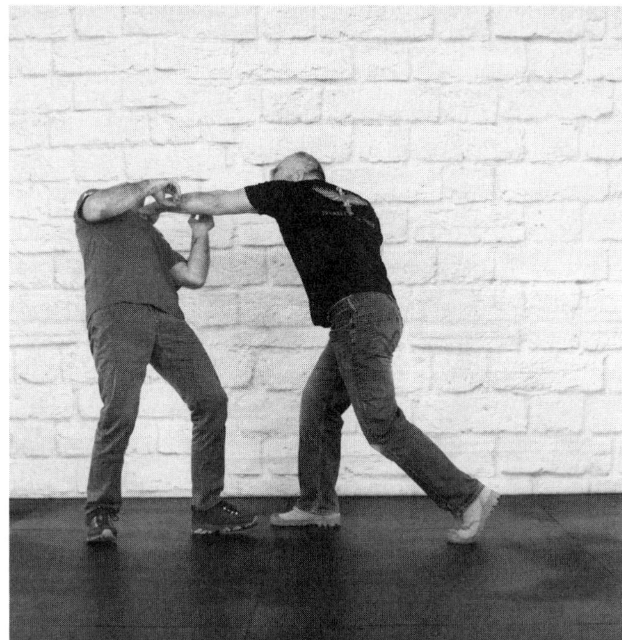

Straight punch.

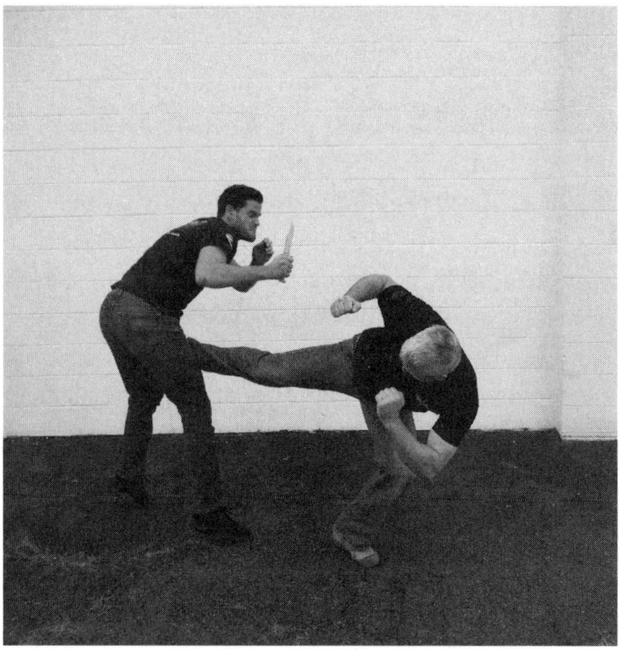

Ball-of-the-foot roundhouse kick.

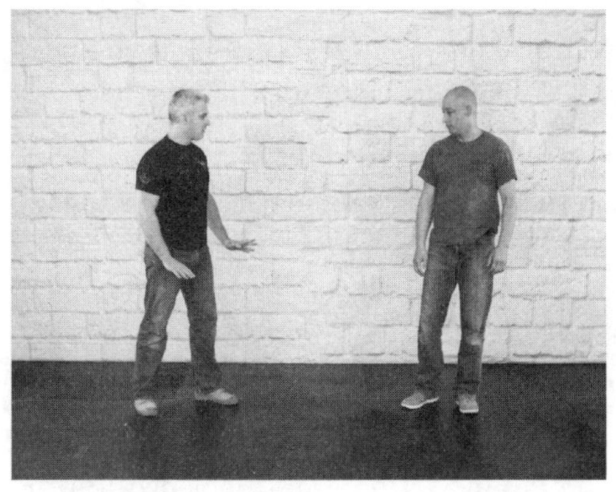

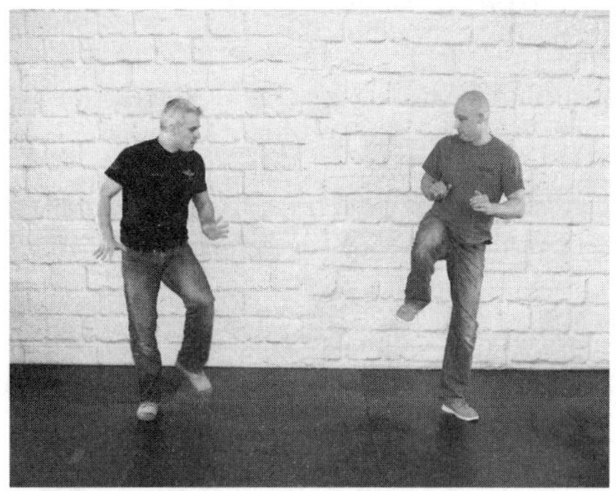

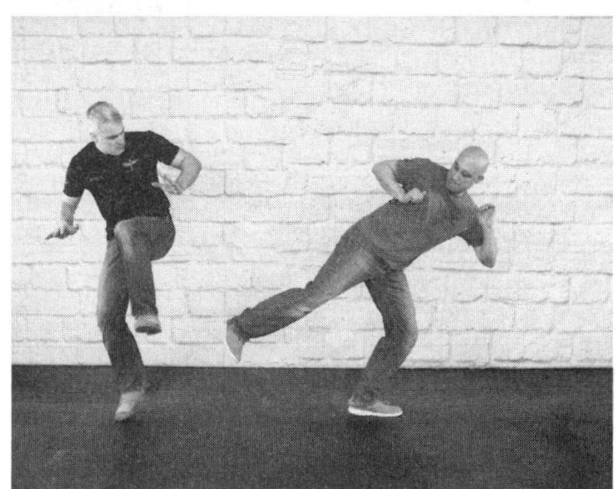

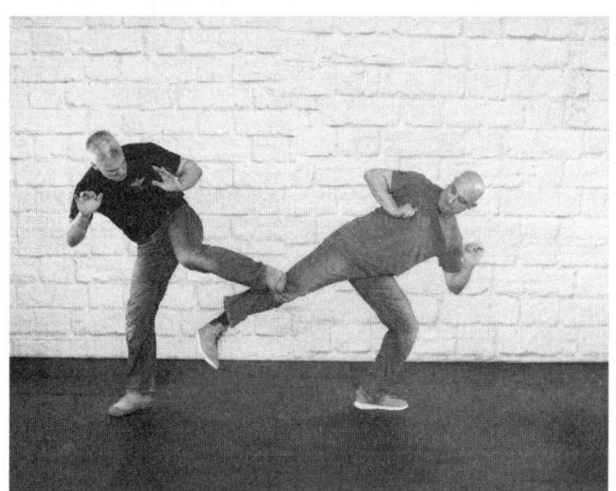

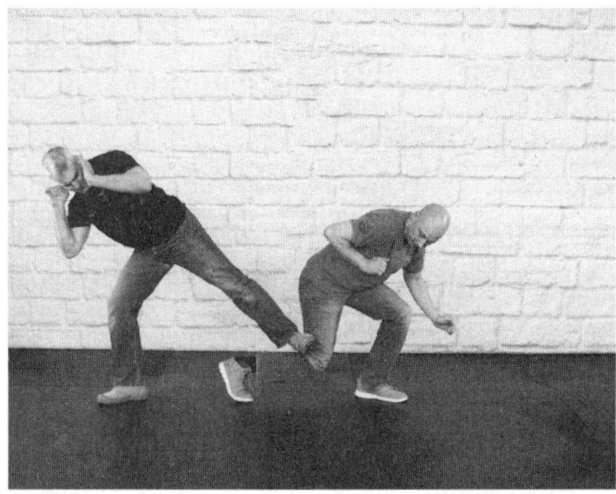

This series depicts a side kick defense using a counter side kick. Such an example exemplifies the requirements of self-defense: recognition, timing, balance, and anatomical targeting, coupled with optimized power.

Strategies to Floor an Adversary

Krav maga is designed to overcome any disparities in size or strength, especially if you need to unbalance an adversary. You can put an assailant on the ground in three ways:

1. *Undermine his balance.* Combatives include strikes and throwing.
2. *Undermine his support.* Combatives include strikes, trips, and leg sweeps, especially on the front leg as he moves forward and shifts his weight.
3. *Lock his joints to force him down.* When the defender is still standing, a heel hook is especially effective. The heel hook is best applied by using your hip and core, not just your leg. As you move your hip, drag your leg with you to ensnare the leg, while knocking his torso off balance.

Keep in mind that a defender often falls to the ground with an assailant because the assailant grabs or locks on to him while falling. Flailing and grabbing are natural instincts when falling to the ground. Do both of these strategically and tactically to attack his vulnerabilities—eyes, throat, groin. To control an adversary's center of gravity, a push or pull move is usually used. This type of combative is best employed when perpendicular to the adversary's center of gravity when neither of his legs can easily recover to restore his balance. The goal is to remove both his support and balance simultaneously. Takedowns, sweeps, and throws displace an opponent's foot or shift his center of mass away from a remaining support leg or even both legs.

Note: If you floor someone and subsequently apply a control hold or joint lock, the aggressor may immediately understand that you are offering to de-escalate. The flip side is that he may fear that being on the ground puts him in a vulnerable position and, consequently, do everything he can to resist you and to rise to his feet. The obvious solution is to reason with him or talk him down, while exerting unequivocal control over him. Similar to all de-escalation reasoning, you must communicate with him in simple straight-forward language, as the human nervous system can only process so much, especially when under stress. Here are a few additional key points to taking an opponent down:

- As soon as you disrupt the attack, you should immediately redirect it into a throw or takedown, using gravity and the ground to further neutralize the threat. A strong combative will stun the assailant, allowing you to close on him to continue injurious combatives, including unbalancing him so you can complete the takedown or throw.
- An unbalanced adversary is obviously easier to displace than a balanced one. Even if your initial throw or takedown is unsuccessful and the assailant maintains partial balance, continue your retzev, applying a subsequent combative or series of combatives to keep attacking the threat. Always attempt to keep your retzev seamless, transitioning from one technique to another in a logical manner.
- Should an assailant attempt to throw you, by the very nature of movement and tactics he is creating an opening for you to counterattack, especially with a counter-

throw. This is true of all combatives, including kicking, punching, and striking with the knees and elbows. A good fighter will minimize his openings or vulnerabilities, but they are still there to be exploited if the defender is skilled enough to recognize the opportunity and execute the counter-technique properly.

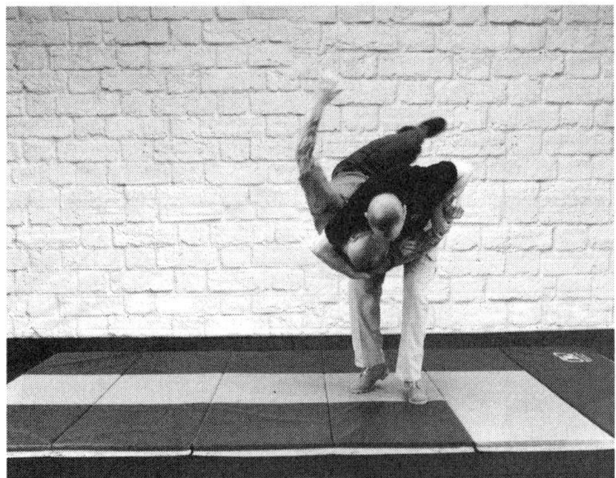

Koshi guruma throw.

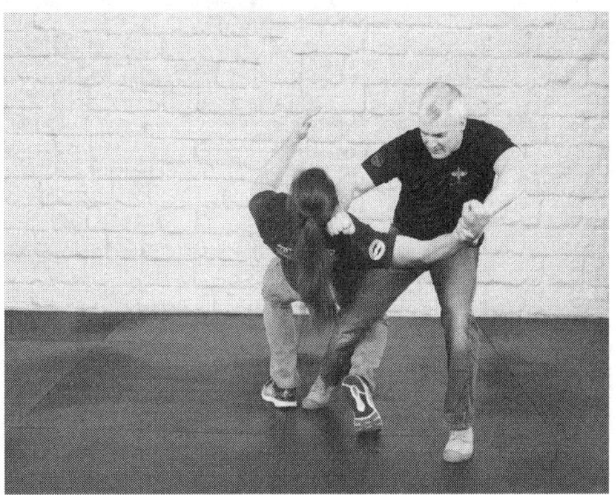

Osoto-gari takedown.

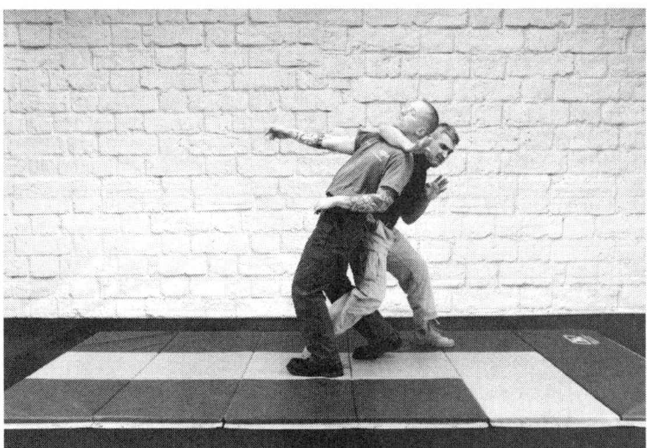

Combined arimi and osoto-gari takedown.

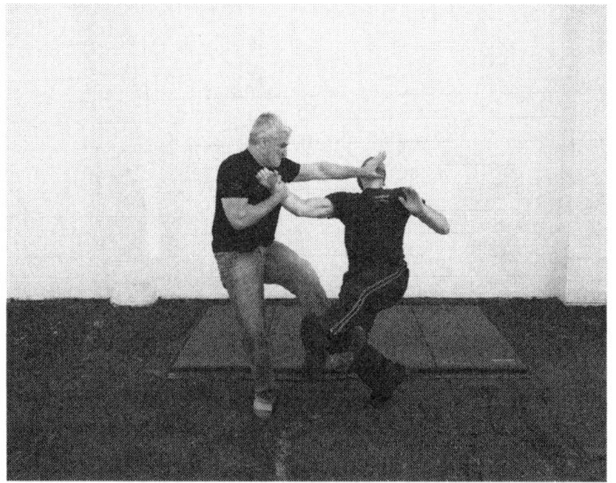

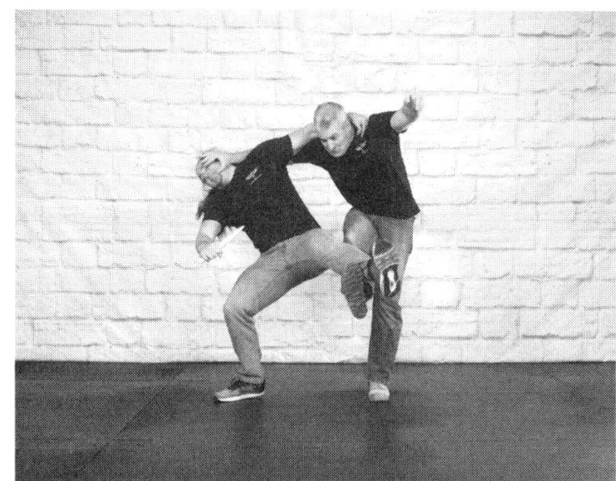

Combined strike and foot sweep takedown.

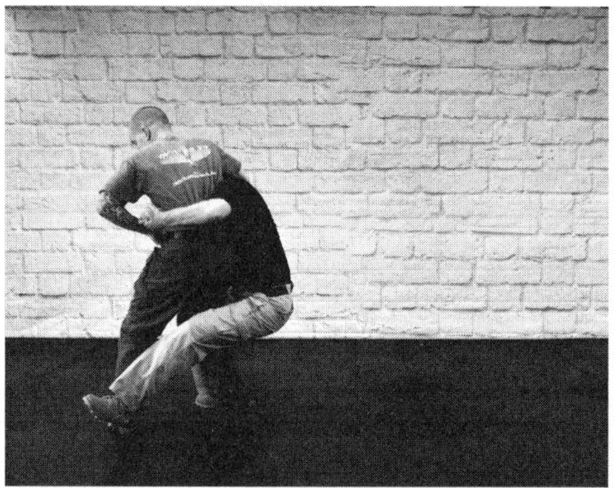

Tani otoshi (valley drop) takedown.

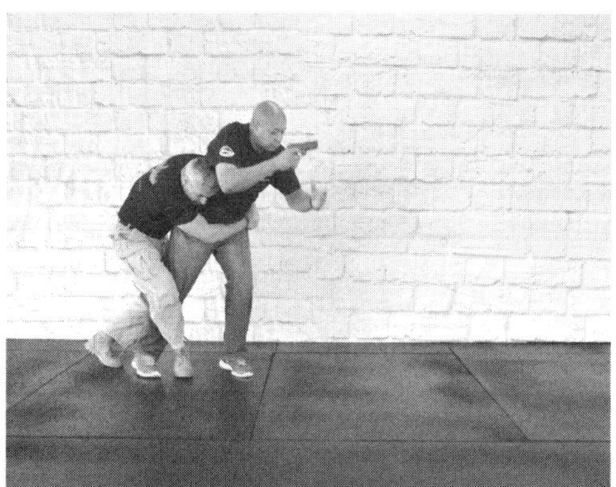

Kosoto gake active shooter takedown.

The Strategy of Retzev

Firearms usage legend Col. Jeff Cooper once said, "The only acceptable response to the threat of lethal violence is immediate and savage counterattack. If you resist, you just may get killed. If you don't resist you almost certainly will get killed. It is a tough choice, but there is only one right answer." Israeli Krav Maga, as taught by Grandmaster Haim Gidon, uses retzev to overwhelm an assailant to complete a defense. When combined with simultaneous defense and attack, retzev is a seamless, decisive, and overwhelming counterattack, forming the backbone of the Israeli fighting system. A defender may have different strengths and capabilities. To adopt and streamline the krav maga method, you must personalize the techniques and make them your own. This begins conceptually as you decide to physically overwhelm your opponent with an instinctive counterattack and ends tactically as you use your preferred combatives directed as the opponent's exposed anatomy dictates. Of course, choose the combatives that are most instinctive and will give you the best chance of debilitating the attacker. Targeted, devastating, and seamless counterviolence leads to a conclusive result: the scale of physical power tilts in your favor. Keep in mind that firepower improperly directed—even when massive—is a waste of precious time and effort.

Retzev is the most effective strategy to keep your opponent paralyzed in the action-reaction OODA Loop, overwhelming his ability to recognize the myriad attacks he faces while breaking down his ability to resist. For retzev, simply ask yourself which logical combative you are most comfortable with executing. Such a strategy allows you to minimize time and streamline the tactics. With practice, you can optimize your preferred tactics without thinking because they have become first nature. Developing this trained fluidity that builds on your body's now-honed instinctive movements improves retzev's effectiveness. Wherever your limbs happen to be, you can strike without chambering and without any other type of preparation that leads to wasted movement, vulnerability, and fatigue.

Retzev requires your four limbs to function like well-coordinated pistons. As one limb extends, another retracts, creating seamless coordinated movement. The goal is to seamlessly integrate each tactic into the next one so that one tactic prepares for the next. In developing explosive, non-telegraphed and seamless movements, you gain a crucial advantage: hampering your adversary's recognition and response time against your counterattack minimizes his ability to successfully respond.

Only well-trained people hit both fast and hard. Most people can do one or the other, but combining the two creates an optimum combative. Your violent intent governs your ability to inflict visceral counterviolence. As noted, true self-defense focuses not simply on survival but rather on how to savagely injure, cripple, maim, and—if necessary and justified, and in the most extreme cases—kill.

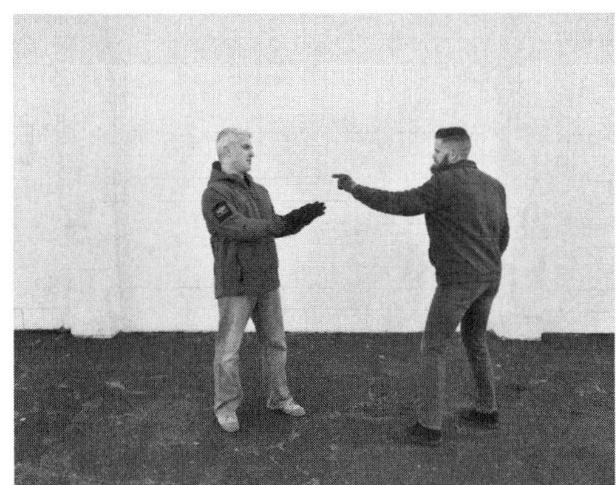

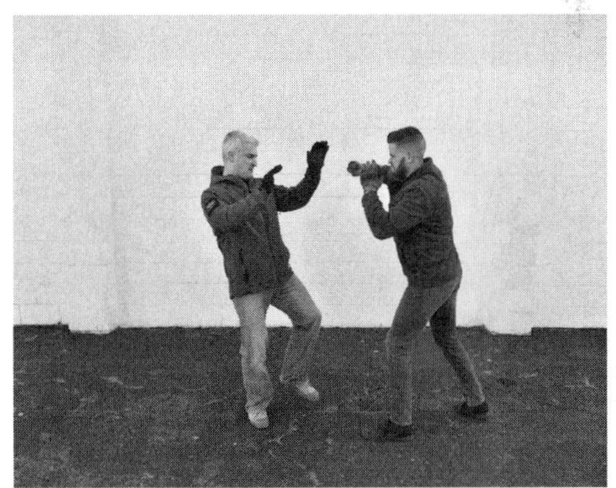

series continued on next page …

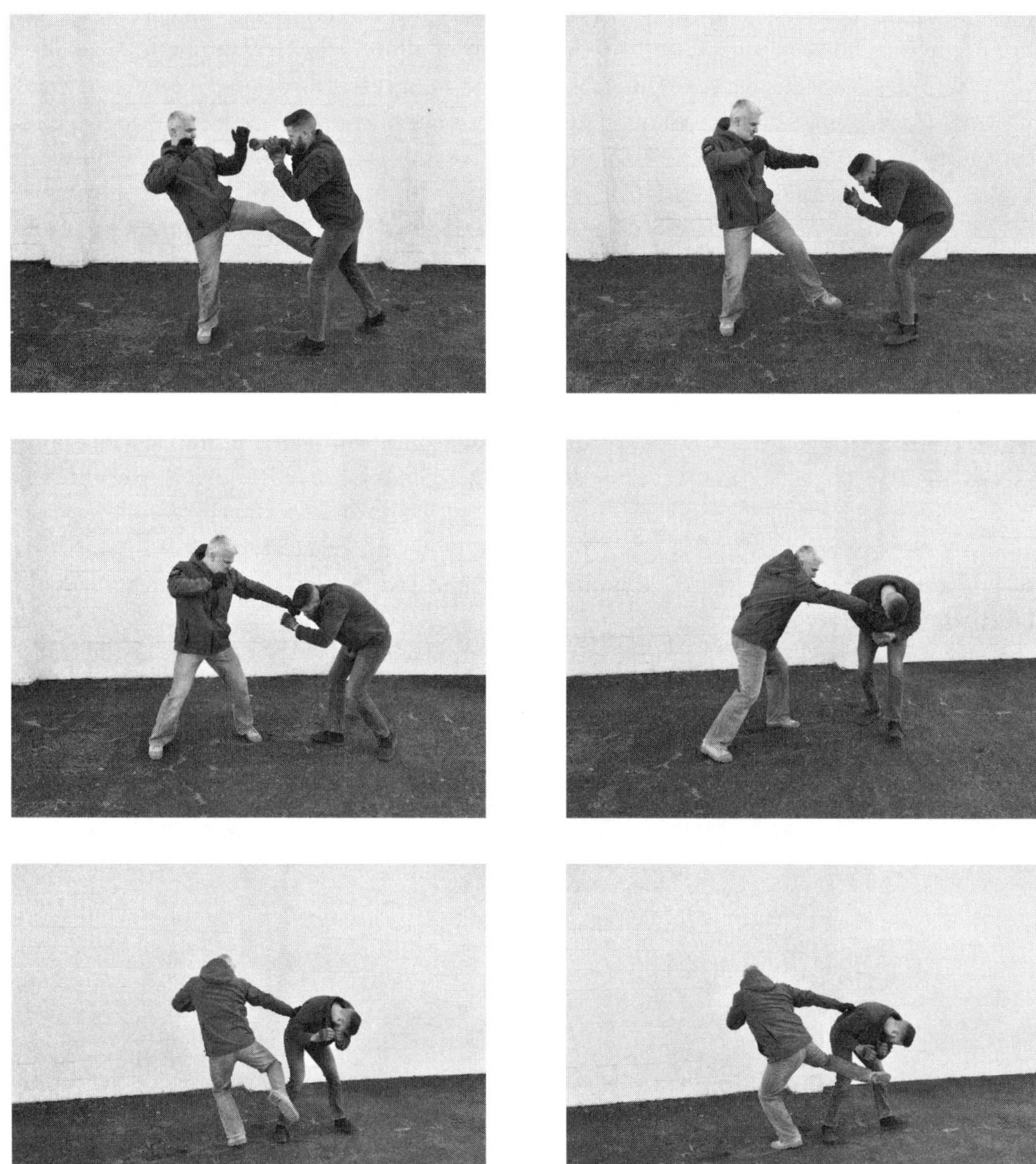

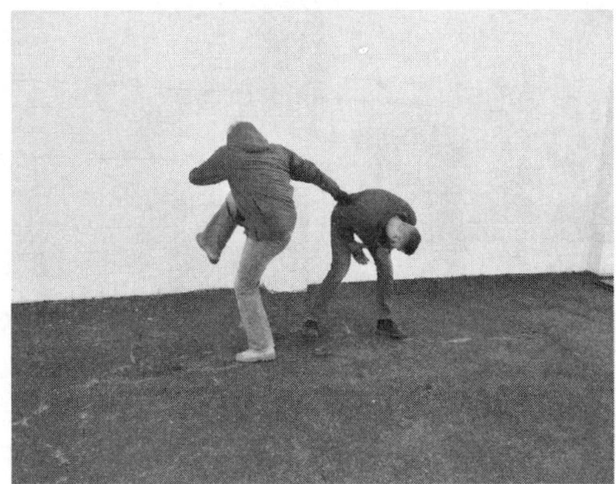

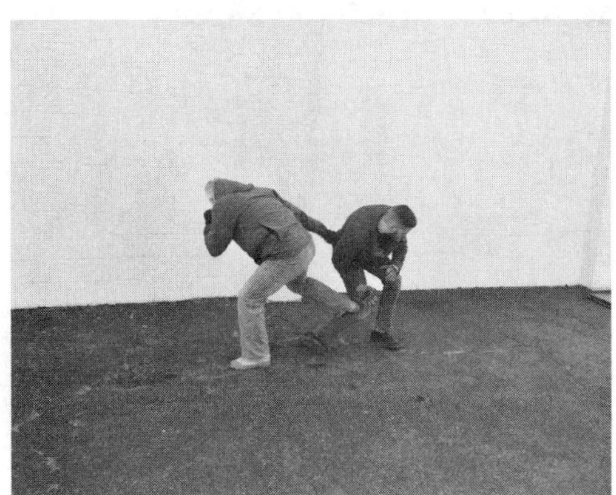

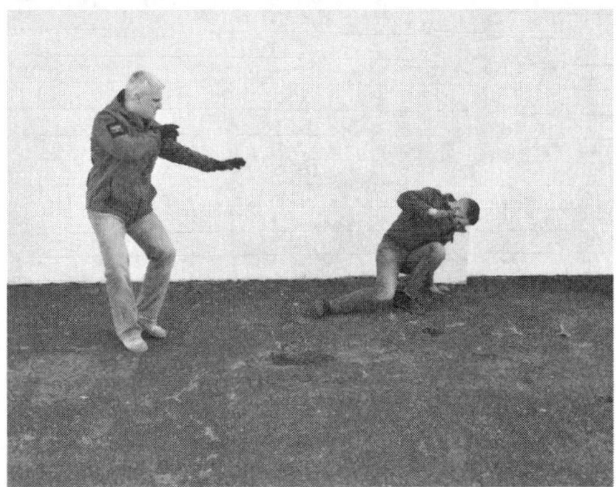

This is a retzev counterattack defense against a straight punch attempt. It shows a timing straight lead kick followed by a straight lead punch (before the kicking leg touches the ground), then a rear straight punch, a rear roundhouse kick, and then a same-side side kick to the knee. Disengage and contact the police.

The Strategic Recognition of Three Primary Types of Attack

There are three primary types of attacks to be aware of:

1. timing
2. feinting
3. overwhelming by brute force

Accordingly, the success of an attack depends on correct timing and selection of the combative.

Self-Defense Fight Timing Strategy

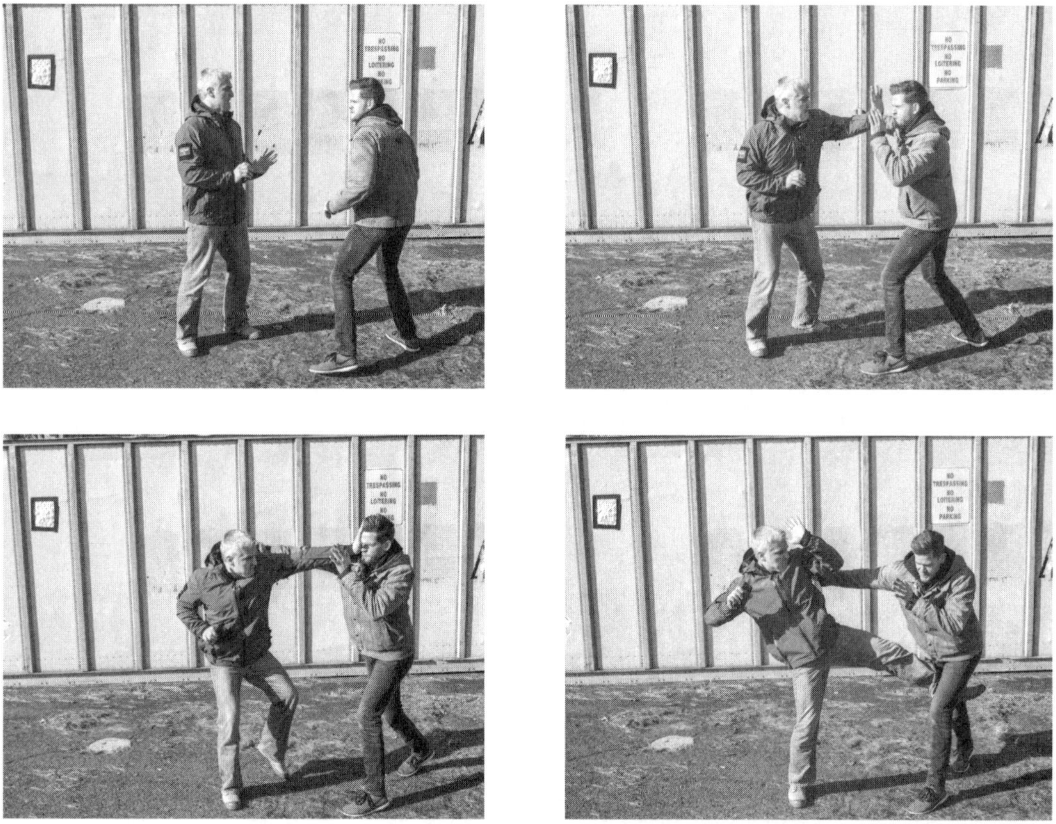

This series depicts a straight palm-heel strike timing defense against a hook punch.

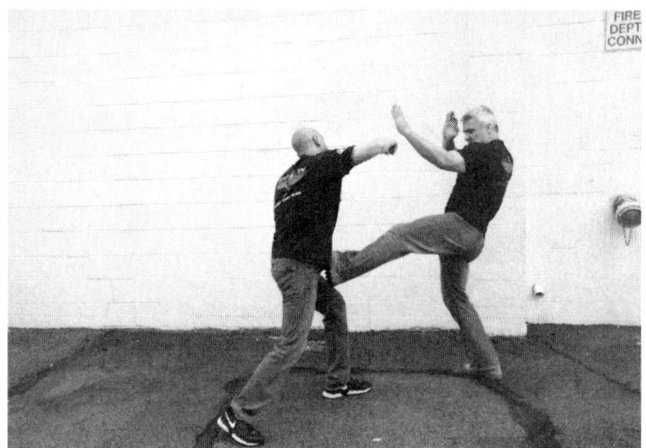

This photo depicts a timing straight kick against a straight punch attempt.

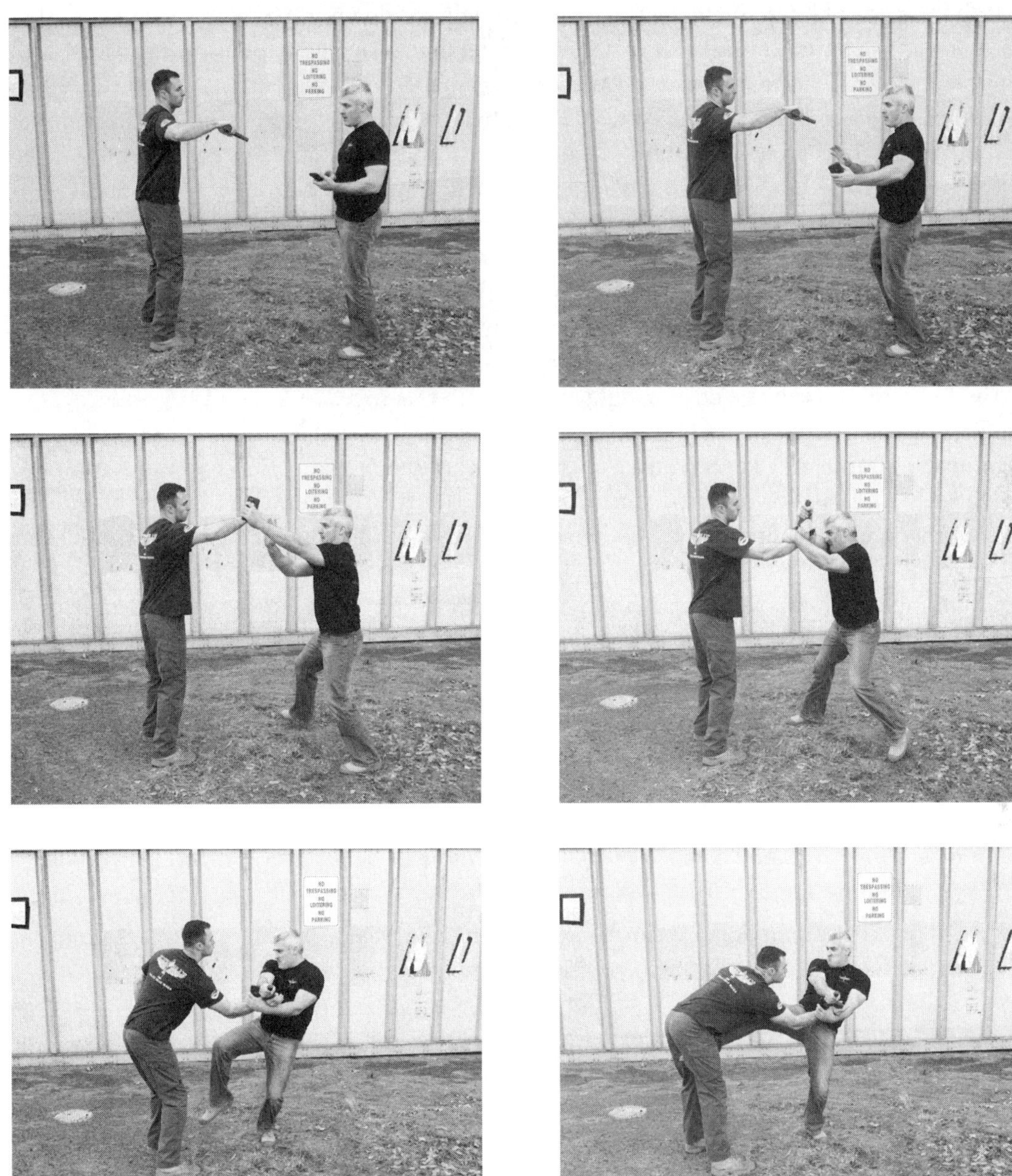

This series depicts a handgun defense #2 disarm with your mobile device still in hand while moving off the line of fire. (Unless you train to drop your device, your extensor reflex will clamp your hand down on it in an emergency situation. Moreover, we condition ourselves regularly not to drop our devices. Therefore, you must be able to fight with your device in your hand until you strategically drop it.)

Grandmaster Gidon distills self-defense and fighting down to one overall word: timing. Effective self-defense timing is essential for a defender to survive an encounter. Haim and another top krav maga instructor (who unsuccessfully vied to become Imi's successor) disagreed whether fight timing could be taught. Haim's competitor argued that timing cannot be taught; one has the ability or one doesn't. Haim explained that timing could be taught. Observing the discussion, Imi agreed with Haim. Fight timing is synonymous with knowing when to counterattack, where to counterattack, and which personal weapon to use. The paramount goal of timing is to orchestrate the right tactic at the right time.

Timing further requires an understanding of what tactic to utilize and when to execute it based on your positioning and weight distribution. Mastering weight distribution enables you to counterattack faster to avoid additional stop-starts using muscle contractions. Timing is the most important aspect of a fight, trumping even speed. Along with possessing the ability to recognize when and how an aggressor presents vulnerable anatomy susceptible to a debilitating counterattack, you must also have the confidence and patience to wait for him to make such a mistake or misstep. When this opportunity arises, however briefly, counterattack with unreserved prejudice. The better your timing, the less chance you will sustain damage.

Fighting could simply be explained as the art of moving advantageously and decisively at the correct time. Fight timing may be broadly thought of as the ability not just to physically defend yourself but also to verbally de-escalate a situation with interjections such as, "You're absolutely right in one sense . . ."

Here are some essential self-defense and fight timing concepts and tactics:

- Correct timing means using an appropriate tactic at the correct time. It is essential to a successful defense.
- Krav maga relies on economy of motion to eliminate wasted movement, which, in turn, improves speed.
- Successful counterviolence can be executed in two ways involving timing: (1) you decide when to preempt or (2) your opponent's movement dictates when you must counterattack.
- Fight timing is also the ability to harness instinctive body movements to either capitalize on a window of opportunity offered by the adversary or to create your own injurious opportunity by using instinctive tactics. An attacker exposes himself when he commits to his preferred initial movement. Avail yourself of this opportunity which will be easier than creating a new opportunity that solely depends on your movement. In other words, let him do the work for you as you exploit his anatomical vulnerability.

Strategic footwork lets you control an adversary to create timing opportunities to injure him while diminishing his opportunity to damage you. In short, superior footwork is a must for any fighter who wants to avail himself of fight timing either by exploiting an opponent's mistake when he presents a physical vulnerability or creating a vulnerability through superior violence of action.

- Timing must be developed and sharpened with realistic training with the objective of trying to simulate a real-speed, concerted attack.
- Simple movements enhance timing as they are faster to execute and usually more direct.
- The faster you can intercept by parrying, blocking, or closing by defensive evasion, the more capable you'll be of taking advantage of the vulnerability created by the opponent's attack.
- While fight speed is not timing, speed can deliver a decisive advantage when the defender moves more quickly than the assailant.
- Timing is a critical source of power for the acceleration of combatives. As far as timing is concerned, a straight-line movement will trump a circular movement.
- Attack an aggressor as he aggressively moves toward you. Harvest your forward momentum and his forward momentum to create a massive impact with whatever target you choose for an initial debilitating strike.
- If you can master distance and closing times, you can prevail against a faster, stronger adversary.
- When possible, avoid an incoming strike while counterstriking *at the same time.* In other words, as he misses, you are simultaneously counterattacking. Optimally timed counterstrikes result when the attacker's combative comes close to actually hitting the defender but misses. As the attacker closes in on you, he is subject to a counterblow while moving forward. Your counterstrike is amplified by your opponent's missing and his momentum carrying him into your combative.
- A successful counterstrike requires precise timing and recognition to correctly read the opponent's attack movement. For example, a counterattack to the knee depends on the element of surprise so you catch the opponent weight bearing and off guard. Catching him off guard requires you to counterstrike as he initiates his attack and is not thinking about a defensive counter-measure such as lifting up his leg to protect his weight-bearing vulnerable knee.
- A crucial concept with weapon defenses is that the attacker expects you to move away rather than close the distance to engage him and control the weapon.
- Keep in mind that humans move faster from the outside in (toward one's center line), requiring a shorter, more economical arm movement, than from inside out, using a longer extended arm movement (away from one's center line). In other words, an inside rotational parry will be faster than an outside rotational parry.

Enhanced Strategies to Improve Reaction Speed Based on Preparation in Training

To be sure, reacting to an attack sooner than later provides a distinct advantage. Perception may be considered the first element of fight reaction speed. The sooner you perceive the threat or incoming attack (including its trajectory/angle), the faster your response will be. The second element of fighting speed is your response time or immediate reaction (without thinking). Our eyes have a more difficult time tracking straight movement toward our face than movement that is oblong or circular, cutting across our field of vision. This means that straight punches and straight kicks—or any linear strike—are more difficult to discern than circular ones.

Colonel Boyd's OODA Loop is crucial to timing and self-defense. (Whoever is more capable of completing the OODA Loop is more likely to prevail. Using a decisive, overwhelming counterattack literally and figuratively keeps your opponent off balance and incapable of catching up with the action-reaction curve. Through superior realistic training, you can cut down on the OODA Loop to close the action-reaction curve. Stated differently, through realistic training you develop early recognition of attack movements, especially with the most common attacks such as hook and linear punches, sucker punches, grabs, kicks, and takedowns as well as common armed threats. Your mind is therefore instantaneously capable of prescribing your preferred response: you have been there and done that courtesy of your conditioned training responses. In short, you are not caught off guard and are thus able to circumvent the OODA Loop through your previous experience handling such a situation or a very similar one. Training against typical attacks allows instantaneous recognition and action to reduce the observation, orientation, decision, and action steps you must take to successfully defend yourself.

Reaction is a two-part phenomenon that includes how you react to a physical stimulus and the time it takes for your body to defensively respond to the stimulus. Reflexes and instinct work in tandem. Reflexes occur when your body receives a stimulus that indicates danger. Importantly, this reflex action emanates from the spine not the brain. Instinctive reactions are natural, and hence faster. Accordingly, if you actively contemplate multiple responses, you cannot react quickly (Hick's Law).[55] For example, in defending a straight punch that an attacker throws with either arm, you might consider using six defenses:

1. Use a timing kick such as a straight or side kick against the attacker's midsection, groin, or knee before he can fully launch the punch. (See retzev example.)
2. Parry the strike with your same-side hand (or an elbow gunt) while delivering a straight kick to the attacker's midsection, groin, or knee.
3. Step off the line with a simultaneous scoop and counterpunch.
4. Step off the line with a sliding over-the-top punch.

55. Hick's Law is paramount for self-defense training as opposed to becoming a martial artist with myriad techniques and tactics that can defeat a single type of threat. It is a psychological principle which states that the more options are available to a person, the longer it will take for him or her to make a decision about which option is best. Source: https://whatis.techtarget.com/definition/Hicks-law

5. Step off the line with a sliding parry and half-hook counterpunch.
6. Step off the line with a double-arm parry and modified roundhouse knee to the attacker's midsection, groin or thigh.

Which counter-tactic you choose will likely be determined by: (1) the point at which he recognized the incoming attack (defense 1 described above would be available), (2) whether or not you are within leg or kicking range (defense 1 would be available), and (3) whether or not you are prepared for the attack (defenses 1–6 would be available) with your hands up or you were ambushed (defenses 4–6 would be available). So, with six options available, what would be your preferred defense if you know all six defenses as described above? The simple answer is whichever defense is most comfortable for you and you have the greatest confidence in based on your preparation in training. Preventing Hick's Law from taking effect involves a balancing act between your preference and your most instinctive response to such an attack, two things that have been determined long before the incident unfolds.

Here are some essential body-reaction tactical concepts:

- Instinct assumes control over cognitive reasoning.
- An attack launched by surprise or an ambush will force you to react from an unprepared state. Therefore, your self-defense reaction must be instinctive and reflexive. Reactive speed may be understood as deflecting or using body defense to make the attacker miss, combined with a simultaneous or near-simultaneous counterattack.
- Once you recognize the attack, the greatest obstacle to speed is how much you slow yourself down (by exerting muscular tension in your limbs performing the strike prior to initiating the strike).
- Relaxation is paramount for optimum speed. In a physical altercation it is certainly difficult to remain relaxed. This can only come from training and experience.
- Importantly, *sub-optimal* instantaneous defensive movement may be superior to *optimal thought-out* movement that requires more time.

When and How to Counterattack Strategy

Counterattacking is essential to thwart an aggressor. To counterattack optimally, you must observe the adversary's body movements and positioning, especially after you deliver your opening combatives. Instead of simply aiming your combatives at whatever attack points you happen to be able to reach, instantaneously evaluate his anatomical vulnerabilities during your observation. In other words, for example, you do not want to batter the top of his skull or bludgeon his arms that are shielding his head. Rather, if his arms are in a protective shield, his lower body will be open to debilitating counterattacks (and his vision is likely to be obscured, too). When possible, do not waste combatives against invulnerable targets, especially that might damage your hands—primarily the top of the skull or his elbows.

The bottom line is to know when to attack with overwhelming firepower using adaptive targeting. Deliver your combatives with precision and correct timing utilizing as much power as you can harness while delivering your counterattacks at the most advantageous moment.

Attack when the opponent advances or changes his position toward you. Many of the below points can also be found in the preceding photo examples in this book. Here are some essential counterattack concepts and tactics:

- What you do instinctively you will do faster.
- Someone who *accidently* invades your private space or startles you will usually freeze. You must recognize this tendency in the milliseconds before launching a counterattack.
- You can preempt or counterattack when he is distracted; when he changes his stance or position, including when he drops his hands; when his feet are parallel; as he retracts his initial attack; or when he is speaking.
- The optimum moment to counterattack is often (but not always) when an opponent aggressively advances toward you. A notable exception is if the assailant is standing in place and attempting to deploy a projectile weapon where you must close the distance to preempt the weapon's deployment.
- Successfully timed counter-strikes (sometimes combined with body evasions) take advantage of an opponent's (1) extended commitment and (2) slight pauses or gaps between follow-on combatives.
- For untrained people the more power they invest in a combative, the more overextended they are likely to be, giving you ample opportunity to decisively counter-strike. (Note: A trained striker accelerates his combative and retracts it often equally as fast.)
- It does not matter how the attacker has initiated, since every attack movement exposes some anatomical vulnerability. Exploit it and use retzev to neutralize the threat.
- The lead leg or arm probably accounts for a majority of initial attacks in a skilled fight.
- Retzev applies this maxim: an overwhelming offense is the best defense. Developing sound combatives allows your mind to concentrate on tactics and fight strategy.
- Try to parry or deflect no more than necessary, focusing immediately on transitioning to retzev counterattack.
- Combatives' power derives from the correct use of speed, acceleration, and body weight.

- In real attacks, the defender is often ambushed. The attacker's combative has a good chance of landing since his victim is likely to be untrained. The defender can only parry or avoid it if he is quick enough in both recognition and reaction to counter them.
- When an attacker misses the mark, especially in an ambush, there may be a momentary pause on his part. He may, in fact, be surprised at his lack of initial success, providing you with the opportunity to mentally and physically dominate him with your counterattack. If you moved off the line, you are also not where he expected you to be. In addition, the miss may throw him off balance, enhancing your ability to counterattack.
- When an attacker misses his first salvo, he will pull back, try to reorient, and then press another attack. Don't let him regroup; counterattack immediately to exploit his misses and turn the tables.
- Do not quit your counterattack until you render the aggressor non-functional (with proportional use of force, of course).

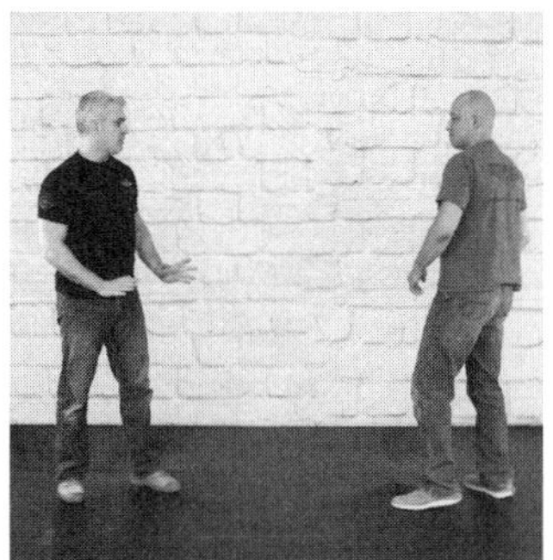
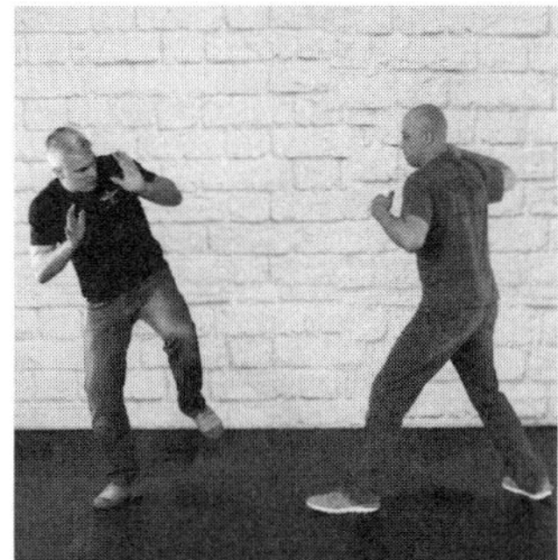
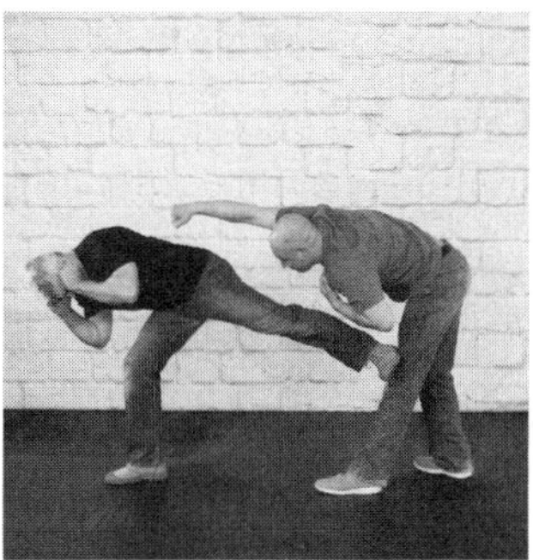

This series shows recognition of an incoming attack and a timing low-line side kick counterattack.

Some additional key ingredients on how and when to move in on an opponent include:

- Switching to a secondary target when the primary targeted attack fails.
- Closing or creating distance to one's advantage.
- Attacking the edge or periphery of his body including, for example:
  - — Catching and breaking his fingers
  - — Impeding his hands
  - — Using an inside slap or axe kick to trap his hands and attack using an upper-body combative targeting his now-exposed neck or head

If you become involved in a self-defense situation that devolves into a fight (when your initial counterattacks did not disable him and you were unsuccessful in closing on him), and you both separate into standing fighting positions, some fight strategies include:

- Attacking with body movements (do not stay in one position).
- Changing your rhythm from fast to slow or slow to fast to interfere with his reads of you.
- Limiting his hands, legs, and head from moving by catching and trapping.

When you and your opponent are in such standing fighting positions facing off, remember that:

- If his feet are parallel, controlling him is easier, since he is in a weak stance.
- If he drops his hands, you can control him more easily, because his arms are in a weak position.
- If he moves back, you can generally move forward faster and with better balance than he can move back.
- If he is an amateur fighter and does not immediately retract his attacking limb, it is extended and more vulnerable to control.

Deceptive Fighting Strategies

Using deception is often essential to gain a decisive advantage against a skilled opponent or multiple opponents. Here are some essential deceptive fight concepts and tactics:

- Do not stare at any one point on your opponent; no single-point focus.
- Deceptive combatives are often the key against a skilled adversary. Retzev combatives and feints are combined so that the two are indistinguishable. The opponent is kept literally and figuratively off balance.
- The success of an attack depends on correct timing with an instantaneous selection of the combative most likely to find initial success, opening the door to decisive, lightning-fast, follow-up combatives through retzev.

Chapter 6

Strategies for Defending an Ambush

Krav maga understands that it is in an ambush situation or the "–5" (you are at a significant disadvantage) where you can successfully use a specific defensive tactic designed to counter a particular threat or attack. In other words, by necessity, the ambushed defensive party reacts first defensively, which could involve a preemptive strike but will more likely involve a deflection or shield against the attack to immediately transition to the counterattack. Conversely, when engaged in mutual combat, offensive capabilities take priority and come to the fore. As emphasized, the one who first imposes a debilitating injury and then follows through with additional combatives is usually the one who prevails. An analogy might be a well-placed bullet from a semi-automatic weapon followed by going fully automatic with that weapon to finish the threat. When facing a potential lethal encounter, every counter-violent combative should focus on inflicting injury or damage to render the aggressor incapable of further aggression. Examples of counter-ambush tactics while texting may be found in my book *Krav Maga Defense*.[56]

The Elements of an Ambush

There are five general elements of an ambush:

1. When an ambush is executed, the victim is usually distracted, complacent, outnumbered, and caught in a state of maximum unpreparedness –5.
2. The chances of escape for the victim are minimized or nonexistent, as the attacker has chosen the site and circumstances.
3. The attacker often acts from concealment or closes on the unwitting victim.
4. The attacker affords himself the chance and avenue for escape.
5. The attacker possesses the intent—and usually the capability—to physically dominate the victim.

56. David Kahn, *Krav Maga Defense: How to Defend Yourself against the 12 Most Common Unarmed Street Attacks* (New York: St. Martin's Griffin, 2016), 106–107, 119–120, 123–125.

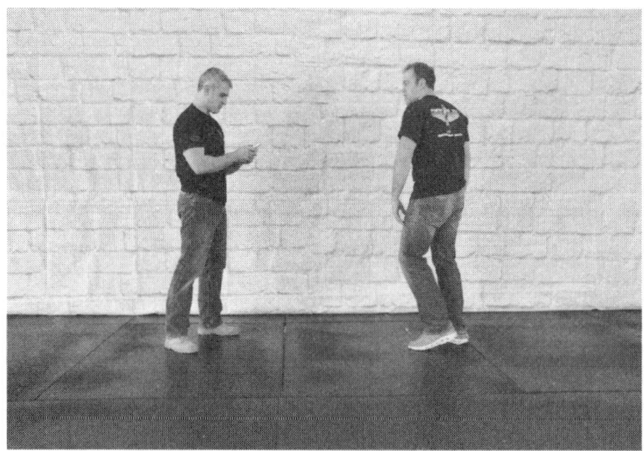

An ambush while you are texting.

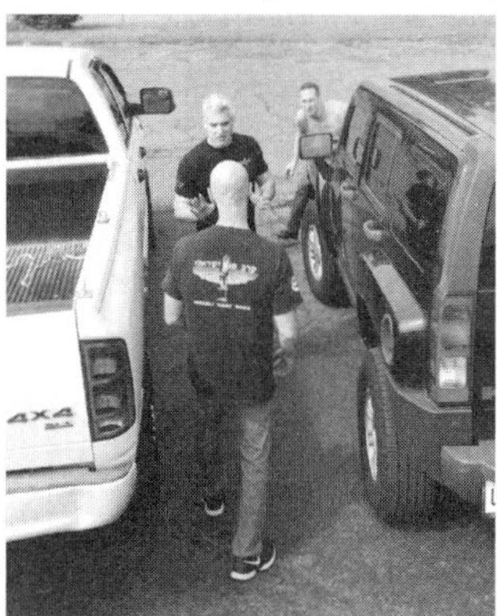

A parking lot ambush.

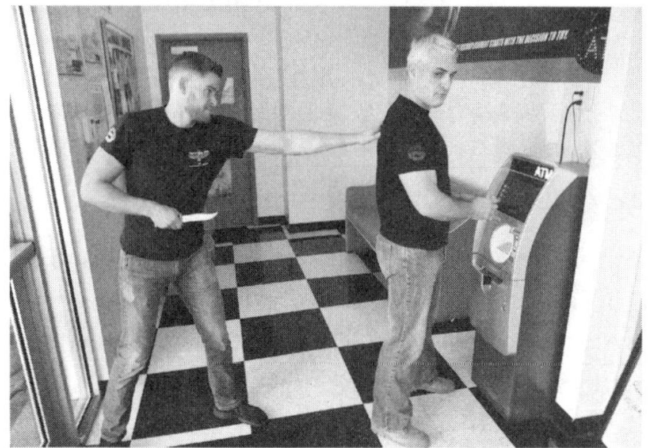

An ATM robbery ambush.

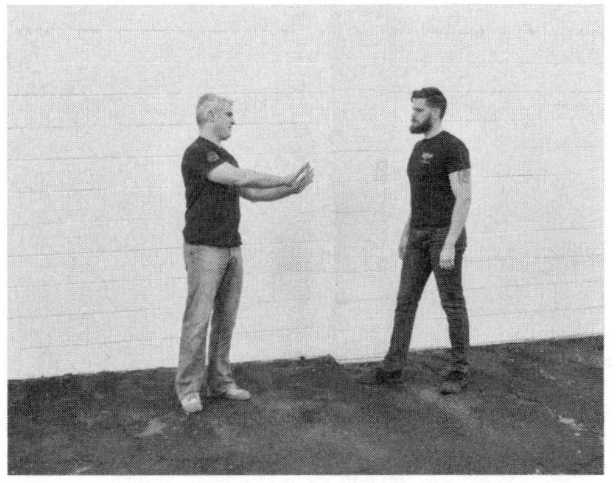

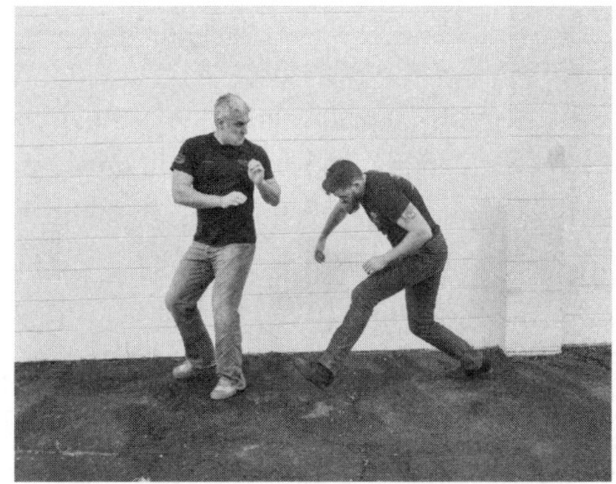

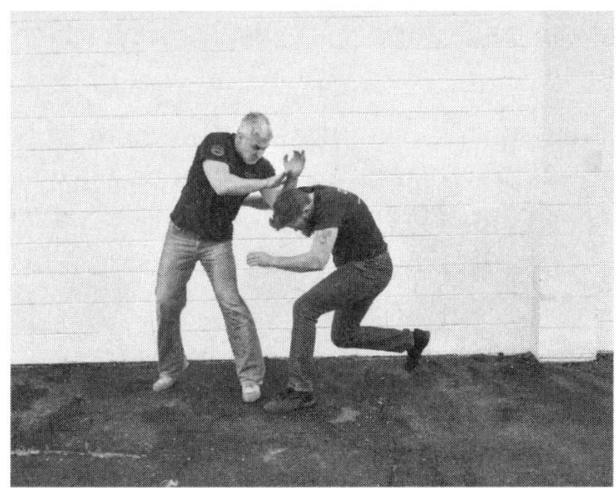

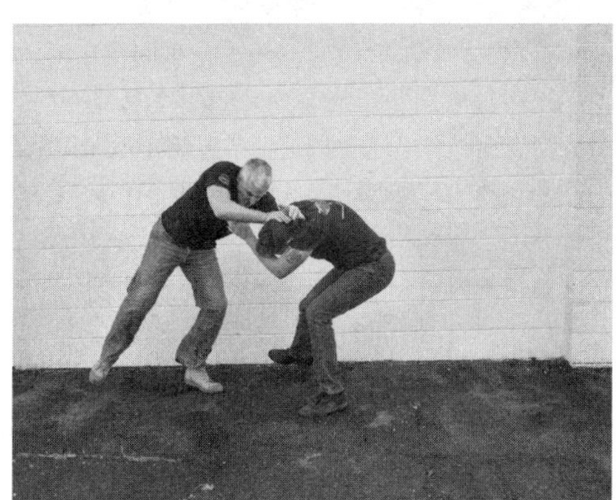

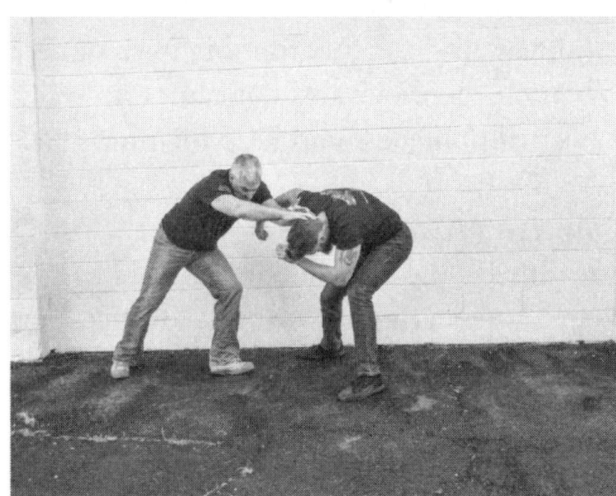

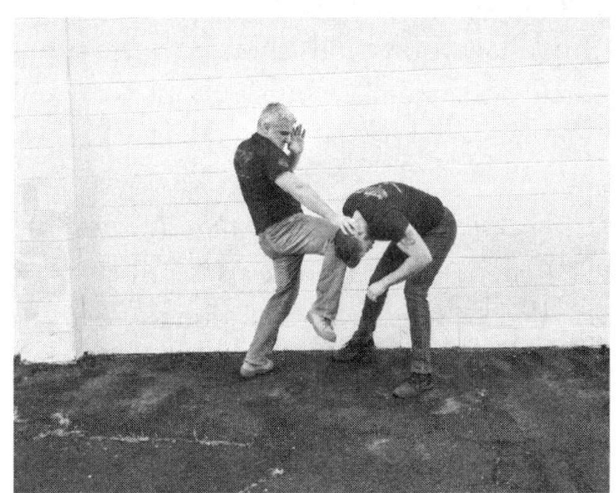

This series depicts an attempt to de-conflict and de-escalate a situation by trying to walk away. Yet, despite what may seem to be a temporary truce, your de-escalation reasoning did not work. Unappeased, the aggressor attempts a rear tackle against you. Note that if someone has shown aggression, you should not turn your back. Always disengage with an eye on the potential threat until you are a safe distance away. Nevertheless, if you were to turn and try to walk away, the aggressor may decide the situation is not over and try to attack you from the rear, in this case using a rear takedown tackle. As noted, you will have to react from whatever position you find yourself in, using combined preemptive and evasion principles.

Human Predatory Strategies

In an ambush or surprise attack, the attacker avails himself of a victim's shock and temporary paralysis to gain the advantage. The attacker chooses the time, place, and conditions most opportune for him to put a victim in the –5. A few key points to keep in mind:

- Criminals position themselves to attack in one of four ways: (1) surprise, (2) surrounding, (3) closing, and (4) cornering.
- A favored method is to corner a victim by trapping the victim (or a group) in a confined space with no escape.
- Similar to animal predators stalking their prey, human predators often wait in ambush. As with animals, humans can also sense danger and fear in their victim.
- Criminals often work in groups to surround, herd, surprise, distract, or simply overwhelm a victim.
- Attackers may close on a victim immediately to orchestrate a surprise violent ambush. Alternatively, an attacker may use ingratiating pseudo-charm to gain proximity and then attack.

Counter-ambush Strategies

To reiterate, a surprise attack will force you to react from an unprepared state. You need to recognize a trap or an inchoate ambush. If a stranger springs out of nowhere, he may have an accomplice flanking or lurking behind you. Train yourself with the mind-set of an attacker. Think how you would ambush yourself at any given moment and use that training to recognize potential dangers as you go about your daily life. When on the move and noticed or accosted by someone who arouses your suspicion, once again discard politeness and keep moving.

Using Objectively Reasonable Counterforce in a Surprise Ambush

Reacting to a surprise attack likely allows more latitude in the use of counterforce because you do not have time to rationally or reasonably analyze the situation. In other words, you are reacting instinctively and defensively and do not have time to calibrate your response. Krav maga's goal is just that: to have you react instantaneously without thinking. Once again, the overriding essence of krav maga is to neutralize an assailant immediately using objectively reasonable force. Nevertheless, the instant you are deemed safe, any additional defensive actions may, in fact, become offensive actions. If you continue to injure an assailant who is no longer a threat, you could face civil and criminal charges—especially if you deliberately turn the assailant's weapon on him.

Human vision is limited by blind spots. You cannot see what is behind you; hence the effectiveness of rear ambushes. Therefore, if an adversary gets too close, he can deliver a knee strike without your seeing it, consequently giving you no time to react. Whenever possible, check your rear or six o'clock position.

As an example of a potential ambush tactic, even when looking straight ahead, you cannot see your feet. Accordingly, a low-line kick or uppercut-type strike may come in under the visual radar. Human vision is also limited in judging the speed of an attack coming straight on versus recognizing the speed of something traveling against a static background. Therefore, tactically, straight attacks are more difficult to defend from a recognition standpoint. Oblong attacks such as hooks and roundhouse kicks are, accordingly, more recognizable. In addition, by their nature these looping types of attacks have a longer distance to travel than does a linear attack.

Most advantageously, a kravist will automatically move quickly to a superior and dominant position relative to his adversary—the deadside. Achieving deadside positioning usually provides a decisive tactical advantage, especially when the defender can deploy a cold or hot weapon in addition to his bodily weapons. Your finishing strategy should revolve around your capabilities and preferred tactics involving long, medium, and short-range combatives combined with evasive maneuvers and weapon deployment. Positioning becomes even more important when facing multiple adversaries. As mentioned earlier, to optimally defend against any attack, you must remain on the balls of your feet. Placing your weight on the balls of your feet allows for instantaneous movement, as you do not have to shift your weight from either heel. This weight positioning allows you to move defensively or offensively (which can be the same, since the best defense may be a superior offense). An aggressor uses a victim's obliviousness and usually some form of concealment to launch a surprise attack. Here are some points to keep in mind to avoid placing yourself in a vulnerable position:

- An ambusher sizes up your every move. If he sees your awareness and preparedness, he will likely hesitate or desist. You can overtly show your awareness by locking your focus on him or covertly by subtle observation. Keep in mind it is best to do your preparation in your own mind to avoid possibly provoking anyone.
- Recognizing an incipient ambush is a combination of elements, including body positioning, eye movement, facial expressions, body lean, and hand placement or hand movement.
- Many attackers rely on violence of action rather than a honed skill set.
- The average person can unleash four or more blows per second.
- Always consider the possibility of another attacker intervening against you as you contend with an initial aggressor.

Rear Naked Choke Ambush Defense

A preferred rear ambush tactic is a choke. This is why tactile-feel training is so important—you must react without seeing or contemplating an impending attack. In short, you must act instinctively, debilitate him, and position him in front of you as a barrier to the other attacker, giving you time to prepare for your next course of action.

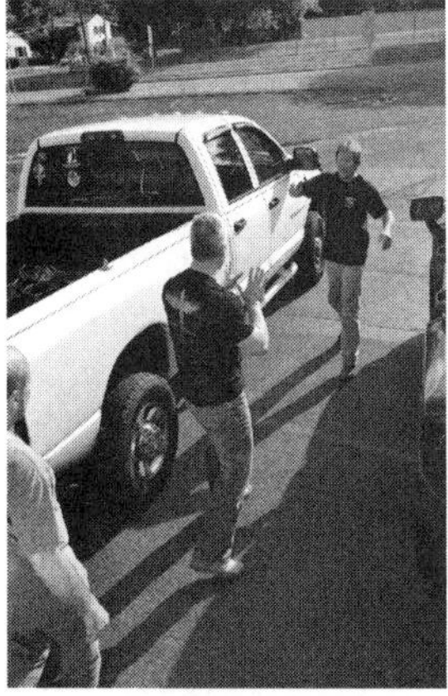
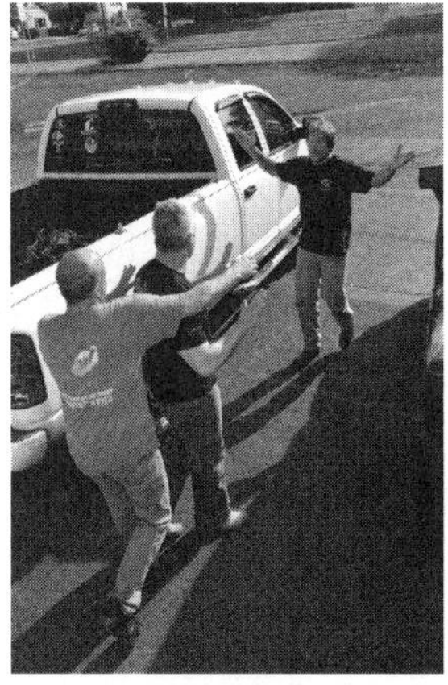
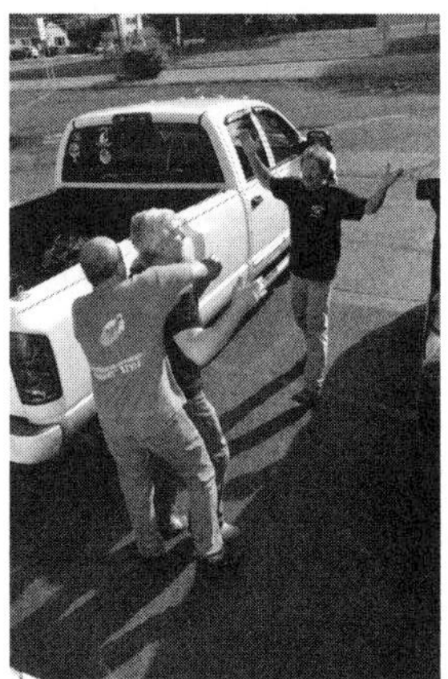
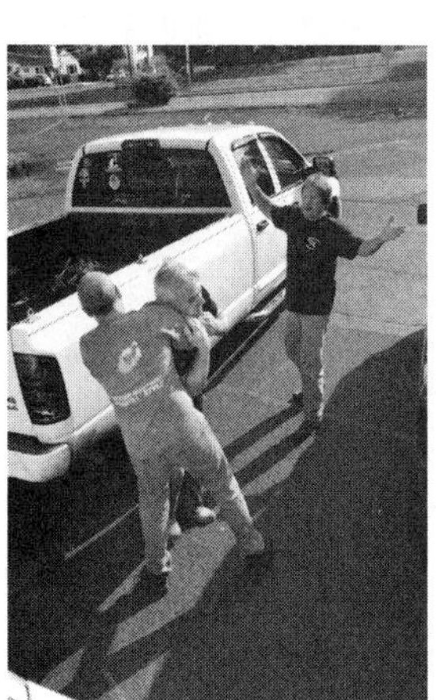
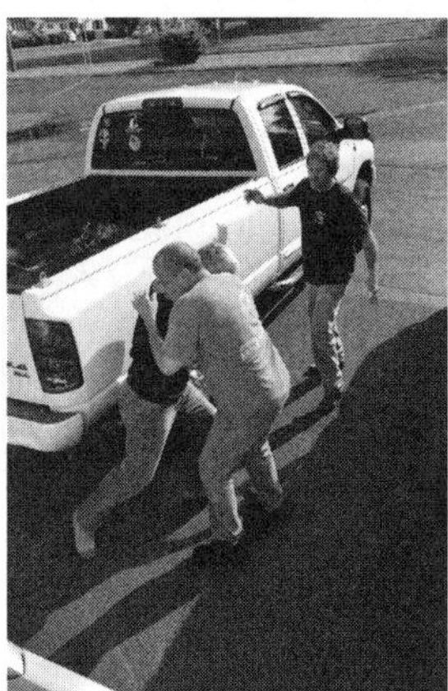
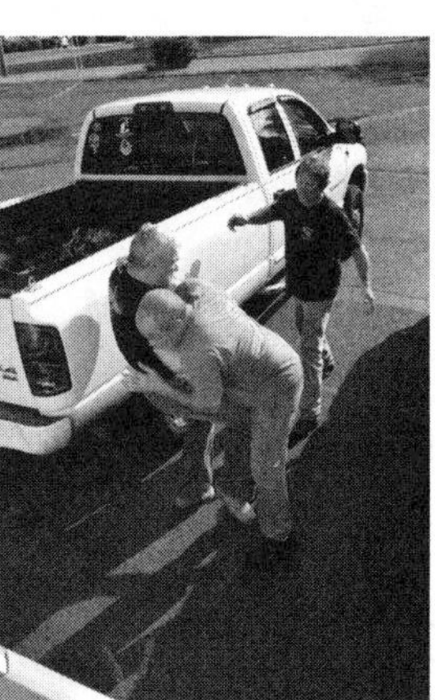

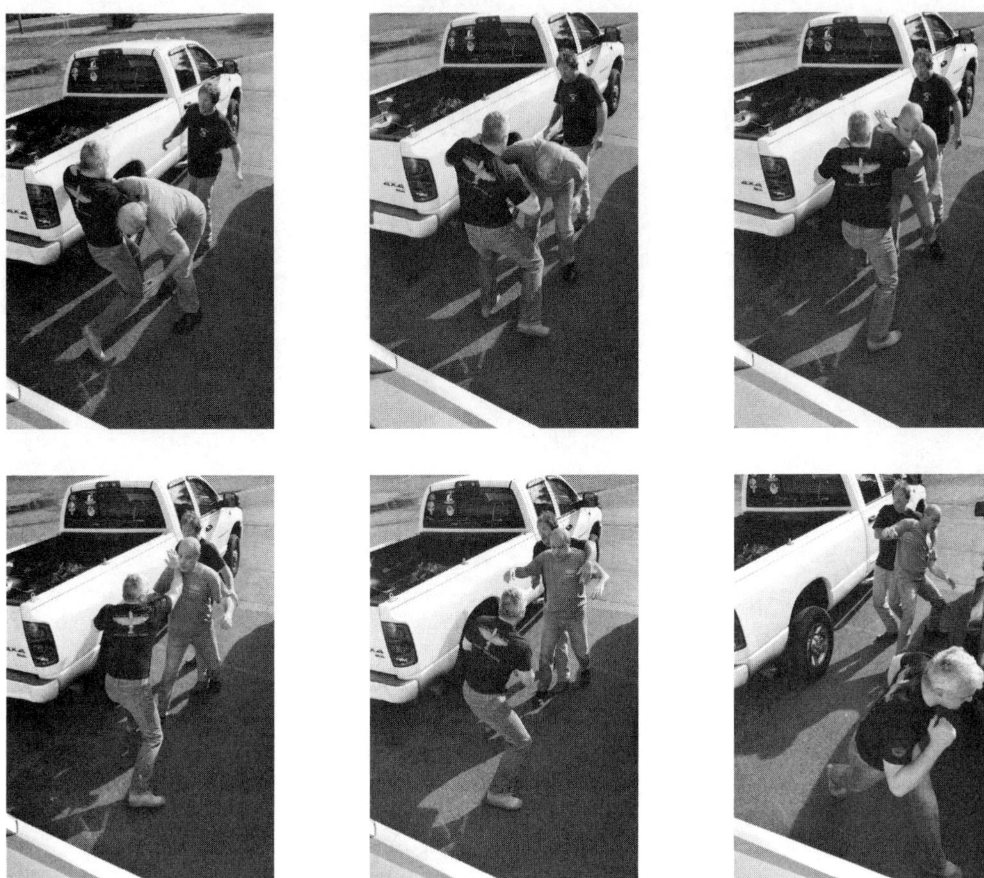

This series depicts defending a rear naked choke ambush between two vehicles. Note the strategic footwork (as previously discussed) where you have trained to turn only one way to defeat the choke. The footwork enables you to about-face into the initial attacker and ram him into the second attacker to make your escape.

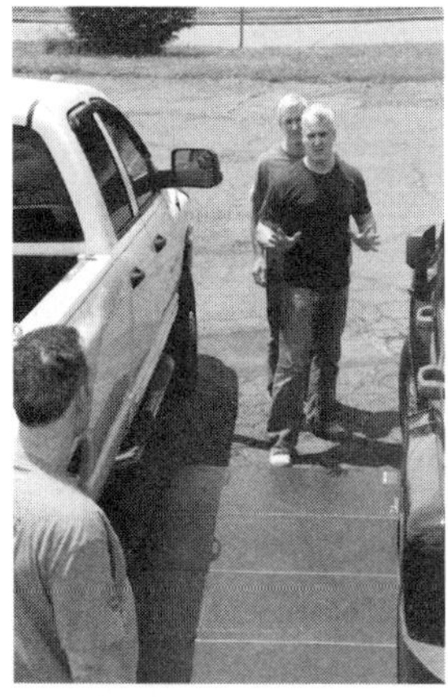
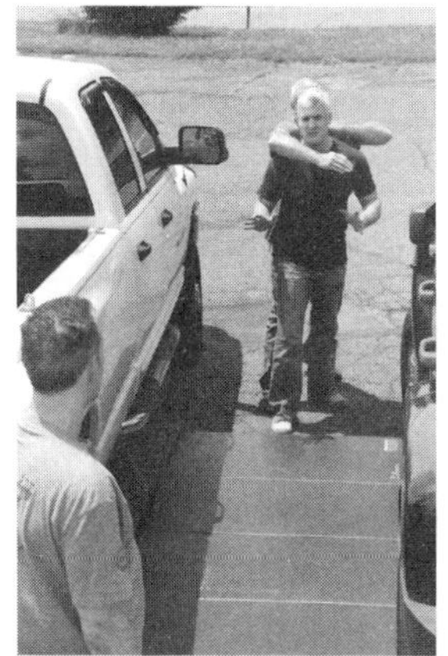
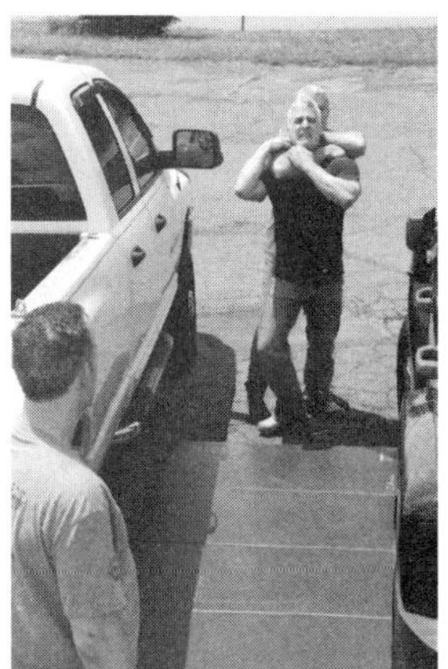
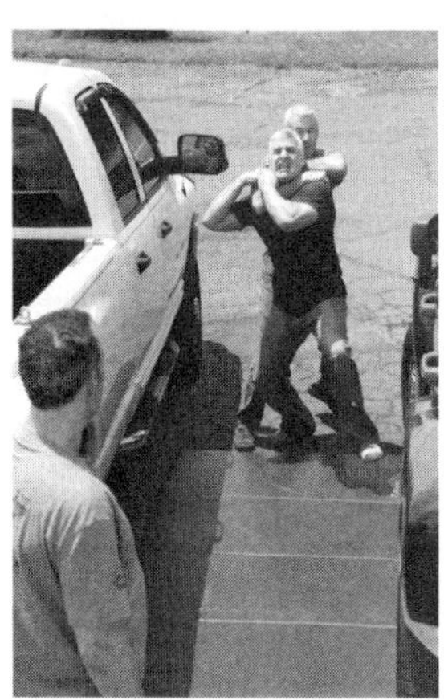
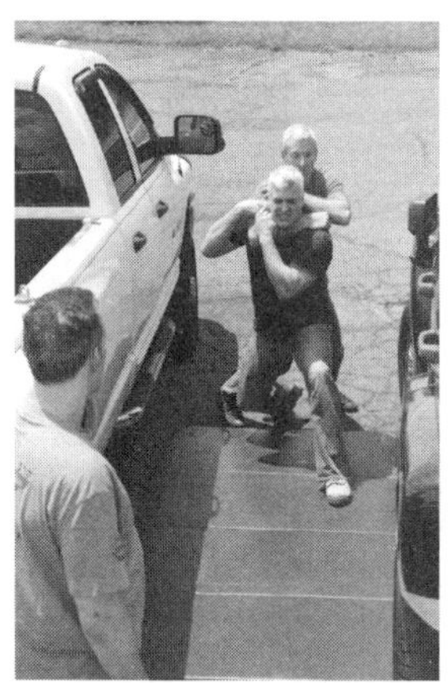
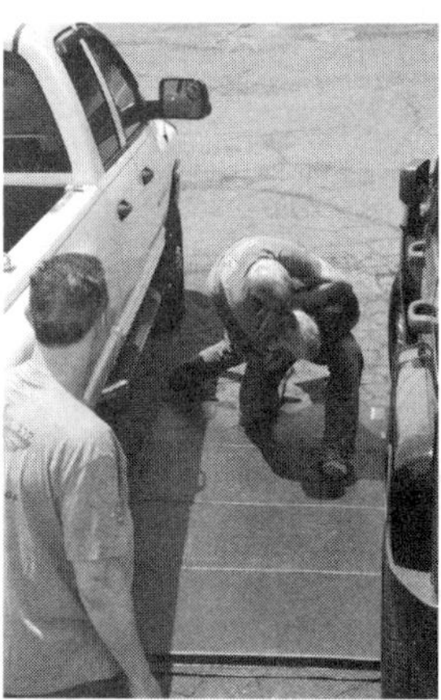

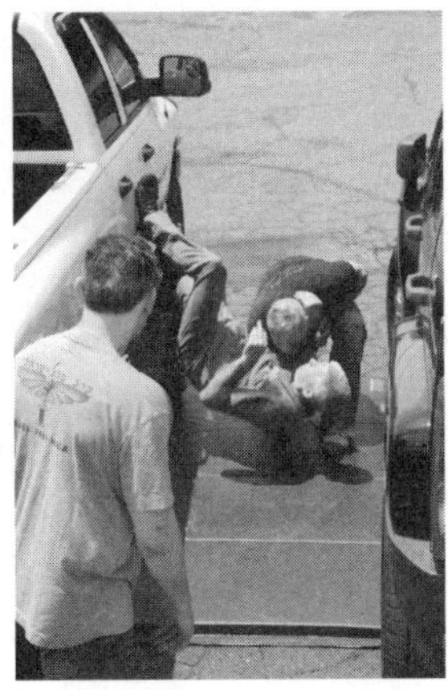
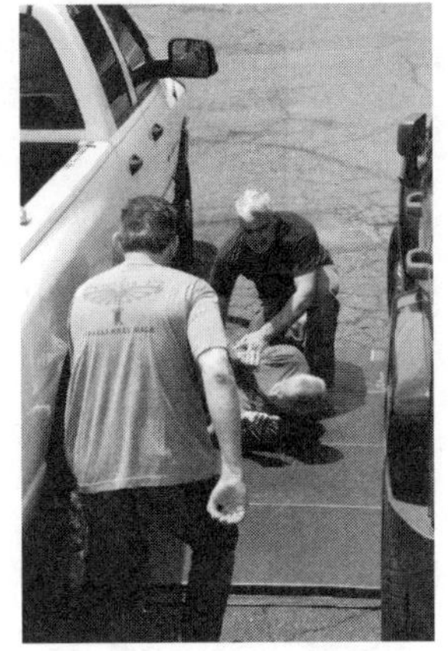
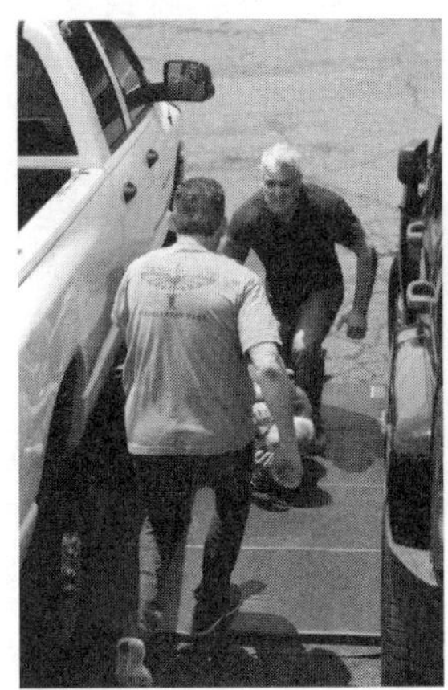
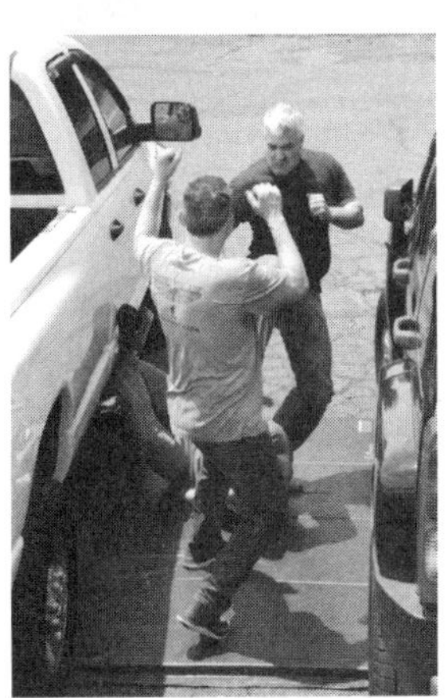
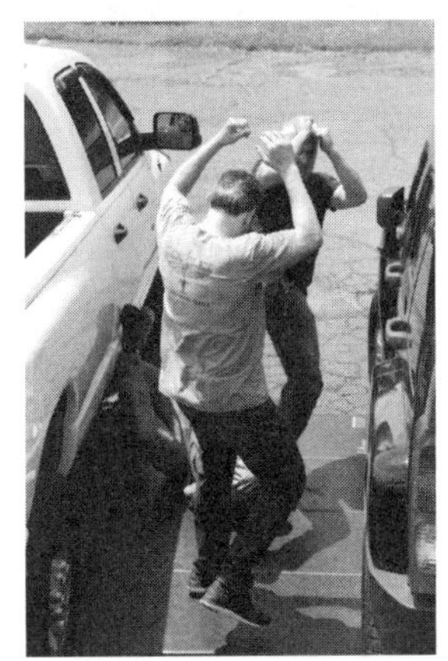
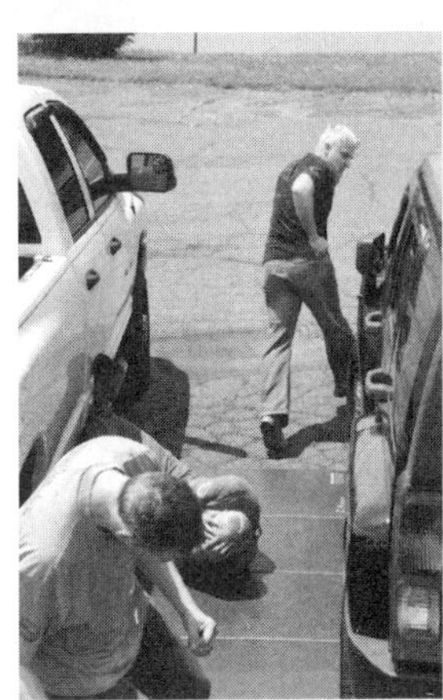

This series depicts defending another type of rear naked choke ambush between two vehicles. In this case the rear attacker drives you forward with the choke. Strategically and instinctively, you should harness the attacker's momentum to execute a drop seo nage throw. Take advantage of your forward movement to immediately kick the second attacker in front of you and make your escape.

Chapter 7

Preemptive Linear Strike and Breaking-Up-a-Fight Strategies

When and How to Preempt an Attack

If you cannot avoid an imminent attack or use de-escalation communication tactics to control both the distance and an escalating verbal interchange, you should seek to preempt your adversary's imminent attack. While you could wait for him to expose his anatomical vulnerabilities as he attacks, I advocate that you instead take the fight to him. Remember, you must be able to articulate why you, as a reasonable person, knew that an imminent attack on your person was about to happen.

Therefore, with a preemption strategy in mind, target any anatomical vulnerability he exposes that he cannot readily defend because he is in motion. In other words, the opponent, even when skilled at delivering his attack, briefly leaves himself open to counterattack. For example, as the opponent delivers a straight punch, he shifts his weight forward, offering you the opportunity to deliver a side kick to damage his front knee. In short, preemption and fight timing are an instantaneous fusion of instinct and decision-making.

Two key elements are at work regarding when and how to initiate a preemptive counterattack:

1. You deprive the opponent of the ability to change his position and defensive posture fast enough to thwart your attack.
2. You strike when the opponent commits to a step and momentary weight transfer, commits himself to a combative (example: straight kick or punch), or tries to deploy a weapon. In other words, the optimum moment to preemptively attack is as the opponent is preparing his attack. The opponent is, for a fraction of second, concentrating on his attack rather than defense and, therefore, is vulnerable to a preemptive counterattack. A counterattack might be opportune when he:

- Leans or steps forward
- Uses footwork to prepare for an attack
- Tries to feint
- Reaches for a weapon
- Is speaking

A preemptive attack is *not an attack into the opponent's attack* (incorrect timing). For example, a preemptive long-range kick is one of krav maga's most versatile and useful tools, providing you with an all-important preemption capability prior to the full initiation of an attack or the active deployment of a weapon. The instant you recognize an aggressive action, you can launch a straight kick or side kick targeting the opponent's vulnerable anatomy, principally his groin or forward knee. These kicks can use *glicha* sliding or *secoul* crossover step footwork to cover distance and place your entire body weight and momentum behind the strike. This is particularly true if the opponent raises his hands, signifying an aggressive action, or sequesters one or both arms behind his back, suggesting he is hiding a weapon. In other words, you should not end up squaring up with someone to fight; as he assumes a fighting stance or any type of aggressive posture, you should kick him. After landing a preemptive kick, follow up with additional retzev combatives as necessary. Your goal should be to thwart an assailant's freedom of action by recognizing the warning signs of impending violence, allowing you to physically stop an attack at its inception.

The Preemptive Straight Kick

A straight kick may be administered using either the front or rear leg. Strike the opponent's vulnerable anatomy with the ball of your foot. Usually the midsection, groin, or knee provide the best targets. Any type of kick may be used, but the straight kick is easy, fast, and instinctive, often flying under the radar. The key to the straight kick (and side kick) is using a sliding glicha step executed with your non-kicking base leg to close the distance while delivering maximum reach and power.

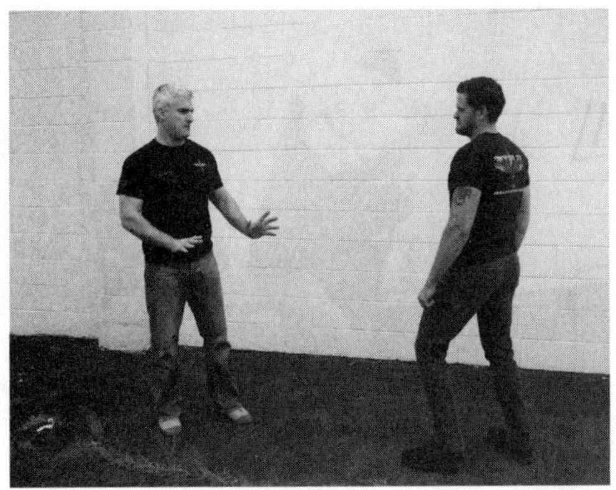

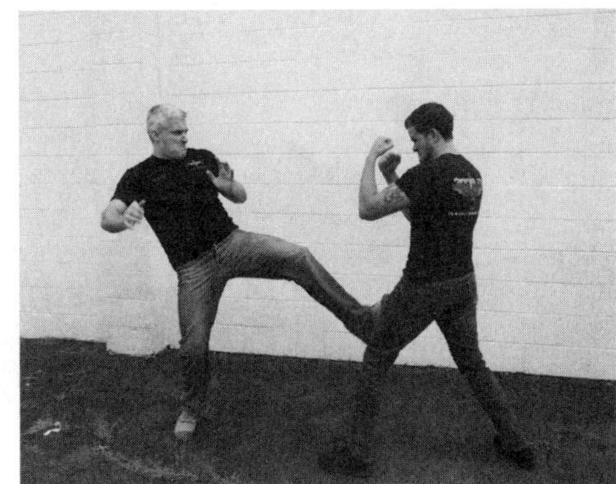

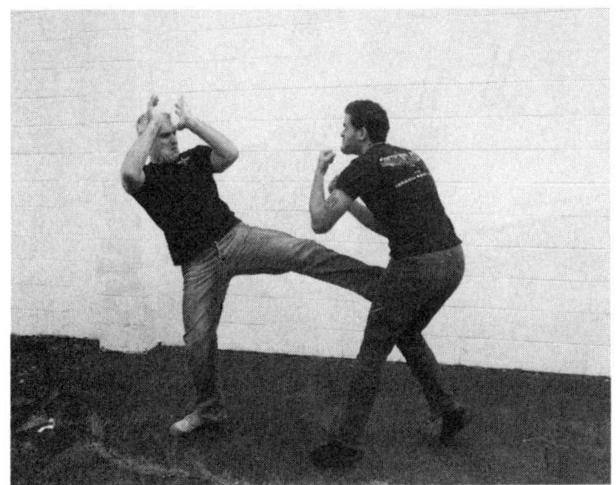

This series depicts a linear preemptive front straight kick.

The Preemptive Side Kick

A side kick must be administered using your front leg. If you were to use your rear leg, it would take too much time, as you would have to switch your stance, giving the opponent ample room to react. Strike the opponent's vulnerable anatomy with the heel of your foot. Usually the knee is the best target; however, you can strike anywhere on the body, including the stomach, ribs, or solar plexus. A glicha sliding step or a secoul crossover step is instrumental in delivering maximum reach, range, and power.

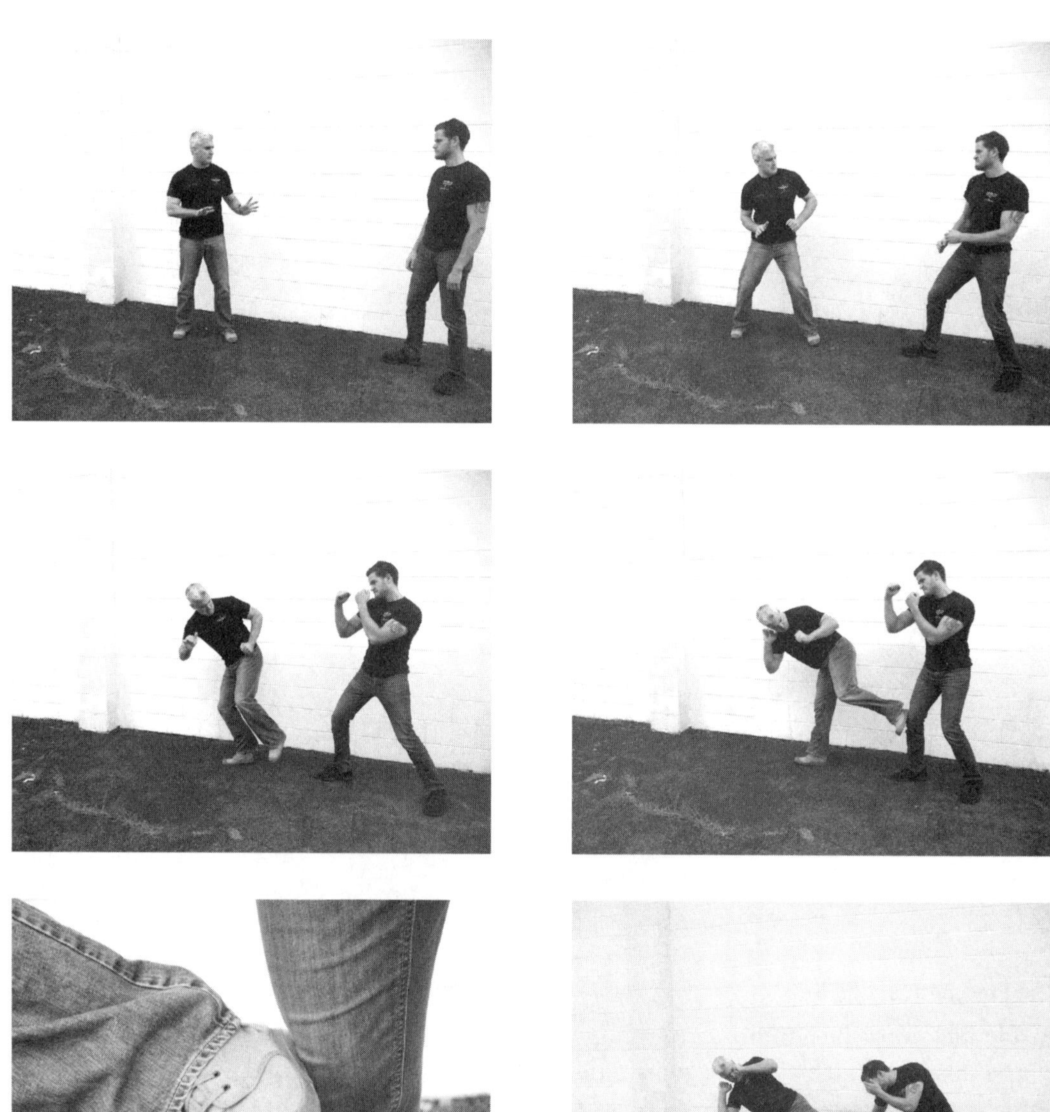

This series depicts a preemptive linear side kick.

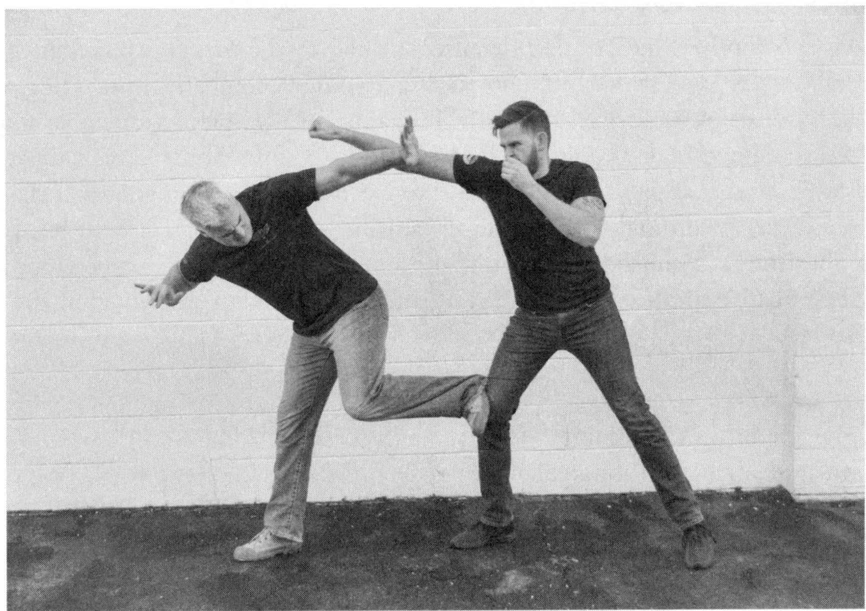

This photo depicts a linear defensive side kick and simultaneous arm block, when the attacker launches a straight punch.

Preemptive Linear Upper-body Strike

Upper-body preemptive linear timing defenses, similar to the previous preemptive straight and side-kick preemptive strikes, rely on timing a straight combative, including a punch, palm strike, heel strike, eye strike, or web strike against an adversary's vulnerable anatomy to preempt his looping punch attempt. A looping hook or roundhouse punch must travel a longer distance than a straight punch requires to reach its target, particularly if the attacker winds up his arm. Accordingly, if an attacker launches a hook punch at your head and you recognize the attacker's impending or initial movement, you can launch a preemptive linear or straight combative to the attacker's head or throat. Finish with additional retzev combatives as required.

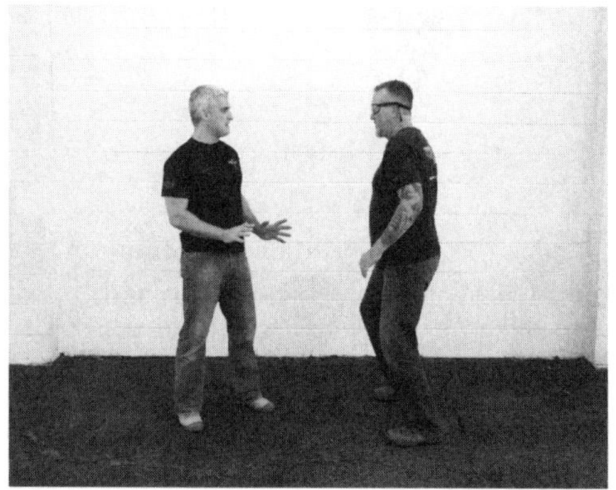

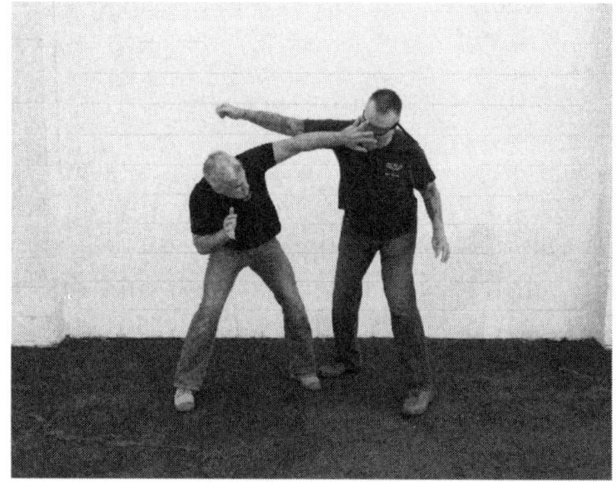

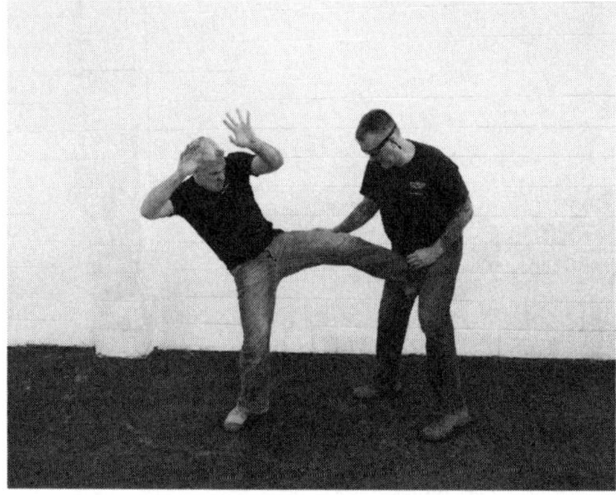

This series depicts a timing defense showing a linear eye strike against a hook punch attempt.

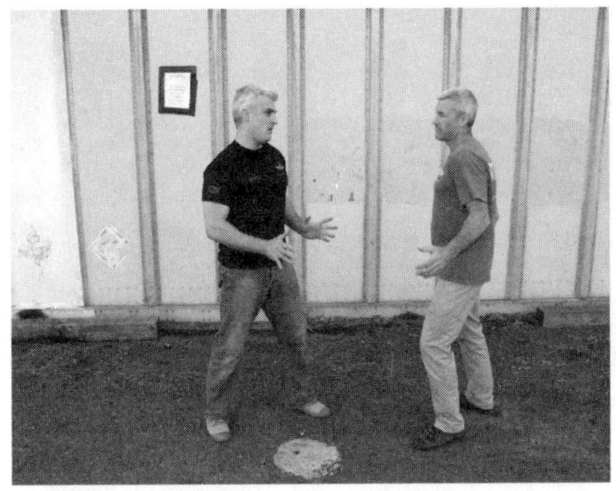

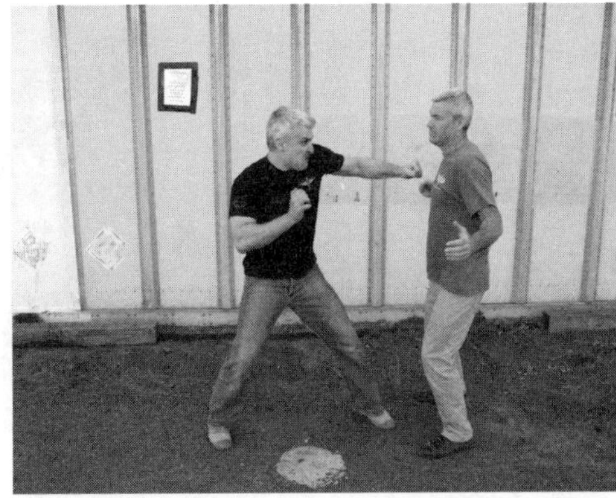

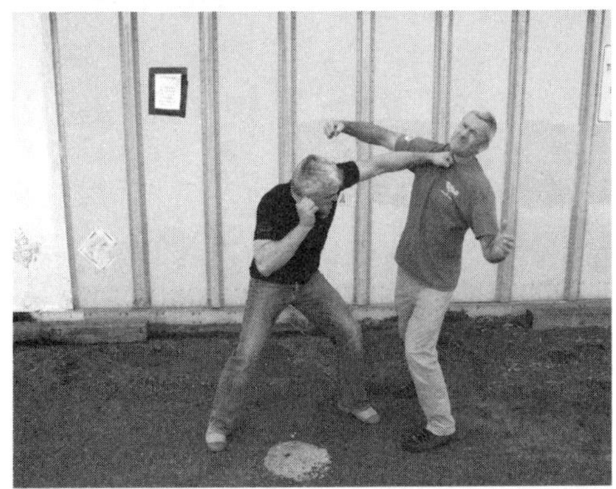

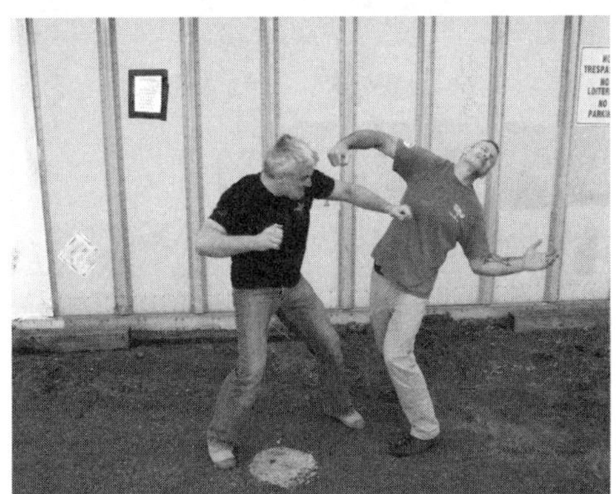

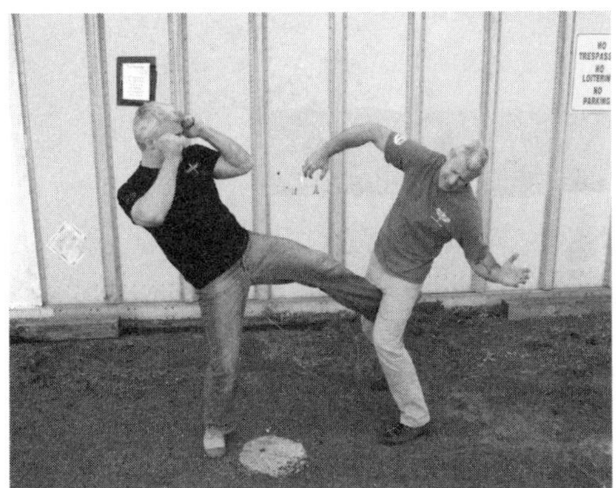

This series depicts a timing defense showing a linear punch to the throat against a hook punch attempt.

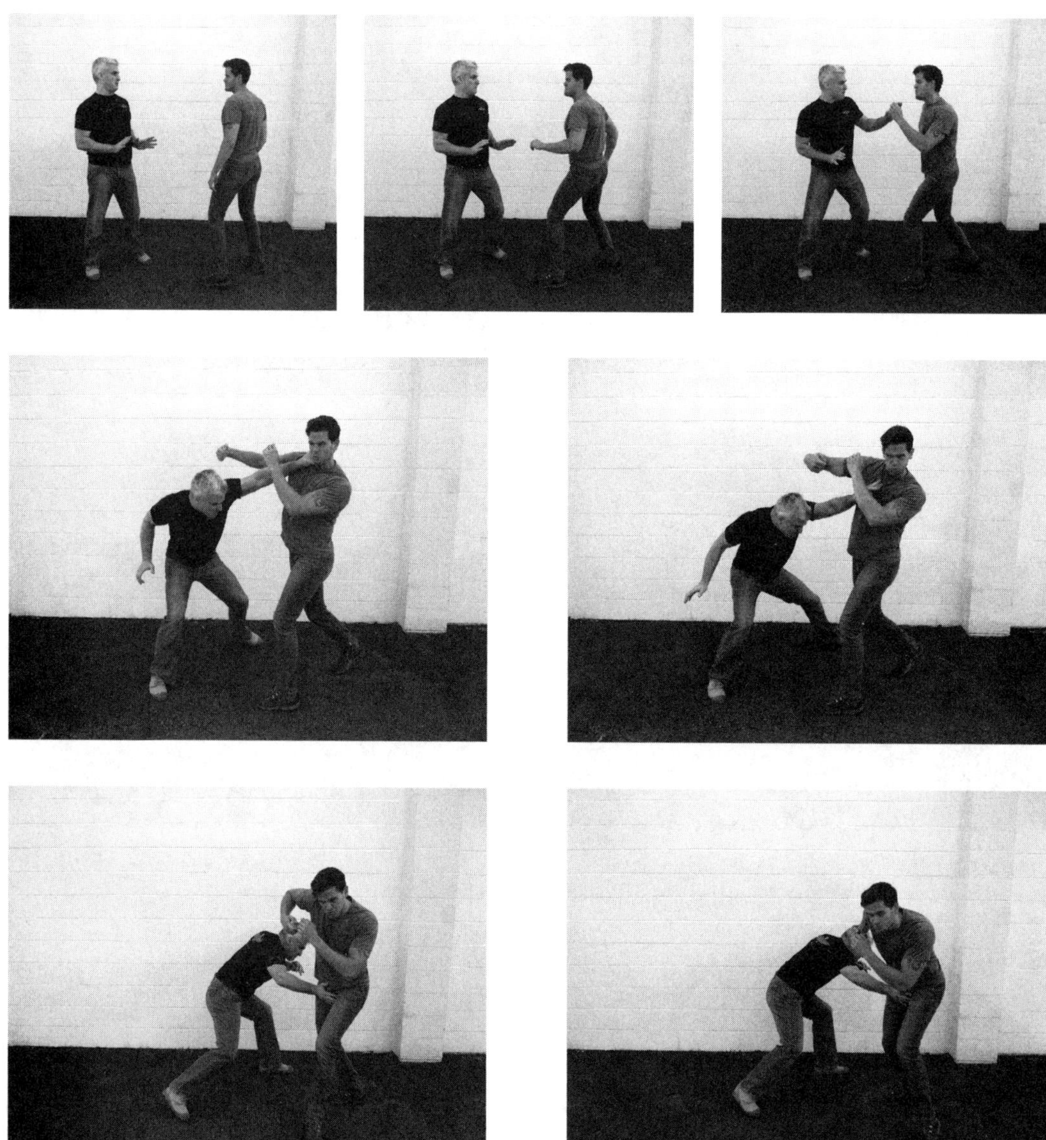

This series depicts a timing defense showing a linear web strike to the throat against a hook punch.

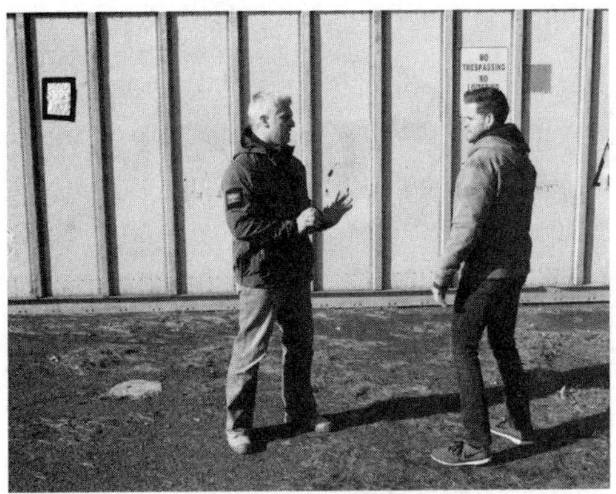

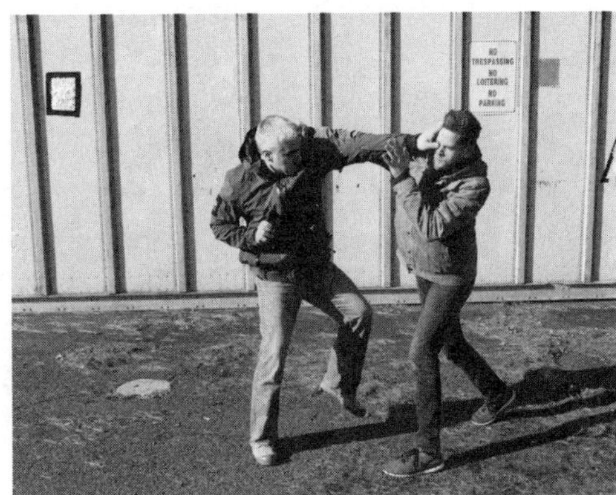

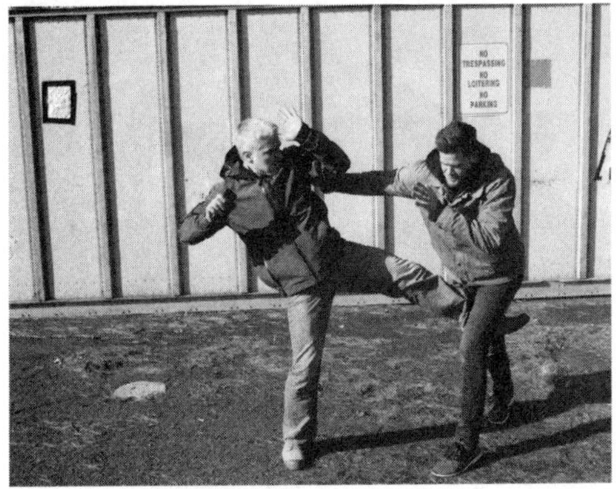

This series depicts a timing defense showing a linear eye strike thumb gouge timing defense against a hook punch.

Third Party Sucker Punch Defensive Strategies When Engaged in an Ambush

A favorite street attack is sucker punching or ambushing a victim with a blindside punch to the head. This often happens when one thug comes to the aid of a confederate who may be already fighting with you. To defend, obviously, you must recognize the incoming attack, using your peripheral vision. The challenge is that you are engaged in a fight, and tunnel vision—focusing exclusively on the threat in front of you—might have set in. While tunnel vision may threaten to hijack your observation skills, you must do a cursory but encompassing visual sweep of the immediate area for other potential aggressors (and for weapons of opportunity you can employ that may be employed against you).

An immediate straight or side kick to preempt or intercept the attack is usually the best answer. However, you may be late in your recognition and have to resort to an outside defense or 360-degree arm interception. (Please also see my *Krav Maga Defense* for additional examples.)[57] Training tip: to practice for such scenarios, you should work with at least two partners. One partner should attack you with speed and power, forcing you to defend. Another partner then should attempt to sucker punch you.

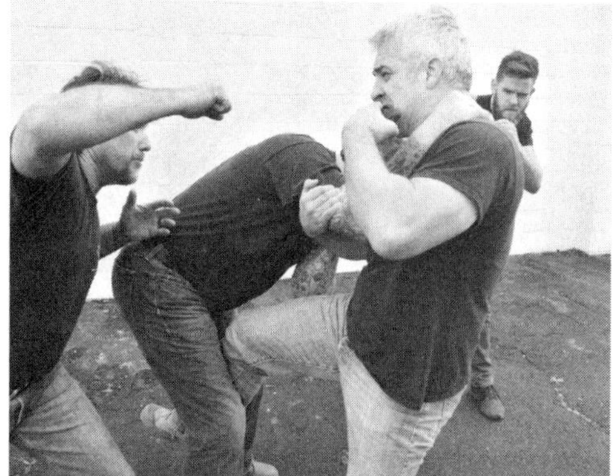

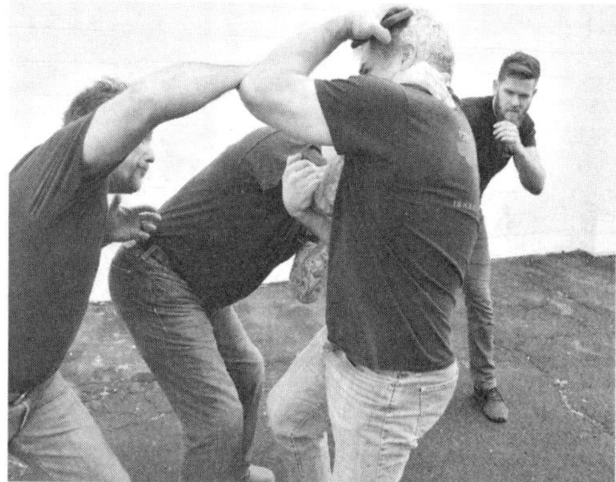

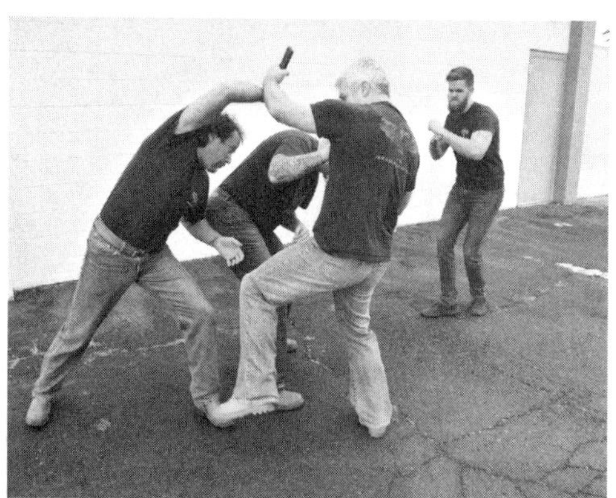

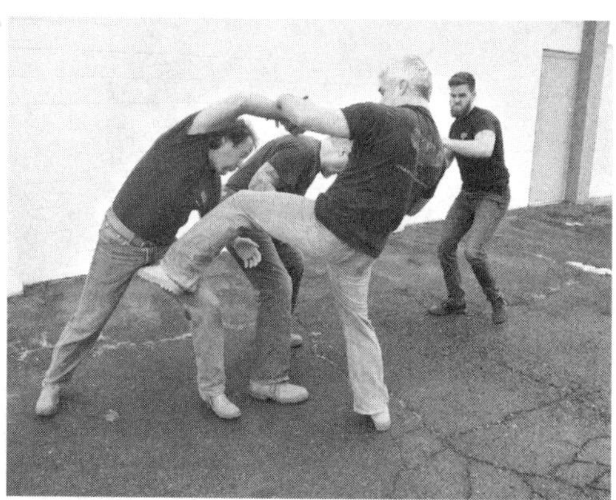

This series depicts a multiple opponent engagement where you are fighting with one adversary while another adversary attempts a sneak attack. Tunnel vision is a real danger. And you must try to debilitate one opponent as quickly as possible regardless of whether you face a single attacker or multiple attackers.

57. Kahn, *Krav Maga Defense*, 103–104, 106-107, 119–120, 123–125.

Breaking-Up-a-Fight Strategy

Krav maga incorporates a few options to break up a fight. Security professionals will note that one option is to let the combatants exhaust themselves and then intervene. Yet you may have to break up a fight before anyone gets hurt or injured. Krav maga uses a modification of a two-arm stabbing impact-weapon defense to literally drive a wedge (or two wedges in this case) between the assailants. It is crucial to tuck your head and use a high diving motion to place your arm wedge above the respective assailants' arms to secure them. As soon as you secure the arms, be sure to firmly pin them to the aggressor's body so that you are not struck. Be careful as you separate the parties using a command voice to cease fighting as they could easily knee or otherwise attack you. Be forceful with your command voice accompanied by your physical intervention to signal that you are there to help and not to provoke.

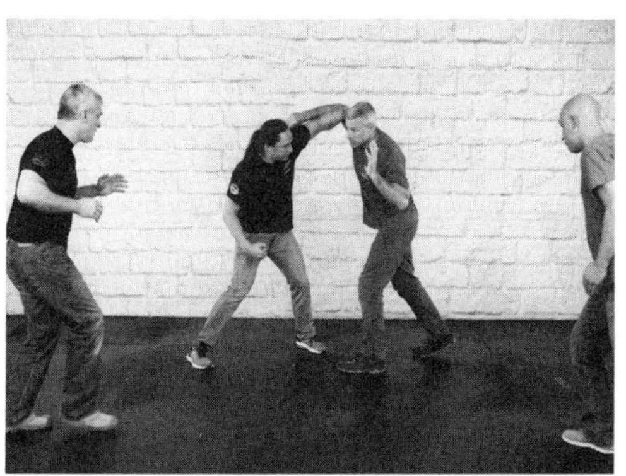

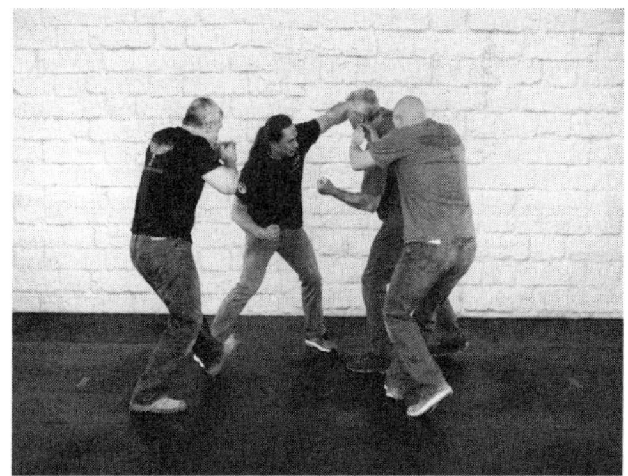

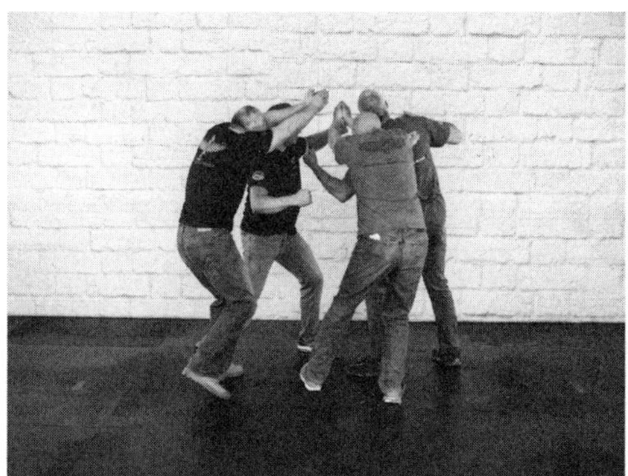

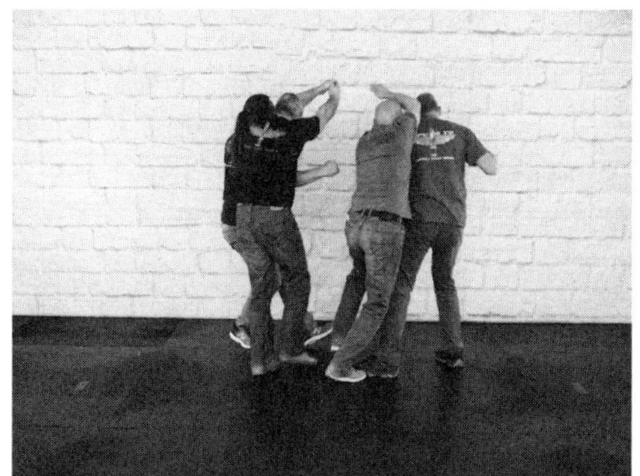

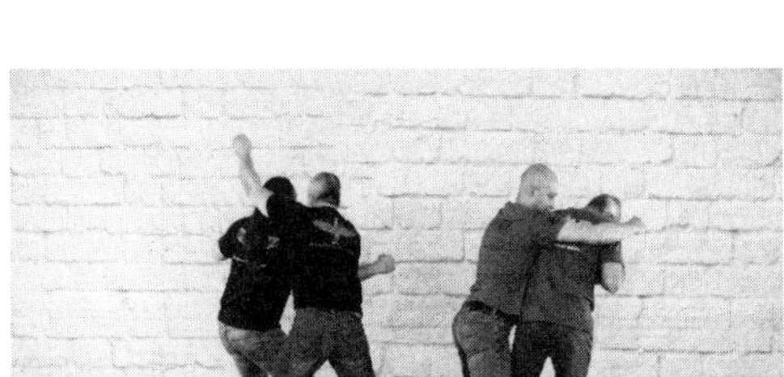

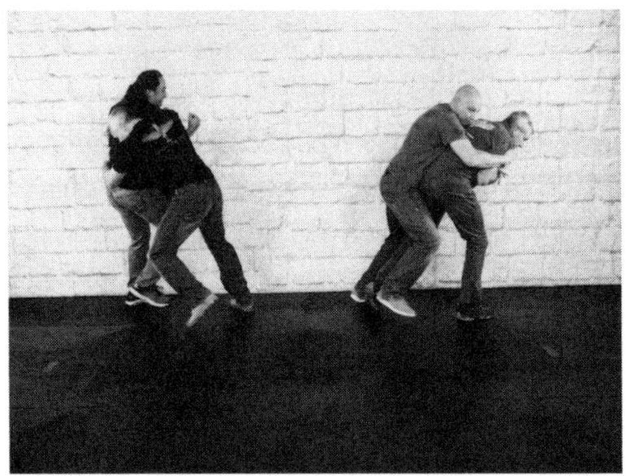

This series depicts breaking up a fight. Both good Samaritans use arm wedges to separate the combatants and then steer them clear, while immediately attempting verbal de-escalation. Be sure to protect yourself, as the person you are separating may turn his aggression on you instinctively or because he simply wants to fight even as you attempt to de-escalate him.

Conclusion

Israeli Krav Maga's pledge is that it can teach nearly anyone to successfully defend against proximate violence. It is my hope and goal that the practical, battle-tested stratagems discussed in this book and our other written and video materials are applicable across the spectrum of martial-arts and fighting systems. No two situations will be the same. You must develop an adaptable strategy supported by a few tried-and-true defensive combatives and tactics coupled with sound defensive principles to deliver you from harm's way.

The krav maga I represent in each of my books is designed to conform to your strengths. This material should be used for big-picture thinking to take you to the next level of krav maga expertise or that of another preferred self-defense discipline. Be sure to have a thorough understanding of reasonable force parameters and the critical legal justifications you must have when using counterforce. You must be able to articulate what you did and why you did it. Sharpen your thinking about where and when you must (and must not) use your krav maga skills.

So whatever your martial-arts or defensive-tactics background, the material in this book can add additional defensive solutions to your repertoire—additional arrows for your quiver. In short, Israeli Krav Maga is designed to synergize with any previous professional self-defense knowledge to enhance your personal survival blueprint. Remember, good tactical minds typically think alike—so welcome aboard. Train well and be well. Here's to everyone's safety …

BECAUSE NOT ALL KRAV MAGA IS THE SAME® …

Notable Biographies

Grandmaster Haim Gidon

Grandmaster Gidon, tenth dan and Israeli Krav Maga Association President, heads Israeli Krav Maga (Gidon System) from the IKMA's main training center in Netanya, Israel. Haim was a member of krav maga founder Imi Lichtenfeld's first training class in the early 1960s and was awarded his eighth dan by Imi in a public ceremony in 1996, making Haim krav maga's highest-ranked instructor in the world. Along with Imi and other top instructors, Haim Gidon cofounded the IKMA. In 1995, Imi nominated Haim as the top authority to grant first dan and higher krav maga black belts. Haim represented krav maga as the head of the system for five years when Wingate Institute, Israel's National Center for Physical Education and Sport, maintained its professional martial arts committee. For the last four decades, Grandmaster Gidon, whose professional expertise is in worldwide demand, has taught defensive tactics to Israel's security and military agencies, having personally received a commendation from the Israeli prime minister's office for his contributions to the state. Haim is ably assisted by some of the highest-ranked and most capable krav maga instructors in the world, including Ohad Gidon (sixth dan), Noam Gidon (fifth dan), Yoav Krayn (fifth dan), Yigal Arbiv (fifth dan), Steve Moshe (fifth dan), Eran Buaron (fifth dan), and Aldema Zirinksi (fifth dan). More information is available at www.facebook.com/gidonsystemkravmaga.

Black-Belt Instructor Rinaldo Rossi

Rinaldo Rossi began his krav maga training in 2001 and his advanced training with David Kahn in 2006. Rinaldo completed his instructor certification with Grandmaster Haim Gidon in both the United States and Israel. Rinaldo is one of only a few Americans to complete Grandmaster Gidon's certification course in Israel. Rinaldo also holds black belts in judo and Japanese jiu-jitsu. Rinaldo has instructed at several prestigious locations, including the Naval Advanced Training Command, Marine Corps Martial Arts Center of Excellence (MACE), U.S. Army Combatives School, and the FBI Academy. Rinaldo is responsible for the national rollout of Israeli Krav Maga in the United States along with Don Melnick, in coordination with the Israeli Krav Maga Association.

Senior Instructor Michael Delahanty

Michael Delahanty began his krav maga training in 2007. Mike is a Marine Gulf War I veteran and retired police lieutenant. He received his advanced belt rankings and awards directly from Grandmaster Haim Gidon. Mike completed his instructor certification with Grandmaster Haim Gidon in the United States. He has taught at the New Jersey State Police Academy and the Philadelphia Police Academy. He regularly travels to conduct Police Krav Maga® training seminars. Mike was featured in the books *Krav Maga Weapon Defenses*, *Krav Maga for Professionals*, *Krav Maga: Defending the Most Common 12 Unarmed Street Attacks*, and *Krav Maga Combatives*, along with *Mastering Krav Maga*® DVD Volume, I, II, III, and IV and the *Mastering Krav Maga*® online program.

Senior Instructor Don Melnick

Don began his krav maga training in 2008. Don has trained extensively in Israel, having received his advanced belt rankings and awards directly from Grandmaster Haim Gidon. Don completed his instructor certification with Grandmaster Haim Gidon in both the United States and Israel, and is one of only a few Americans to complete Grandmaster Gidon's certification course in Israel. He has taught at the New Jersey State Police Academy and the Philadelphia Police Academy and regularly travels to conduct training seminars. As co-owner of Israeli Krav Maga Cherry Hill, Don manages day-to-day operations, serves as the coordinator for Civilian and Law Enforcement training programs, and spearheads a number of krav maga pro bono training programs. Don was featured in the books *Krav Maga Weapon Defenses*, *Krav Maga for Professionals*, *Krav Maga: Defending the Most Common 12 Unarmed Street Attacks*, and *Krav Maga Combatives*, along with *Mastering Krav Maga*® DVD Volumes, I, II, III and IV and the Mastering Krav Maga® online program.

Senior Instructor and Photographer Paul Karleen

Paul began his krav maga training in 2012 and received his advanced belt rankings and awards from David Kahn. Paul completed his instructor certification with Grandmaster Haim Gidon in the United States. Paul has taught at the New Jersey Transit Counter-Terror Training Center and the Philadelphia Police Academy, and regularly travels to help conduct Police Krav Maga® training seminars. Paul was featured in and took many of the photos for *Krav Maga Combatives* and for this book. Paul also volunteers as a technical editor for David Kahn's writing.

Senior Instructor Jeff Gorman

Jeff began his krav maga training in 2005. Jeff received his advanced belt rankings and instructor certifications directly from Grandmaster Haim Gidon in the United States. Jeff was featured in the books *Krav Maga Weapon Defenses*, *Krav Maga Professional Tactics*, and *Krav Maga Combatives*, along with *Mastering Krav Maga*® DVD Volumes I, II, III and IV, and the Mastering Krav Maga® online program.

Senior Instructor Frank Colucci

Frank began his krav maga training in 2007. Frank received his advanced belt rankings and awards directly from Grandmaster Haim Gidon. He completed his instructor certification with Grandmaster Haim Gidon in the United States and Israel. Frank was featured in the books *Krav Maga Weapon Defenses*, *Krav Maga Professional Tactics*, *Krav Maga: Defending the Most Common 12 Unarmed Street Attacks*, and *Krav Maga Combatives*, along with *Mastering Krav Maga*® DVD Volumes I, II, III and IV and the Mastering Krav Maga® online program.

Senior Instructor Sean Hoggs

USAF Maj. Sean Hoggs, Ret., began his krav maga training with David Kahn in 2013. Sean completed his instructor certification along with additional intense training with Grandmaster Haim Gidon in the United States. Sean teaches at the Hamilton, NJ, training center, and has also achieved Military Instructor status, being granted the first Military Krav Maga™ belt, #001. Sean served in the 353 Special Operations Group as a Black Hat, a 421 Ground Combat Readiness Instructor, and a Line Combatives Instructor. A renowned public speaker, Sean authored the acclaimed book *Bastard Child* and is the host for *Let's Talk about It* on BKS 1 Radio. Sean will appear in several forthcoming krav maga books.

Senior Instructor Ronald E. Jacobs

USMC MSgt. Ronald E. Jacobs, Ret., is both the former chief instructor of the Marine Corps Martial Arts Program and a lead East Coast Combatives Instructor for Naval Special Warfare. Ron, a former Scout Sniper, is an expert in close quarters battle and marksmanship. He is currently a contract subject matter expert for the United States government. Ron holds a sixth-degree black belt in MCMAP along with high-ranking belts in numerous other martial-arts systems, including a black belt in Israeli Krav Maga and black belts in both Brazilian and Japanese jiu-jitsu in addition to being Muy Thai Kru (master instructor). Ron was featured in the books *Krav Maga Professional Tactics* and *Krav Maga Combatives.*

Senior Instructor Joseph Drew

Trooper Joseph Drew began his krav maga training in 2010 and received his advanced belt rankings and awards directly from David Kahn. Joe completed his instructor certification with Grandmaster Haim Gidon in the United States and advanced law enforcement instructor training with David Kahn. Joe as a Police Krav Maga® instructor has taught defensive tactics at the New Jersey Transit Counter-Terror Training Center, Philadelphia Police Academy and the PA Game Commission Training Center. Joe was featured in the *Mastering Krav Maga®* DVD Volumes II and III, along with the Mastering Krav Maga® Online Program

Additional Israeli Krav Maga Instructors

Mike McElvin, John Papp, Bill Dwyer, Clay Hamil, Anne Mennen, Jonathan Sabin, Rich VanCamp, Dan Rednor, Kevin Scozarro, Rich Kahl, Brandon Druker, Dion Privett, Kathryn Badger, Marc Schneiderman, and Andre Kwon have all trained extensively with David Kahn and Grandmaster Gidon. Each highly capable instructor is instrumental in assisting in the day-to-day classes in the New Jersey Israeli Krav Maga training facilities.

Senior Instructor Albert "Poodie Carson"

Officer Al "Poodie" Carson began his Police Krav Maga® training in 2015 under David Kahn and his instructor training with Grandmaster Haim Gidon in Israel in 2017. Poodie received both his Civilian Level I and Law Enforcement Levels I & II Israeli Krav Maga Association teaching certifications from the United States Chief Instructor. He is an active law enforcement officer having served as a SWAT team leader for the past two decades with the benefit of having received special training from Navy SEAL CQB instructors. He is instrumental in the David Kahn Krav Maga Football Combatives program and has trained dozens of NFL players, including NFL Defensive MVPs Aaron Donald and Khalil Mack along with many other top college and NFL prospects. Poodie teaches in Western Pennsylvania.

Senior Instructor Martin "Het" Hetman

Het, a US Air Force veteran, began his krav maga training in 2015 and received his advanced belt rankings and awards from David Kahn. He completed his instructor certification with David Kahn and was featured in the Mastering Krav Maga® online program.

Training Resources

Asian World of Martial Arts
9400 Ashton Road
Philadelphia, PA 19114
(800) 345-2962
www.awma.com

Aries Fight Gear
(800) 542-7437
www.punchingbag.com

Mancino Mats
1180 Church Road
Lansdale, PA 19446
(800) 338-6287
www.mancinomats.com

Authentic Israel Army Surplus
P.O. Box 31006
Tel Aviv 61310
Israel
U.S. Local Phone: (718) 701-3955 Toll Free Number: (888) 293-1421
Israel: (972) 3-6204612; Fax: (972) 9-8859661
www.israelmilitary.com

To read more about *krav maga* and its history:

Israel Defense Forces
Homepage: www.idf.il/en/

Israeli Special Forces Krav Maga
Homepage: www.ct707.com

Israeli Krav Maga Association (Gidon System)
Homepage: www.israelikrav.com and www.kravmagaisraeli.com

Index

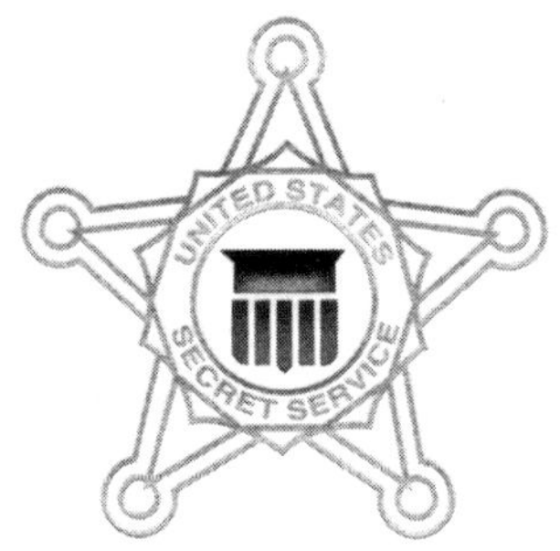

United States Secret Service

Certificate of Appreciation

Presented to

David Kahn
U.S. Chief Instructor
Israeli Krav Maga Association

in special recognition of your efforts and superior contributions to the law enforcement responsibilities of the United States Secret Service.

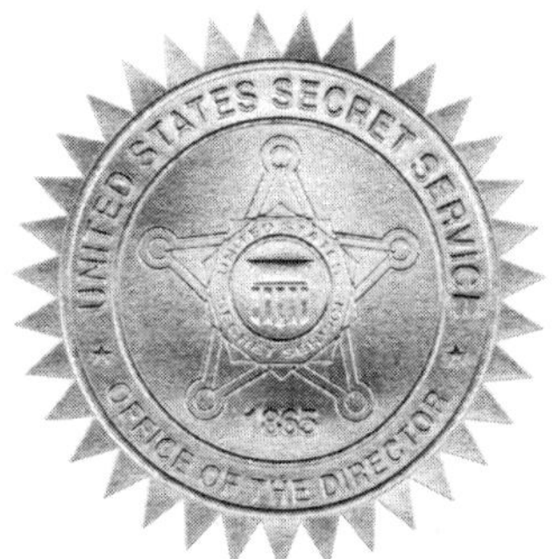

Issued in the city of Washington, D.C.
Given under my hand and seal in the Year

2020

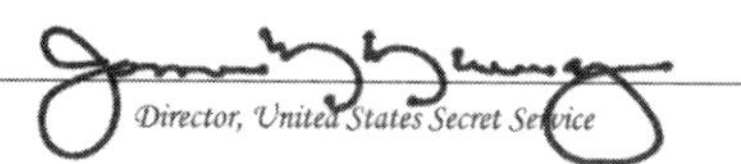

Director, United States Secret Service

About the Author

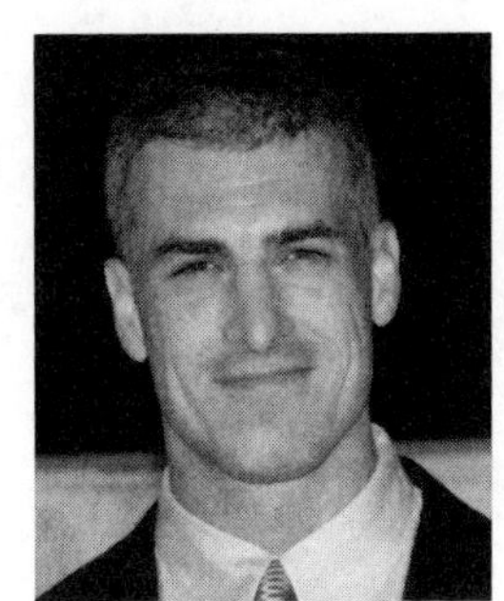

David Kahn, IKMA United States Chief Instructor, received his advanced black-belt teaching certifications from Grandmaster Haim Gidon and is the only American to sit on the IKMA board of directors. The United States Judo Association also awarded David a fifth-degree black belt in combat jiu-jitsu. David has trained all branches of the U.S. military, the Royal Marines, in addition to federal, state, and local law enforcement agencies. David has been invited to teach at many respected hand-to-hand combat schools, including the Naval Special Warfare Advanced Training Command and TRADET 2, the Marine Corps Martial Arts Center of Excellence (MACE), U.S. Army Combatives School, the FBI Academy, U.S. Secret Service Academy, and the New Jersey State Police Academy. David serves as the lead Police Krav Maga® instructor certified by the State of New Jersey Police Training Commission. David has created a program for marquee NFL and collegiate football players, including his alma mater Princeton University, utilizing modified krav maga tactics for the sport of American football. David is regularly featured in major media outlets, including *Men's Fitness, GQ, USA Today, Los Angeles Times, The Washington Post, The New Yorker, Penthouse, Fitness, Marine Corps News*, Armed Forces Network, Special Operations Report, and Military.com. David is the author of *Krav Maga, Advanced Krav Maga, Krav Maga Weapon Defenses, Krav Maga Professional Tactics, Krav Maga Defense,* and *Krav Maga Combatives.* To date, he has won five national book awards. He also produced the *Mastering Krav Maga®* DVD series, Volumes I, II, III and IV, along with the Mastering Krav Maga® online program. This unique learning offering includes 500+ lessons, or more than forty-two hours of online lessons covering approximately 90 percent of the krav maga civilian curriculum. Please visit: www.masteringkravmaga.com and www.davidkahnkravmaga.com for more information.

David and his partners operate several Israeli Krav Maga training centers of excellence. For more information contact info@israelikrav.com or the following:

Israeli Krav Maga U.S. Main Training Center
127 Highway 206
Hamilton, NJ 08505
(609) 585-MAGA
www.israelikrav.com

Israeli Krav Maga Association (Gidon System)
POB 1103
Netanya, Israel

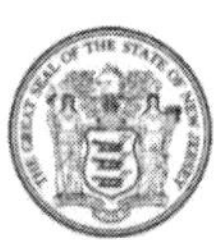

State of New Jersey

OFFICE OF THE ATTORNEY GENERAL
DEPARTMENT OF LAW AND PUBLIC SAFETY
DIVISION OF STATE POLICE
POST OFFICE BOX 7068
WEST TRENTON, NJ 08628-0068
(609) 882-2000

PHILIP D. MURPHY
Governor

SHEILA Y. OLIVER
Lt. Governor

GURBIR S. GREWAL
Attorney General

PATRICK J. CALLAHAN
Colonel

August 30, 2019

David Kahn, IKMA U.S. Chief Instructor
Israeli Krav Maga LLC
860 US Hwy 206
Bordentown, NJ 08505

Mr. Kahn,

Another outstanding response from the 35 participants you provided training to during the New Jersey State Police Fundamentals of Executive Protection Course. The Israeli Krav Maga, Gidon System close quarter defensive tactics and disarming training instruction and practical exercises are a perfect tool for Executive Protection.

The participants in the training were from Eleven U.S. State Police agencies including Arkansas, Arizona, Illinois, Kentucky, Maryland, Massachusetts, New York, New Jersey, Rhode Island, Virginia, Vermont. Also in attendance were the U.S. Federal Air Marshals, local police officers from New Jersey including the Newark Police Department, Essex County Sheriff's Office and the Rumson Police Department. All 35 participants gave the close quarter defensive tactics and disarming training instruction and practical exercises a perfect "ten" (ten being the highest grade). In the evaluation narratives, the words "outstanding", "excellent", "practical", "simple and highly effective" appeared multiple times.

Since the NJ State Police Executive Protection Bureau's first exposure to Israeli Krav Maga, Gidon System in 2003, all of our members over the last 16 years have appreciated the simple, highly effective, and concise techniques. The close quarter disarming techniques are a perfect fit for the environments we work in daily where we always consider innocent third party bystanders and public safety while neutralizing threats and other unwanted behaviors from people who want to cause destruction, harm and embarrassment.

All the training and instruction you and your staff including Joe Drew and Paul Karleen provided this past training, gave the participants effective techniques to be used in an unpredictable and increasing dangerous world. We look forward to future Israeli Krav Maga training opportunities and appreciate your tremendous generosity of your time and willingness to share your expertise with us.

Thank you,

Lt. Louis J. Maniace #6327
New Jersey State Police, Office of Executive Protection

"An Internationally Accredited Agency"

New Jersey Is An Equal Opportunity Employer
Printed on Recycled Paper and Recyclable

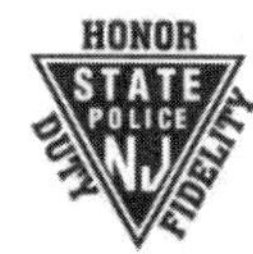

BOOKS FROM YMAA

101 REFLECTIONS ON TAI CHI CHUAN
108 INSIGHTS INTO TAI CHI CHUAN
A SUDDEN DAWN: THE EPIC JOURNEY OF BODHIDHARMA
A WOMAN'S QIGONG GUIDE
ADVANCING IN TAE KWON DO
ANALYSIS OF SHAOLIN CHIN NA 2ND ED
ANCIENT CHINESE WEAPONS
ART AND SCIENCE OF STAFF FIGHTING
ART AND SCIENCE OF STICK FIGHTING
ART OF HOJO UNDO
ARTHRITIS RELIEF, 3D ED.
BACK PAIN RELIEF, 2ND ED.
BAGUAZHANG, 2ND ED.
BRAIN FITNESS
CARDIO KICKBOXING ELITE
CHIN NA IN GROUND FIGHTING
CHINESE FAST WRESTLING
CHINESE FITNESS
CHINESE TUI NA MASSAGE
CHOJUN
COMPLETE MARTIAL ARTIST
COMPREHENSIVE APPLICATIONS OF SHAOLIN CHIN NA
CONFLICT COMMUNICATION
CUTTING SEASON: A XENON PEARL MARTIAL ARTS THRILLER
DAO DE JING
DAO IN ACTION
DEFENSIVE TACTICS
DESHI: A CONNOR BURKE MARTIAL ARTS THRILLER
DIRTY GROUND
DR. WU'S HEAD MASSAGE
DUKKHA HUNGRY GHOSTS
DUKKHA REVERB
DUKKHA, THE SUFFERING: AN EYE FOR AN EYE
DUKKHA UNLOADED
ENZAN: THE FAR MOUNTAIN, A CONNOR BURKE MARTIAL ARTS THRILLER
ESSENCE OF SHAOLIN WHITE CRANE
EVEN IF IT KILLS ME
EXPLORING TAI CHI
FACING VIOLENCE
FIGHT BACK
FIGHT LIKE A PHYSICIST
THE FIGHTER'S BODY
FIGHTER'S FACT BOOK
FIGHTER'S FACT BOOK 2
FIGHTING ARTS
FIGHTING THE PAIN RESISTANT ATTACKER
FIRST DEFENSE
FORCE DECISIONS: A CITIZENS GUIDE
FOX BORROWS THE TIGER'S AWE
INSIDE TAI CHI
JUDO ADVANTAGE
JUJI GATAME ENCYCLOPEDIA
KAGE: THE SHADOW, A CONNOR BURKE MARTIAL ARTS THRILLER
KARATE SCIENCE
KATA AND THE TRANSMISSION OF KNOWLEDGE
KRAV MAGA COMBATIVES
KRAV MAGA FUNDAMENTAL STRATEGIES
KRAV MAGA PROFESSIONAL TACTICS
KRAV MAGA WEAPON DEFENSES
LITTLE BLACK BOOK OF VIOLENCE
LIUHEBAFA FIVE CHARACTER SECRETS
MARTIAL ARTS ATHLETE
MARTIAL ARTS OF VIETNAM
MARTIAL ARTS INSTRUCTION
MARTIAL WAY AND ITS VIRTUES
MASK OF THE KING
MEDITATIONS ON VIOLENCE
MERIDIAN QIGONG EXERCISES
MIND/BODY FITNESS
MINDFUL EXERCISE
MIND INSIDE TAI CHI
MIND INSIDE YANG STYLE TAI CHI CHUAN
NATURAL HEALING WITH QIGONG
NORTHERN SHAOLIN SWORD, 2ND ED.
OKINAWA'S COMPLETE KARATE SYSTEM: ISSHIN RYU
PAIN-FREE BACK
PAIN-FREE JOINTS
PRINCIPLES OF TRADITIONAL CHINESE MEDICINE
PROTECTOR ETHIC
QIGONG FOR HEALTH & MARTIAL ARTS 2ND ED.
QIGONG FOR LIVING
QIGONG FOR TREATING COMMON AILMENTS
QIGONG MASSAGE
QIGONG MEDITATION: EMBRYONIC BREATHING
QIGONG MEDITATION: GRAND CIRCULATION
QIGONG MEDITATION: SMALL CIRCULATION
QIGONG, THE SECRET OF YOUTH: DA MO'S CLASSICS
QUIET TEACHER: A XENON PEARL MARTIAL ARTS THRILLER
RAVEN'S WARRIOR
REDEMPTION
ROOT OF CHINESE QIGONG, 2ND ED.
SAMBO ENCYCLOPEDIA
SCALING FORCE
SELF-DEFENSE FOR WOMEN
SENSEI: A CONNOR BURKE MARTIAL ARTS THRILLER
SHIHAN TE: THE BUNKAI OF KATA
SHIN GI TAI: KARATE TRAINING FOR BODY, MIND, AND SPIRIT
SIMPLE CHINESE MEDICINE
SIMPLE QIGONG EXERCISES FOR HEALTH, 3RD ED.
SIMPLIFIED TAI CHI CHUAN, 2ND ED.
SOLO TRAINING
SOLO TRAINING 2
SPOTTING DANGER BEFORE IT SPOTS YOU
SPOTTING DANGER BEFORE IT SPOTS YOUR KIDS
SUMO FOR MIXED MARTIAL ARTS
SUNRISE TAI CHI
SURVIVING ARMED ASSAULTS
TAE KWON DO: THE KOREAN MARTIAL ART
TAEKWONDO BLACK BELT POOMSAE
TAEKWONDO: A PATH TO EXCELLENCE
TAEKWONDO: ANCIENT WISDOM FOR THE MODERN WARRIOR
TAEKWONDO: DEFENSE AGAINST WEAPONS
TAEKWONDO: SPIRIT AND PRACTICE
TAI CHI BALL QIGONG: FOR HEALTH AND MARTIAL ARTS
TAI CHI BALL WORKOUT FOR BEGINNERS
THE TAI CHI BOOK
TAI CHI CHIN NA: THE SEIZING ART OF TAI CHI CHUAN, 2ND ED.
TAI CHI CHUAN CLASSICAL YANG STYLE, 2ND ED.
TAI CHI CHUAN MARTIAL POWER, 3RD ED.
TAI CHI CONCEPTS AND EXPERIMENTS
TAI CHI CONNECTIONS
TAI CHI DYNAMICS
TAI CHI FOR DEPRESSION
TAI CHI IN 10 WEEKS
TAI CHI PUSH HANDS
TAI CHI QIGONG, 3RD ED.
TAI CHI SECRETS OF THE ANCIENT MASTERS
TAI CHI SECRETS OF THE WU & LI STYLES
TAI CHI SECRETS OF THE WU STYLE
TAI CHI SECRETS OF THE YANG STYLE
TAI CHI SWORD: CLASSICAL YANG STYLE, 2ND ED.
TAI CHI SWORD FOR BEGINNERS
TAI CHI WALKING
TAIJIQUAN THEORY OF DR. YANG, JWING-MING
TAO OF BIOENERGETICS
TENGU: THE MOUNTAIN GOBLIN, A CONNOR BURKE MARTIAL ARTS THRILLER
TIMING IN THE FIGHTING ARTS
TRADITIONAL CHINESE HEALTH SECRETS
TRADITIONAL TAEKWONDO
TRAINING FOR SUDDEN VIOLENCE
TRUE WELLNESS
TRUE WELLNESS: THE MIND
TRUE WELLNESS FOR YOUR GUT
TRUE WELLNESS FOR YOUR HEART
WARRIOR'S MANIFESTO
WAY OF KATA
WAY OF SANCHIN KATA
WAY TO BLACK BELT
WESTERN HERBS FOR MARTIAL ARTISTS
WILD GOOSE QIGONG
WINNING FIGHTS
WISDOM'S WAY
XINGYIQUAN

VIDEOS FROM YMAA

ADVANCED PRACTICAL CHIN NA IN-DEPTH
ANALYSIS OF SHAOLIN CHIN NA
ATTACK THE ATTACK
BAGUA FOR BEGINNERS 1
BAGUA FOR BEGINNERS 2
BAGUAZHANG: EMEI BAGUAZHANG
BEGINNER QIGONG FOR WOMEN 1
BEGINNER QIGONG FOR WOMEN 2
BEGINNER TAI CHI FOR HEALTH
CHEN STYLE TAIJIQUAN
CHEN TAI CHI CANNON FIST
CHEN TAI CHI FIRST FORM
CHEN TAI CHI FOR BEGINNERS
CHIN NA IN-DEPTH COURSES 1—4
CHIN NA IN-DEPTH COURSES 5—8
CHIN NA IN-DEPTH COURSES 9—12
FACING VIOLENCE: 7 THINGS A MARTIAL ARTIST MUST KNOW
FIVE ANIMAL SPORTS
FIVE ELEMENTS ENERGY BALANCE
INFIGHTING
INTRODUCTION TO QI GONG FOR BEGINNERS
JOINT LOCKS
KNIFE DEFENSE: TRADITIONAL TECHNIQUES AGAINST A DAGGER
KUNG FU BODY CONDITIONING 1
KUNG FU BODY CONDITIONING 2
KUNG FU FOR KIDS
KUNG FU FOR TEENS
LOGIC OF VIOLENCE
MERIDIAN QIGONG
NEIGONG FOR MARTIAL ARTS
NORTHERN SHAOLIN SWORD : SAN CAI JIAN, KUN WU JIAN, QI MEN JIAN
QI GONG 30-DAY CHALLENGE
QI GONG FOR ANXIETY
QI GONG FOR ARMS, WRISTS, AND HANDS
QIGONG FOR BEGINNERS: FRAGRANCE
QI GONG FOR BETTER BALANCE
QI GONG FOR BETTER BREATHING
QI GONG FOR CANCER
QI GONG FOR DEPRESSION
QI GONG FOR ENERGY AND VITALITY
QI GONG FOR HEADACHES
QI GONG FOR HEALING
QI GONG FOR THE HEALTHY HEART
QI GONG FOR HEALTHY JOINTS
QI GONG FOR HIGH BLOOD PRESSURE
QIGONG FOR LONGEVITY
QI GONG FOR STRONG BONES
QI GONG FOR THE UPPER BACK AND NECK
QIGONG FOR WOMEN
QIGONG FOR WOMEN WITH DAISY LEE
QIGONG FLOW FOR STRESS & ANXIETY RELIEF
QIGONG MASSAGE
QIGONG MINDFULNESS IN MOTION
QI GONG—THE SEATED WORKOUT
QIGONG: 15 MINUTES TO HEALTH
SABER FUNDAMENTAL TRAINING
SAI TRAINING AND SEQUENCES
SANCHIN KATA: TRADITIONAL TRAINING FOR KARATE POWER
SCALING FORCE
SHAOLIN KUNG FU FUNDAMENTAL TRAINING: COURSES 1 & 2
SHAOLIN LONG FIST KUNG FU: ADVANCED SEQUENCES 1
SHAOLIN LONG FIST KUNG FU: ADVANCED SEQUENCES 2
SHAOLIN LONG FIST KUNG FU: BASIC SEQUENCES
SHAOLIN LONG FIST KUNG FU: INTERMEDIATE SEQUENCES
SHAOLIN SABER: BASIC SEQUENCES
SHAOLIN STAFF: BASIC SEQUENCES
SHAOLIN WHITE CRANE GONG FU BASIC TRAINING: COURSES 1 & 2
SHAOLIN WHITE CRANE GONG FU BASIC TRAINING: COURSES 3 & 4
SHUAI JIAO: KUNG FU WRESTLING
SIMPLE QIGONG EXERCISES FOR HEALTH
SIMPLE QIGONG EXERCISES FOR ARTHRITIS RELIEF
SIMPLE QIGONG EXERCISES FOR BACK PAIN RELIEF
SIMPLIFIED TAI CHI CHUAN: 24 & 48 POSTURES
SIMPLIFIED TAI CHI FOR BEGINNERS 48
SIX HEALING SOUNDS
SUN TAI CHI
SUNRISE TAI CHI
SUNSET TAI CHI
SWORD: FUNDAMENTAL TRAINING
TAEKWONDO KORYO POOMSAE
TAI CHI BALL QIGONG: COURSES 1 & 2
TAI CHI BALL QIGONG: COURSES 3 & 4
TAI CHI BALL WORKOUT FOR BEGINNERS
TAI CHI CHUAN CLASSICAL YANG STYLE
TAI CHI CONNECTIONS
TAI CHI ENERGY PATTERNS
TAI CHI FIGHTING SET
TAI CHI FIT: 24 FORM
TAI CHI FIT: FLOW
TAI CHI FIT: FUSION BAMBOO
TAI CHI FIT: FUSION FIRE
TAI CHI FIT: FUSION IRON
TAI CHI FIT: HEART HEALTH WORKOUT
TAI CHI FIT IN PARADISE
TAI CHI FIT: OVER 50
TAI CHI FIT OVER 50: BALANCE EXERCISES
TAI CHI FIT OVER 50: SEATED WORKOUT
TAI CHI FIT OVER 60: GENTLE EXERCISES
TAI CHI FIT OVER 60: HEALTHY JOINTS
TAI CHI FIT OVER 60: LIVE LONGER
TAI CHI FIT: STRENGTH
TAI CHI FIT: TO GO
TAI CHI FOR WOMEN
TAI CHI FUSION: FIRE
TAI CHI QIGONG
TAI CHI PUSHING HANDS: COURSES 1 & 2
TAI CHI PUSHING HANDS: COURSES 3 & 4
TAI CHI SWORD: CLASSICAL YANG STYLE
TAI CHI SWORD FOR BEGINNERS
TAI CHI SYMBOL: YIN YANG STICKING HANDS
TAIJI & SHAOLIN STAFF: FUNDAMENTAL TRAINING
TAIJI CHIN NA IN-DEPTH
TAIJI 37 POSTURES MARTIAL APPLICATIONS
TAIJI SABER CLASSICAL YANG STYLE
TAIJI WRESTLING
TRAINING FOR SUDDEN VIOLENCE
UNDERSTANDING QIGONG 1: WHAT IS QI? • HUMAN QI CIRCULATORY SYSTEM
UNDERSTANDING QIGONG 2: KEY POINTS • QIGONG BREATHING
UNDERSTANDING QIGONG 3: EMBRYONIC BREATHING
UNDERSTANDING QIGONG 4: FOUR SEASONS QIGONG
UNDERSTANDING QIGONG 5: SMALL CIRCULATION
UNDERSTANDING QIGONG 6: MARTIAL QIGONG BREATHING
WATER STYLE FOR BEGINNERS
WHITE CRANE HARD & SOFT QIGONG
YANG TAI CHI FOR BEGINNERS
YOQI QIGONG FOR A HAPPY HEART
YOQI QIGONG FOR HAPPY SPLEEN & STOMACH
YOQI QIGONG FOR HAPPY KIDNEYS
YOQI QIGONG FLOW FOR HAPPY LUNGS
YOQI QIGONG FLOW FOR STRESS RELIEF
YOQI SIX HEALING SOUNDS
WU TAI CHI FOR BEGINNERS
WUDANG KUNG FU: FUNDAMENTAL TRAINING
WUDANG SWORD
WUDANG TAIJIQUAN
XINGYIQUAN
YANG TAI CHI FOR BEGINNERS

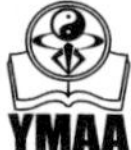